This book is dedicated to:
Peggy, whom I love, cherish, and respect in my
mind, in my heart, and in my soul.

Our Sisters, Ann, Ruby, and Mary
for continued love and friendship.
—Gayle

My understanding and patient "Tucker."
—Sandy

Student Nurse Handbook
DIFFICULT CONCEPTS MADE EASY

Second Edition

B. Gayle Twiname, PhD, RN
Associate Professor of Nursing (Retired)
Lamar University
Beaumont, Texas

Sandra M. Boyd, MS, RN
Assistant Professor of Nursing
Lamar University
Beaumont, Texas

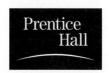

Prentice
Hall

Upper Saddle River, New Jersey 07458

Library of Congress Cataloging-in-Publication Data
Twiname, B. Gayle.
    Student nurse handbook : difficult concepts
made easy / B. Gayle Twiname, Sandra M.
Boyd—2nd ed.
        p. ; cm.
    Includes bibliographical references and index.
    ISBN 0-13-041712-2 (alk. paper)
    1. Nursing students—Handbooks, manuals, etc.
2. Nursing—Study and teaching—Handbooks,
manuals, etc. I. Boyd, Sandra M. II. Title.
    [DNLM: 1. Nursing. 2. Nursing Care.
WY 16 T973s 2002]
RT73.T94   2002
610.73—dc21

                                2001041110

Publisher: Julie Alexander
Executive Editor: Maura Connor
Acquisitions Editor: Nancy Anselment
Editorial Assistant: Mary Ellen Ruitenberg
Development Editor: Elisabeth Garofalo
Director of Manufacturing and Production: Bruce Johnson
Managing Editor: Patrick Walsh
Production Editor: Linda Begley, Rainbow Graphics
Manufacturing Manager: Ilene Sanford
Manufacturing Buyer: Patrick Brown
Marketing Manager: Nicole Benson
Creative Director: Cheryl Asherman
Design Coordinator: Maria Guglielmo
Cover Design: Joseph Sengotta
Composition and Interior Design: Rainbow Graphics
Printing and Binding: RR Donnelley and Sons

Pearson Education LTD.
Pearson Education Australia PTY, Limited
Pearson Education Singapore, Pte. Ltd
Pearson Education North Asia Ltd
Pearson Education Canada, Ltd.
Pearson Educación de Mexico, S.A. de C.V.
Pearson Education–Japan
Pearson Education Malaysia, Pte. Ltd

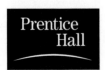

10 9 8 7 6
ISBN 0-13-041712-2

Contents

SECTION III

Universal Issues 107

SECTION IV

Understanding Difficult Concepts 243

SECTION V

Knowledge Building 327

Preface

Wow! You are a nursing student. What a challenge! During our years as nursing faculty we have seen many successful students. This text is our way of helping you to successfully graduate from nursing school.

The second edition of our book incorporates some new chapters and some revised chapters. We made these changes based on input from students and others who reviewed our book. Here are some of the changes:

1. **Learning Styles** and information on **Web Courses** have been added (Chapter 1).
2. We have included a new chapter on **Time Management** (Chapter 2).
3. **Ethics and delegation** have been added to the chapter on Legal/Ethical Concerns (Chapter 9).
4. Another new chapter has been added on **Alternative Therapies** (Chapter 21).
5. All of the Web addresses have been updated and more have been added (Chapter 35).

Do not expect this to be a typical text on a specific nursing area. Rather, it is a resource for some of the more difficult foundation material generally covered in early nursing courses: knowledge that is used in multiple nursing settings. This book will not be able to replace detailed textbooks or class attendance. You will still need to read your textbooks, participate in the learning laboratory, and put time and energy into written assignments.

We anticipate, however, that this book will help you by presenting the highlights of these challenging, yet essential, topics. You will notice that this book is different from course texts in three additional ways.

1. The format is flexible: some material is in typical narrative format, some is in question and answer format, and some is in outline or bulleted (list) format.
2. Many areas are written in "conversation" style, as if we were with you in a learning environment.
3. Some chapters are very short.

In addition to the difficult topics, we have also included guidance in some areas that tend to be stumbling blocks to success.

As with many professions, knowledge learned today in nursing is often outdated by tomorrow. New technology and research is occurring at an alarming pace. So what does this mean for you? Well, several things. First, you must understand this phenomenon and accept it. Second, when research supports new knowledge and techniques, you must be able to release "old" knowledge and ways of doing things. Third, you must keep on top of these current changes through multiple means: reading your professional journals, attending conferences, and searching the Internet for credible new information and technologies.

We believe that this book will help as you progress through nursing school. We would love to hear from you through our publisher, Prentice Hall. How has our book helped you? Are there some other things you would like to see in future editions?

Nursing is a rich and rewarding career. We are very proud of the "nurse" in us and pleased that we may share a small part of building the "nurse" in you. We wish you the best in your nursing career!

Reviewers

The authors and publishers gratefully acknowledge the reviewers whose comments and suggestions have been incorporated in this second edition of the *Student Nurse Handbook*:

Arlene M. Coughlin, RN, MSN
Holy Name Hospital School of Nursing
Teaneck, New Jersey

Jan G. Overman, RN, MSN
Caldwell Community College and Technical Institute
Boone, North Carolina

Elaine Williams
School District of Hillborough County—Learey Technical Center
Tampa, Florida

Acknowledgments

The authors would like to thank the following people:

➤ The Students, Nurses, and Faculty who saw the first edition, bought it, and gave such wonderful positive feedback! We appreciate it!

➤ Peggy Reed: For reading and critiquing our multiple drafts and all the grammatical corrections!

➤ The editorial and production staff of Prentice Hall.

➤ Elisabeth Church Garofalo: For her friendship and continued support of this project.

➤ The current and former students at Lamar University in Beaumont, Texas: For allowing us to travel the road of education with them.

➤ Our family and friends for their encouragement.

➤ And last but not least, to each other: For the commitment to complete this project and have fun at the same time!

Dr. B. Gayle Twiname

Sandra M. Boyd

1

How to Learn, Study, and Take Tests

Learning Styles

We all learn in different ways. Some of us have to physically practice a skill in order to grasp it. Others of us can watch a video and replicate a skill almost immediately. Still others do better listening to an instructor or videotape describe how a skill is done. It is essential that you figure out how you learn best. There are many theories on learning and learning styles. According to Barsch (1996) there are four primary ways in which we interpret our environment or learn. They are:

- Visual
- Auditory
- Tactile
- Kinesthetic

Visual learners make pictures in their heads. They have to "see" something in order to learn. They respond well to overhead transparencies, videotapes, and writings on a blackboard as well as handouts. Using colorful highlighters and writing things out for a quick review can help visual learners when taking notes.

Auditory learners have to hear in order to understand. Often, an auditory person can be heard reading or repeating directions out loud. Auditory learners do well taping classes and listening in class and then summarizing on an audiotape.

Tactile learners are hands on. They have to feel and touch in order to be able to comprehend. They need to take and keep lecture notes and may need to rewrite them several times.

Kinesthetic learners learn best by actually using their bodies to perform a task. If you can perform some type of movement, it can help while you try to memorize your lecture materials.

Most of us use more than one type of learning and sometimes switch from one to another, although one is usually more dominant than another. As you take the following self-test, you may need to keep in mind that you will have a primary learning style. However, you will also have a secondary learning style that might be of use to you when you are in class or studying.

Tactile and kinesthetic learners may have a tough time using their primary mode of learning in a classroom setting. This author (a visual learner) can see the nursing faculty response to students' performing dances or singing during a lecture! As you read further, you will begin to see that primary kinesthetic and tactile learners may need to rely on a secondary mode of learning (visual or auditory) in the classroom environment.

Barsch (1996) developed a self-evaluation tool to help you discover what your learning style is (Figure 1–1). There are 32 questions; the test is not timed, so take your time and answer each question as honestly as you can.

Once you complete the inventory and total your responses, you will have a good indication of what your primary learning style is. If several of your scores are within 4 or 5 points of each other, it means that you can use any of those senses for learning tasks. If you were in a hurry, it would be best for you to use your primary mode of learning. However, if you have some extra time it might behoove you to work on developing those sensory areas that you are less likely to use.

◼ Making the Most of Study Time

Studying is not new to you. We know that you have been studying for quite a long time now. Studying in nursing school may be a bit more difficult, but not any different from what you have already experienced. You may already be well aware of what works and doesn't work for you when you are studying. Whether you need to find a new way to study, enhance the way you already study, or stick with the tried and true method you've used in the past, find a system that works for you and stick with it.

The best way to find a system that works for you is trial and error. Here are some ideas that might speed the process along.

Place a check on the appropriate line after each statement.

	5 pts Often	3 pts Sometimes	1 pt Seldom
1. I can remember more about a subject through listening than reading.			
2. I follow written directions better than oral directions.			
3. Once shown a new physical movement, I perform it quickly with few errors.			
4. I bear down extremely hard with a pen or pencil when writing.			
5. I require explanations of diagrams, graphs, or visual directions.			
6. I enjoy working with tools.			
7. I am skilled with and enjoy developing and making graphs and charts.			
8. I can tell if sounds match when presented with pairs of sounds.			
9. I can watch someone do a dance step and easily copy it myself.			
10. I can understand and follow directions on maps.			
11. I do better at academic subjects by listening to lectures and tapes.			
12. I frequently play with coins or keys in my pocket.			
13. I enjoy perfecting a movement in a sport or in dancing.			
14. I can better understand a news article by reading about it in the paper than by listening to the radio.			
15. I chew gum, smoke, or snack during studies.			
16. I feel the best way to remember is to picture it in my head.			
17. I enjoy activities that make me aware of my body's movement.			
18. I would rather listen to a good lecture or speech than read the same material in a textbook.			
19. I consider myself an athletic person.			
20. I grip objects in my hands during learning.			
21. I would prefer listening to the news on the radio rather than reading about it in the newspaper.			
22. I like to obtain information on an interesting subject by reading relevant materials.			
23. I am highly aware of sensations and feelings in my hips and shoulders after learning a new movement or exercise.			
24. I follow oral directions better than written ones.			

Figure 1–1. Barsch Learning Style Inventory (Jeffrey R. Barsch, EdD). *Source:* Academic Therapy Publications, Barsch Learning Style Inventory, Barsch, J. R. *(Continued)*

25. It would be easy for me to memorize something if I could just use body movements at the same time. _____ _____ _____

26. I like to write things down or take notes for visual review. _____ _____ _____

27. I remember best when writing things down several times. _____ _____ _____

28. I learn to spell better by repeating the letters out loud than by writing the word on paper. _____ _____ _____

29. I frequently have the ability to visualize body movements to perform a task, e.g., correction of a golf swing, batting stance, dance position, etc. _____ _____ _____

30. I could learn spelling well by tracing over the letters. _____ _____ _____

31. I feel comfortable touching, hugging, shaking hands, etc. _____ _____ _____

32. I am good at working and solving jigsaw puzzles and mazes. _____ _____ _____

Scoring Procedures:

Place the point value on the line next to its corresponding item number. Next, add the points to obtain the preference scores under each heading.

VISUAL		AUDITORY		TACTILE		KINESTHETIC	
No.	Pts.	No.	Pts.	No.	Pts.	No.	Pts.
2	_____	1	_____	4	_____	3	_____
7	_____	5	_____	6	_____	9	_____
10	_____	8	_____	12	_____	13	_____
14	_____	11	_____	15	_____	17	_____
16	_____	18	_____	20	_____	19	_____
22	_____	21	_____	27	_____	23	_____
26	_____	24	_____	30	_____	25	_____
32	_____	28	_____	31	_____	29	_____
VPS =		APS =		TPS =		KPS =	

VPS = Visual Preference Score
APS = Auditory Preference Score
TPS = Tactile Preference Score
KPS = Kinesthetic Preference Score

How to Use This Information:

This form is to be used in conjunction with other diagnostic tools to help you determine some of the ways you are best able to learn. Discuss your scores with someone who is qualified to interpret them in order to make the best use of the time and effort you have invested.

Figure 1–1. *(Continued)*

Finding a System That Works

The best way to find a system that works for you is trial and error. Here are some ideas that might speed the process along.

1. **Most people prefer a designated study place.** Some people prefer to study in absolute quiet. Others find that background noise actually increases their concentration. Be sure that you have adequate lighting, comfortable seating, and all of the supplies that you need to avoid frequent interruptions.
2. **Avoid marathon study sessions.** It is essential that you take breaks, get up, walk around, and stretch (Figure 1–2). You need to keep your blood moving, and you need to give your mind a break. It is much easier to study for shorter intervals and it will probably increase your comprehension. If you study consistently from the beginning of the course to the end, and review prior content, you shouldn't have to resort to marathon studying or cramming for exams.

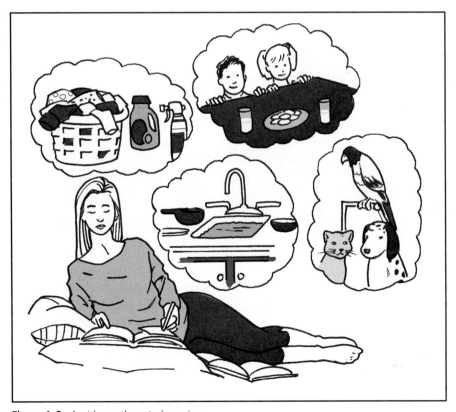

Figure 1–2. Avoid marathon study sessions.

3. Focus on what you are reading.
- If you are worried about something, take the time to deal with it, or put it in the back of your mind until you take a break.
- If you have to, write down the things that distract you from your studying.
- Sometimes, the "I forgot to . . ." pops into your mind. Keep a list of these things so you can move on and get back to your reading.
- If you have a major personal problem that is interfering with your studying, you may need to seek outside help.

If you discover that no matter what you do and how you study, you continue to have problems understanding the material and/or passing exams, consider the following:

- Seek help at the campus counseling center.
- Most counseling centers will provide:
  - Learning style assessments
  - Ways to conquer test anxiety
  - Tutoring
  - Study skills assessment
  - Career counseling

Students who try to cover up major difficulties often end up failing courses because of them. Find someone you can talk with and, if you are comfortable, let your faculty know. Nursing faculty has dealt with many a problem, and will know what resources are available to help you. If you are not comfortable with the faculty, seek out a friend, counselor, family member, minister, priest, rabbi, or family physician. Find someone that you trust and get help. Is it worth potentially destroying your career to keep your silence?

Making the Most of Your Learning Style When You Study

As you might already have imagined, visual, auditory, tactile, and kinesthetic learners benefit from using a study method that fits with their method of learning. The following information can help you tailor your studying so you get the greatest benefit.

Visual Learner—needs to "see" all study materials.
- Reorganize notes on small cards to carry with you.
- Use bright, eye-catching colors!

- Use charts, maps, notes, and flashcards.
- Frequently review notes for a quick visual snapshot.

Auditory Learner—needs to "hear" all study materials.
- Listen to classes and audiotape them also.
- As you review your notes, summarize them on tape.
- Verbally review lectures with a friend.
- Does well with study groups.
- Read study materials aloud when studying.
- Make flashcards and read them aloud.

Primary Tactile Learner—needs to "feel" study materials.
- Trace words as you say them.
- Write down important facts several times.
- Type your notes or use a word processor.
- Learning sign language will help reinforce tactile skills.
- Keep something malleable in your hand when you study such as Silly Putty or Play Doh.

Primary Kinesthetic Learner—needs to involve the body in learning.
- Play your favorite music while you study and move with the beat.
- Make flashcards and walk while you study them.
- Try dancing, poetry, rap, crafts, or other ways to reinforce learning.
- Ask for assignments that involve experiments or building things.
- Seek group interactions to study.

In addition, here are some general study tips that all learners can use regardless of their learning style:

- Take good lecture notes and reorganize them into flashcards.
- Read an assignment for 25 minutes (after that, you lose 85% of your comprehension).
- After 25 minutes, get up, stretch, relax, or eat a snack—whatever is comfortable for you.
- Underline main points in eye-catching highlighters.
- Review the underlined material.
- Repeat the first five steps and then when done, review all of the underlined material one more time.
- Learn a relaxation technique.
- Use quiet background music with a 4/4 beat, as rhythm is indigenous to each of us. It will help you achieve and maintain relaxation.
- Use your olfactory sense. Our sense of smell is a primary learning mode for all of us. Use a pleasant odor, perfume, peppermint candy, or the like that can be available during exams to help you stimulate the recall process.

- Use natural timing. When studying lists and facts, read them, say them, and count to eight between each item. This will give you time to process and integrate one fact before adding another.

Preparation for Lectures

Nursing courses build on one another. You can't isolate and forget material from one or more courses. For example, if you hated pathophysiology, you can't throw your notes away and never think about it again. Why? Because pathophysiology is found in nearly all nursing courses, so once it is over, you can't forget the material. If you don't believe a course or certain course material is relevant to your education, you will tend to forget the material. It is vital for you to remember that *all* of your courses are important building blocks to graduation.

Class Preparation

1. **Attend all classes.** Most of us have our own way of taking notes in class. Some of us highlight, draw pictures, or scribble in the margins. No one will take notes the way that you do! We also learn through all of our senses. When you get notes from others, you lose a great deal in the interpretation. You will also spend a lot of time trying to decipher someone else's notes. If you have an emergency, ask someone you trust to tape record the class and tell you what they remember from class. Use their notes only as a backup.
2. **If possible, sit in the front of the classroom.** Students who sit up front tend to follow the lectures better and pay attention more. The back of the room usually attracts students who want to be distracting. It is difficult to take adequate notes when the student next to you is providing details about his or her latest "hot date."
3. **Be prepared for class.** It is important to read the required reading prior to class. When you have done the reading, you will be able to concentrate more on what the instructor is saying, and you will be able to ask intelligent questions to clarify anything you didn't understand.
4. **During class, be alert for clues to questions that might appear on exams.** As you listen to lecture listen for words like:
   - "The most important part of . . ."
   - "This would make a good test item."
   - "The main thing to remember is . . ."

- "To repeat . . ."
- "The major emphasis is . . ."

5. **Review your notes as soon after class as feasible.**
    - Be sure to make any corrections or add any important information that you can recall.
    - Highlight any major concepts, and note any areas that you might have missed or need clarification on.
    - Read your text again to see if it can provide the answers to your questions.
    - If you are unable to fill in the blanks or clarify the content, check with your instructor to get the *correct* information.
    - Remember that relying on other students does not always provide accurate information!
    - If you and your instructor have modems, you may be able to e-mail your questions.
    - If e-mail is not available, check for your instructor's office hours, or call the instructor with your questions.

Taping Classes

Some students prefer to tape class lectures in addition to taking notes. Often, class content is delivered so that a lot of material is covered in a short period of time. If you choose to tape your classes, be sure to:

- Check your course syllabus to see if taping is permitted.
- Ask permission of the instructor prior to taping.
- Check to be sure your equipment is in working order.
- Have extra tapes and batteries on hand.
- Remember that you can't interrupt the class in order to change tapes or batteries.
- Be sure that you have a backup plan just in case.

Testing

Testing is a part of all education programs. Most nursing programs use teacher-made exams that are similar to the National Council of Licensing and Examination (NCLEX) test that you will take upon graduation to be eligible for your nursing license. The NCLEX is made up of multiple-choice questions, so most likely you will have a great deal of experience with multiple-choice questions during your nursing education.

Before Exams

1. **Find out what type of exam you will be taking.** Is it multiple-choice, matching, fill-in-the-blank, or essay questions? Find out the expected number of items and approximate length of time allotted for the test.
2. **Clarify any content that you don't understand if you haven't already done so.**
3. **Know your instructor!** Is this the first exam that you have had from this instructor? If so, you may be at a disadvantage. Sometimes, it takes a first test to understand what an instructor expects. It can help you to determine what the instructor focuses on. The focus may vary from instructor to instructor, as they are all individuals.
   - Does the instructor focus on details or on general concepts?
   - Use the textbook only?
   - Use notes only?
   - Rely heavily on outside reading or audiovisuals?
   - Or use some combination of these?
   - Sometimes, only time will tell. It is best to be as prepared as possible for the first exam and use it as a learning experience!
4. **Continue to review the material that will be on the exam.**
   - Remember that studying for an exam begins as soon as new content is introduced following the previous exam.
   - As each new area of content is introduced, review previous material first and then focus on the new content. For example, if the first area of content is anxiety, go over your notes and read the text and any other material. If the next area of content to be introduced is mood disorders, you need to go back and review anxiety and then add information about mood and so on.
   - You should never need to cram for an exam, because you will be ready. This is also a great way to avoid the disasters of feeling ill or having a family emergency the night before an exam. These things do happen and students who have saved up to cram the night before will end up failing an exam.
5. **Be sure to get a good night's sleep the night before the exam.** Do not rely on sleep-enhancing medication as it can interfere with your sleep cycles. If you have been studying on a regular basis, you should only need to review the material, not cram. A good night's sleep will give you the energy you need for the exam!

The Day of the Exam

1. **Eat a meal before the exam.**
   - If you have class from 8 A.M. to 11:30 A.M. and an exam at 11:45 A.M., eat a good breakfast and then eat a snack high in complex carbohydrates, not simple sugars, prior to the exam!

- If you rely on sugar, remember that you will hit a low sometime during the exam!
- Eating the right foods has been shown to increase test performance!

2. **Plan ahead so that you leave yourself plenty of time to get to the exam without the added stress of being fearful that you will be late.**
   - Be sure that your car has gas and air in the tires.
   - Be sure that you leave time for the little things that can keep you from getting to the exam on time.
   - Don't allow too much time though, because it will give you additional time to worry if you are a worrier.

3. **Do not rely on drugs to either stimulate you or relax you prior to the exam.** Medications can have side effects or untoward effects that can interfere with your concentration.

4. **If possible, go to the exam room and sit down.** *Do not* sit around and compare notes or questions with other students at the last second. If a student asks you, "What is that statistical test that is used with a Solomon 4 group design?", it may send you into orbit! Not to mention that it will decrease your concentration and confidence!

5. **It is important that you maintain some anxiety.** Anxiety tends to improve performance as long as it is controlled and minimized. We can remember playing a relaxation tape for students who had problems with test anxiety. The relaxation tape was so good that several of the students fell asleep! The students were so relaxed that they actually did worse on the exam because they had so little anxiety.

6. **Be sure that you follow the directions on the exam and from the faculty.**
   - Check to be sure that you have all of the pages on the exam in the correct order.
   - Be sure that all of the pages are legible and that you have the correct number of test items.

7. **Be sure to fill in the scantron or computerized test form accurately.**
   - Answer all of the questions to the best of your ability unless points will be deducted for wrong answers.
   - Be certain that you have not left a blank on the answer sheet and that all questions correspond to the number on the form. We have had students leave out an entire page of an exam because they were not paying attention to the numbering.

8. **Be careful when changing answers.**
   - Students invariably want to know if they should change answers on an exam.
   - For the most part, we find that students tend to change answers from right to wrong. But, we have had the occasional student who actually does better by changing answers.
   - You know yourself best. Keep track of the answers you have changed and compare them at test review.

- Did you improve your score or not? If you didn't, then make a rule for yourself that you will not change answers on the next exam.

9. **Do not cheat.**
    - It does you no good, and it will affect your patients in the long run.
    - Do not let other students cheat off of you for the same reasons.
      I can recall one of my nursing instructors asking me to think about this scenario. She told me to close my eyes and imagine that I had just awakened in the recovery room after major surgery. Then she said to imagine that the student cheating off me was the one providing my nursing care. Would you be comfortable with this student taking care of you? Think about waking up with that student holding your life in his or her hands. If the student cheated his or her way through school, he or she does not know much.
    - Most schools have a process for making faculty aware of cheaters. It will benefit all of those involved if you could see your way clear to report cheaters and other unethical behaviors.
    - Once students graduate, they don't leave their lack of ethics behind and often jeopardize patients as a result.

10. **Beware of the post-exam autopsy.**
    - This is similar to the pre-exam "did you study X, Y, Z," but focuses on questions that were on the exam.
    - The autopsy usually begins with "What answer did you get for that question about . . . ?"
    - Students tend to form groups and as individuals begin to compare notes.
    - Invariably, some will walk away "knowing" that they have "failed" the exam.
    - Rarely does a student feel better following the exam autopsy.
    - Whether or not you choose to participate is your choice, but we would recommend that you head for home or your next class, or treat yourself to something fun!

Types of Exams

Most schools use multiple-choice exams or some combination of multiple-choice items mixed with matching, fill-in-the-blank, and true or false questions. As stated earlier, this is to prepare the student for the NCLEX exam.

ANATOMY OF A MULTIPLE-CHOICE ITEM

Multiple-choice questions consist of a *stem* and usually four or more *distracters,* or choices.

The chapter you are reading is about?   (Stem)

a. pathophysiology
b. pharmacology   (Distracters)
c. anatomy
d. studying and testing

HOW TO TAKE A MULTIPLE-CHOICE EXAM

Read the entire item including the stem and all of the distracters. Most students can choose two distracters that are wrong—which gives them a 50 percent chance of getting the answer right. There are all kinds of tips for doing well on a multiple-choice test. Examples of the described distracters are indicated by an asterisk. We're not sure how reliable they are but here are some we have heard.

1. The longest distracter is usually the answer.
   One of the primary contributors to heart disease is:
   a. exercise
   b. eating a high-fat diet* (correct answer)
   c. weight loss
   d. vitamin intake
2. If two distracters have the same terms or mostly the same terms, then one of them is probably the answer.
   Skin cancer is most often caused by:
   a. a diet high in vitamin D
   b. long-term sun exposure*
   c. unprotected sun exposure* (correct answer)
   d. swimming
3. If you have no idea what the answer is, choose b or c.
4. If the item lists more than one thing in each distracter, be sure to read the whole list. Avoid choosing answers if any one of the listed items is incorrect.
   In basic life support, ABC stands for?
   a. airway, bleeding, circulation*
   b. anatomy, biology, chemistry
   c. airway, breathing, circulation (correct answer)
   d. anxiety, bleeding, circulation*
5. Be wary of items that state "always," "never," or any other absolutes.
   When confronting a hostile patient, the nurse would:
   a. speak softly (answer)
   b. yell loudly to get the patient's attention
   c. always call for help*
   d. start screaming loudly

As you progress through your nursing courses, you will probably find that the test items tend to get harder over time. This occurs because the instructors are trying to help you apply what you have learned in a variety of settings. Most test questions will reflect leveling. This means that they will be more difficult. Instructors are looking for the following skills:

1. **Knowing**—These items ask you to regurgitate what you have learned. A bit like a parrot, they expect you to repeat what you have heard. For example: What does ABC stand for in basic life support? If you have memorized ABC, you can repeat back airway, breathing, circulation.

2. **Comprehension**—These items ask you to repeat something that you have learned, only in a different way. For example, if you have been told that stress is the major cause of automobile accidents, your instructor may ask a question about two people involved in an automobile accident. The instructor may want to know what is the probability that the accident was stress related. Your answer would be the highest possible number since you were told that stress is the major cause of automobile accidents (therefore, the highest percentage).

3. **Application**—These items ask you to put material you have learned into new situations. For example, you drive up to the scene of a car accident and find that there are two injured people. One is having difficulty breathing and the other is bleeding from a superifical cut on her right knee. Which of these patients would you take care of first? Remember your ABCs and prioritize! You would care for the person having problems breathing first and then the person who is bleeding.

SHORT-ANSWER OR ESSAY QUESTIONS

Most nursing schools use multiple-choice exams to prepare you for the NCLEX exam. You may be given a short-answer or essay question as part of an exam, or in a nursing elective. Essay questions are a great way to determine what a student knows about a particular subject, but they are extremely difficult to grade because it is hard for the faculty to be objective. The primary thing to remember about both short-answer and essay questions is that you need to read and answer what is asked. Many times students read part of the question and start writing an answer without digesting the whole question. It is helpful if you underline the verb in the question. For example, if the question asks you to *describe* how you would triage patients in an emergency room following a bus accident, be sure to **detail** what you would do. On the other hand, if it asks you to *list* the steps taken by a triage nurse following a bus accident, be sure to **list** your answer.

After you read and understand the question and what it is asking, some students choose to do a quick outline to organize their thoughts. Other students prefer to just start writing.

- Do whatever works for you.
- Be sure that you answer in complete sentences using correct spelling and grammar.
- Be sure to be as objective as possible unless the question specifically asks for your opinion about something.
- Be succinct in your answer but include as much information as possible.
- Beware of running on or throwing in as many words as you think the teacher wants to see. (As nursing faculty, we are very good at determining when a student does not really know an answer and is just filling up a page with words.)
- If you have no idea what the question is asking, see if your instructor can provide you with more detail or clarify it for you (some will and some will not).
- If you are not sure of an answer, write down anything that you think relates to the question because you may get partial credit. Many times essay questions have a high point value so it is better to get partial credit than none.

Test Anxiety

Unfortunately, some students experience test anxiety in any testing situation, and it is vital for these students to learn to deal with this disabling anxiety. Most test anxiety results from negative childhood messages that are incorporated into the subconscious. According to Erwin and Dinwiddie (1983), there are several types of unconscious messages that lead to test anxiety.

UNCONSCIOUS MESSAGES THAT CREATE ANXIETY

1. **You are stupid, a dummy, or not very smart.**
   - Basically, the student who heard this message believes that he or she will never do anything right.
   - This message sets the student up for failure by creating a no-win situation.
   - During study time, the student thinks "Why bother, I can't pass the test anyway."
   - Studying becomes a hopeless endeavor and the student does not do well on the exam, which reinforces the message that he or she is "stupid, a dummy, and not very smart."
2. **Be perfect.**
   - Students who have been told that they have to be perfect force themselves to achieve all As because their parents only focused on A grades.
   - If the child had five As and one B, they were punished for receiving the B rather than congratulated for the As that they achieved.
   - This student studies so compulsively that he or she often neglects other needs.

- The student is often so worried about not achieving perfection that he or she tends to be easily distracted during testing.
- If the student doesn't know the answer to one question, the panic tends to snowball and the student believes that he or she will fail the exam.

3. **You are phenomenal.**
   - This child has been told over and over again how bright, intelligent, and amazing he or she is.
   - This child grows up to believe that he or she has to live up to others' expectations.
   - Unfortunately, it is impossible to live up to such high expectations all of the time.
   - The student begins to have doubts and believes that other people will discover that he or she is not as perfect as others believed him or her to be.
   - This sets the student up for failure since he or she feels like an impostor most of the time.

If you believe that you have test anxiety that is interfering with your ability to take and pass exams, please seek help. It is possible to change these messages and many techniques have been found to be useful in controlling test anxiety. Most universities have a testing or counseling center that can help you learn to control your anxiety levels.

Learning how to take exams is an essential component of nursing school. The more exams you take and the more information you have, the more you will succeed. Remember that test taking is a learning experience too. Do the best that you can do and remember that you are more than your grades!

Students with Learning Disabilities or Other Disabilities

Colleges and universities are required by law to meet various specifications. The laws that are vital for you to review are:

- Rehabilitation Act of 1973 (especially section 504)
- Americans with Disabilities Act (ADA) of 1990
- Individuals with Disabilities Education Act (IDEA) of 1990
- Family Educational Rights and Privacy Act (FERPA) of 1974, which protects student records confidentiality

It is also important for you to:

- Be a self-advocate.
- Be prepared to document your disability (this evaluation should be current within the past 2 to 5 years).

- Be certain that you meet the criteria set by the university and program that you are interested in. (Remember, universities are not required to alter admissions requirements, nor are they required to alter programmatic requirements for students with disabilities once they have been admitted).
- Remember, the application form may not require you to disclose whether or not you have a disability. It is up to you whether you want to "disclose" your disability or not.
- Contact or visit the Disability Support Services office on campus.
- Determine what type of accommodations the university provides. The university is required to provide accommodations to qualified students with disabilities, including learning disabilities. Some common forms of accommodation are:
  - Individual test administration
  - Large-print materials
  - Special answer sheets for exams
  - Extended testing time
  - Audiocassette tests
  - Using a computer to write exams or papers
  - Sign language interpreters
  - Volunteer "buddies" to help the disabled

Long Distance Learning

The classroom of the future is upon us. You may currently have, or soon will have, didactic portions of your nursing and non-nursing courses offered in a long distance learning (LDL) format. The two most common methods are courses offered by the video format and courses offered by the Web format; that is, the course is offered online. Like the "live" classes you are accustomed to, long distance methods have some drawbacks. To start, be aware that most LDL methods are *not* correspondence courses in which you can work at your own pace. You will need to read the course syllabus carefully and mark your calendar for due dates: tests, papers, learning activities, class participation, and so on. Also, trips to the library may be necessary.

Here are some hints to help you make your LDL experiences successful.

- Video courses will require that you go to a specific facility in your area where you view the course faculty presenting the class in real time. You will be able to ask questions and participate in other verbal class activity. In some cases, the equipment available may allow the faculty member to also see you. In addition, video courses may have a portion of the course grade derived from attendance and/or class participation. So be prepared to meet specific class attendance requirements.

- Online courses have their own challenges:
  - **Technical requirements**—Online courses have specific hardware, and perhaps software, requirements. Thus, you may need to upgrade your computer. In addition, you may also have to download (usually free) some specific programs to accommodate course material.
  - **Computer literacy**—In addition to using your computer as a word processor, you will need to know how to do such things as use links, send and receive e-mail attachments, enter and participate in course chat rooms, participate in threaded discussions, take exams online, save and move documents, and so on.
  - **Problems**—Be prepared for technical problems (your server goes down during an exam, you cannot get into the required chat that has a grade attached, you cannot download required assignments, material online is poor quality or completely unreadable; the list goes on.). At the *beginning* of the course, find out how to handle such problems!
  - **Learning**—The responsibility for understanding and learning course content shifts in this format. In the classroom, you take notes and can ask questions. In addition, faculty can often tell by your body language when further explanation is needed. *Online courses do not have this element.* So you have the responsibility of contacting faculty when you need help. The method for contact is usually e-mail, but may include fax and/or phone contact. If faculty do not hear from you, they do not know your needs. **Again, you have the responsibility of contacting faculty for help.**

As you can see, taking a course by long distance method has many challenges. If you have a choice between taking a live class or its long distance format, you are cautioned to carefully weigh the options. If you do not learn well outside the traditional setting, LDL may not be for you.

Learning how to study and take tests is vital in order for you to successfully complete your nursing studies. Knowing your particular learning style and understanding the ways that you study best are important. Learn how to take exams, and give yourself some time to figure out specific instructors' ways of asking questions. Give yourself a break if you are not doing well, and if you find yourself in a situation in which you continue to get bad grades or have other difficulties, consider going to the counseling center on campus for some assistance. Remember, you are the only one who can reach out for help when you need it. Learning, studying, and test taking may be a different kind of challenge for you, but you can do well and you can graduate! Just remember, day by day, test by test, and course by course!

2

Time Management

Time Management

Let's face it—most of us don't sit around complaining that we have too much time on our hands with nothing to do. With our current technological capabilities, we spend our lives being available 24 hours a day. Since you are attending nursing school, be prepared to set aside some major blocks of time to:

- Attend classes
- Attend clinical
- Study
- Write papers
- Jump through hoops (okay, we wanted to see if you were paying attention)

The small amount of time you thought you had just got significantly smaller! How will you keep up? What can you do now to plan ahead so that you don't lose sight of the other very valuable things in your life?

- Family
- Work
- Fun
- Exercise
- Spirituality
- Sleep

Time management can help you achieve your goals with a minimum of stress and overreaction.

A CASE IN POINT

> Lori is organized! She has a calendar and fills in when all her papers, projects, and assignments are due as well as when she has classes/clinical, when she will study, and when her exams are scheduled. Although she sometimes feels overwhelmed, she is able to break down all her assignments into smaller pieces in order to accomplish each task. The freedom from worrying about whether or not she is getting things done on time allows her more time to accomplish what she needs to.

One of your primary goals in nursing school is to graduate! Right now, that may seem a long way off, but in order to get to graduation there are many smaller steps involved. Rather than overwhelming yourself by thinking of graduation, concentrate instead on the smaller steps.

1. The courses that you have to take:
   - Check your degree plan.
   - Visit your advisor regularly.
   - Note your visits in your calendar.
   - Make copies of pertinent papers.
2. Individual course requirements:
   - Assignments (papers, projects, debates, etc.)
   - Exams
   - Clinical requirements
   - Point distribution

A CASE IN POINT

> Beatrice was in her first day of nursing fundamentals. She spent the day dreaming about graduation, her diploma, walking across the stage, and her nursing license arriving in the mail. The next class period, when her first assignment was due, she didn't even know she had an assignment and was totally unprepared. Embarrassed and feeling overwhelmed, she spent the whole day crying and worrying about everything else that was due between now and graduation! Her friend, K.C., not only turned in her first assignment on time; she also had a calendar made with all due dates and exams highlighted in various colors. K.C. felt in control and calm. She knew what she had to do and when she had to do it in order to graduate on schedule.

3. Assignments:
- Criteria for completion
- Point distribution

Organization! Most of us would rather be like K.C. than like Beatrice. What is the difference in the two approaches? K.C. is organized and Beatrice is not. So, how does one get organized?

1. Assessment: The first thing you need to know is how are you currently spending your time? Write it down! Account for every 30 minutes in a 24-hour day for a whole week! Doing this will tell you a great deal about where your time is going. It will take some time, but remember sometimes it takes time to save time.

Exercise: Get a spiral notebook and title seven pages with the days of the week. In the top section, write a description of the usual things you do on a daily basis and assign a symbol to it. For example, you will probably have the following categories:

- Work
- Exercise
- Eating
- Play
- Family
- Sleep
- Spiritual/Church
- Add others as needed (music, team sports, etc.)

Write down how you spend your time and at the end of the week total it up! You should be able to figure out where your time is going. This will help you plan in the time needed for nursing school!

2. Planning: Now that you have a general idea of how your time is spent, what do you do? All of us have 168 hours per week—no more, no less. So, you need to prioritize. What activities are the most vital? If you want to graduate, then school will need to be high on your list! You also need to develop a monthly, weekly, and daily schedule (see Figures 2–1a, b, and c).

Be sure that when your calendar is complete you make a copy to post at home to remind you and your family of your schedule. In planning your schedule consider all your roles and activities, not just school! Remember to plan for sleep, exercise, and relaxation. Also plan the "in between" activities. For example, if you have an exam coming up, be sure to plan in study time! Keep in mind your "best" time of the day! Are you a morning person? If so, plan for the majority of your activity or heavy thinking time to occur in the morning. If you are a nighttime person then

February 2001						
Sun	**Mon**	**Tue**	**Wed**	**Thu**	**Fri**	**Sat**
				Pharmacology exam		Joe's birthday
Teach Sunday school class	Clinical St. Mary's	Clinical St. Mary's		Paper due Case Study Nursing 103		Dinner with the Walkers
	Clinical Dr. Creed's Office	Clinical Home Health	Dental Appt. 3:30 pm		Nursing 103 Exam	
Teach Sunday school	Clinical Dr. Eger's office	Clinical Health Dept.	Martin's Birthday			"Our night out"
	Clinical St. Mary's	Clinical St. Mary's	Debate Nursing 106			

Figure 2–1a. Monthly calendar.

don't plan to be doing a lot of studying in the morning. You know yourself best so plan things at a time when you know you will be at your best.

There are a number of ways to develop and keep your calendars up to date. Probably the cheapest option is to purchase a monthly or weekly

A Case in Point

Crystal kept a meticulous schedule, with all of her nursing school information highlighted in various colors. Her day planner included all the papers, projects, exams, and assignments due for the entire semester. Tuesday afternoon after clinical, she frantically searched her backpack only to discover her planner was missing. For two days she was totally lost and had no idea what was due or even where she was supposed to be. Crystal spent many hours trying to reconstruct her schedule. The next day a fellow student called to say he had found her planner in the nurse's lounge at the hospital. Crystal decided that from then on she would make a copy of her calendar "just in case."

February 2001	
Sun 11	Attend church 9:30 am Lunch with family 12:00 noon Review all notes for Nursing 103 exam Friday Make plans for "our night out" on the 25th
Mon 12	Clinical Dr. Creed's office from 8 am to 4:30 pm Meet with Study Group at 5 pm Mary's house—bring some snacks
Tue 13	Clinical Home Health Office "Dress in blue pants/white top and labcoat" Pick up dry cleaning Review notes for Nursing 103 exam
Wed 14	Pharmacology class 9 am Nursing 103 class 10:30 am English 201 class 1 pm Dental Appt. 3:30 pm
Thu 15	Practice IV technique in the lab from 9 am to 10 am Meet with study group at noon in cafeteria Swim with Mattie at 4 pm Spend quality time with family and relax!
Fri 16	Walk with Mom 8 am Nursing 103 exam 10 am—eat a good breakfast! English 201 class 1 pm Meet Joey at school for softball practice 4:30 pm
Sat 17	Family cleaning day—spruce up! Picnic lunch with family noon—our backyard Prepare material for Sunday school class tomorrow

Figure 2–1b. Weekly calendar.

planner available each year at office supply stores. Some students who have a lot to organize may prefer a larger datebook that not only includes a calendar, but also a variety of other things such as expense planner, to-do lists, address books, and the like. This type of day planner usually contains removable sections that can be replaced or added to as needed.

For the technologically minded student, there are numerous computer calendar generating software options, as well as personal digital as-

	Friday, February 16, 2001
6am	Wake up/Breakfast
7am	Meditate/Review notes for exam
8am	Walk with Mom 45 min
9am	Leave for school—bring snack
10am	Nursing 103 Exam
11am	
Noon	Meet with study group—Lunch
1pm	English 201 Class
2pm	
3pm	Pick up dog/cat food
4pm	Meet Joey at school 4:30
5pm	Softball practice (Joey)
6pm	Dinner
7pm	Review next clinical assignment
8pm	Relax with family
9pm	Bath/Kids to bed
10pm	Me to bed!

Figure 2–1c. Daily calendar.

sistants (PDAs) and other electronic date books. Some potential problems with these are:

- Battery failure
- Software glitches
- Failure to print a hard copy of your schedule
- Not having the device with you at all times

What kinds of things belong on your calendar or in your day planner? Here are some ideas:

- Paper, project, and presentation due dates
- Clinical times and locations
- Class times and locations
- Meetings and appointments
- Special occasions, birthdays, anniversaries, social events
- Steps toward long-term goal achievement
- Completion of parts of a larger project
- Increase in exercise from 30 minutes to 45 minutes, working up to your goal of 60 minutes 6 days a week

Students who fail to plan and make schedules often experience overwhelming feelings as they forget, procrastinate, cram, and make poor grades. These students are always trying to catch up, and many of them never do! They also endure more stress and have more difficulty at home, at work, and in their other relationships. Are you sitting there shaking your head saying "no way!" "This author has got to be kidding me, this is too much work!" "Plus, if I schedule myself into a corner, where is my freedom?" "When will I have play time?" "This is too inflexible!" I promise, this will actually give you *more* flexibility. Are you thinking "yeah right!" "I'm too busy to spend time doing all that scheduling, who is she kidding?" "She must have nothing better to do but sit around and make schedules!" Ah! But, I am here to tell you that if you think you don't have the time to spend making up a schedule, then you are the one who needs it the most!

Just remember, if you have been a free spirit all or a procrastinator of your life, it takes time to unlearn behaviors. You will need to use time to make time, and you may need to exercise a lot of self-discipline.

1. **Scheduling time:** The first thing you need to do is establish your priorities. As stated earlier, one of your major priorities has to be nursing school if you are planning to graduate! Obviously, if you have a spouse and children, your family will also be a priority to you. If you don't have a family, spending time with friends may be important to you. Let's compare the priorities of two students, one who is a married adult student with children, the other, a single traditional student (see Table 2–1).

Table 2–1. Comparison of Priorities of a Married Adult Student with Children and a Single Traditional Student

Adult Married/Children	Priority Categories	Single Traditional Student
1. Caring for family	Education/classes	1. Close friends
2. Part-time job	Work	2. Classes/studying
3. Studying/classes	Family	3. School involvement
4. Church/meditation	Friends/relationships	4. Team sports
5. Personal time/wellness	Personal time	5. Exercise/relaxation
6. Relationships/ entertainment	Household tasks	6. Chores/groceries/ errands
7. Household tasks	Extracurricular activity	7. Time with family
	School/community	
	Spiritual life	

Exercise: It is easy to see how these two students' priorities differ. What are your priorities? Number them from 1 to 7 and remember, school needs to be near the top!

One thing that is important to remember is to be flexible! Things change and "stuff" happens. For example, you might have a family emergency or you might find that one of your classes has been canceled. The more that you can "go with the flow," the less anxiety you will experience. If there comes a time when you are feeling particularly stressed and overwhelmed, it may help to refer back to your priority list. Is there something that you are not doing? We tend to let things go as we become more and more stressed. Are you still taking personal time? Spending time with your family and friends? Getting your spiritual needs fulfilled?

Some people enjoy the satisfaction of keeping to-do lists. A to-do list is basically a list of all things that need to be done within a specific time frame, usually a day or a week. This list needs to be prioritized! Some people label their priorities A, B, C or 1, 2, 3. This helps them to know which items need to be done first (A or 1 items), those that can be done next (B or 2 items), and those items that have the least priority (C or 3 items). Knowing that as you complete each item you get to physically cross the item off a list is a great incentive to some people. Be certain that anything left on the list is moved to the top of the next list!

One thing to remember as you develop your schedule and to-do lists is that when you allot time for studying, completing a project, anything, consider Parkinson's law. Parkinson's law states that the time it takes to do a task

A CASE IN POINT

Joseph got the notice to renew his student malpractice insurance on July 30, six weeks before he was due to start clinical. Instead of paying it, he put it in his "to-do" pile. Four weeks later, he found the notice under a stack of "stuff" on his desk and decided to wait until he went to the university to pay it so he "wouldn't waste a stamp." Although Joseph went to the university the following week, he forgot to bring the malpractice insurance forms with him. The day before clinical started, his instructor called him out of class to inform him that unless he paid for his malpractice insurance that day and brought proof to clinical the next morning, he would be unable to continue in the program. Joseph didn't bring his checkbook with him so he now had to make several trips and deal with the embarrassment of being the only student who had not renewed his malpractice insurance. A minor inconvenience was now a major screw-up!

will stretch out to fill whatever time you have assigned to that task (Pauk, 1998). So, be sure to set a realistic time limit in which to complete any task!

2. **Problems with procrastination:** Many individuals procrastinate! They put minor things off until they develop into huge problems.

Here are some of the reasons why people tend to procrastinate:

- Not having goals or having unrealistic ones
- Low self-esteem
- Perfectionism and fear of making mistakes
- Fear of a situation

How can you fight your desire to procrastinate?

- Weigh the benefits of completing a task versus the consequences of putting it off.
- Set reasonable goals
- Do something! Start! Take that first step!
- Break an overwhelming task into smaller easier to accomplish pieces.
- Ask for help! If you don't understand an assignment, ask for an explanation.
- Do not expect perfection!

3. **Delegation:** Another way to deal with the feeling of being overwhelmed by numerous tasks is to learn the art of delegation. Many routine tasks can be delegated to family members or others in order to lighten the load. Many of us have someone in our lives that can willingly help us meet our goals. Is there someone in your life to whom you might delegate some of your activities? Do you have a family member, friend, or perhaps several who can help? Remember, they can't read your mind, so you will have to ask! Even children can help out and they often react well to helping mommy or daddy go to school. Your children can also gain independence by lending a helping hand. Don't forget that it may take a while to teach a new skill, but once learned, the individual will master the skill, gain confidence, and independence.

Delegation requires communication! Have a family meeting. Allow each person to come up with activities that he or she might be able to help with. Suggestions for you to consider include:

- Cook simple meals
- Mow the lawn
- Shop
- Carpool

- Sort laundry
- Clear dishes from the table
- Make own bed
- Wash/dry dishes
- Vacuum
- Car maintenance
- Load laundry into washer/dryer
- Pay bills

There are other things that are specific to your lifestyle that might be delegated. What are they?

Be sure that you occasionally review your time management plan and see how it is working. Are things flowing smoothly? Are your priorities being met? Do you need to delegate more? Is someone ready to learn another new skill?

Writing things down does not mean inflexibility! Take stock of your plan every 3 months or so to see how things are going. Good luck with your time management, organizing, and scheduling!

3

Papers

Guidelines for Writing Papers

Writing papers requires preparation. It is vital that you begin to think about them long before their due date. We would like to provide you with some things to consider when writing papers.

1. **Be certain that you find out what style the papers are to be written in.** Most nursing schools use American Psychological Association (APA) format.
   - Purchase the APA manual or go to the library and read the important sections that relate to citations and references.
   - Be sure that you can access the manual easily, or that someone you know has a copy for those crisis times when you will need to refer to it. Believe us, it is worth the money to buy a copy for peace of mind, ease of access, and the points that you will earn because you are following the format correctly.
2. **Be certain that you obtain the paper criteria from your instructor.**
   - Read all of the criteria first.
   - Clarify any questions you might have immediately.
   - Don't wait until you are at the library gathering information or at home typing.

- Note those areas that have the highest point value and project how long you think the paper might take you to complete.
- Look again at the sections with the most points, project how long these sections might be and how much time they might take you to complete.
- Be careful to distribute your time wisely.
- It makes no sense to write five pages of a paper on a section worth 10 points and one page on a section worth 50 points.

    For example, you are given a paper to write with four sections. Sections I and II are worth 40 points each, and Sections III and IV are worth 10 points each. It is much more important for you to spend the majority of your efforts on Sections I and II, as these sections total 80 points of your grade. If you need to skimp, do so in the last two sections, as they are only worth 20 points. Just think, if you did not even address the last two sections, you could still get an 80 on the paper if everything else was extremely well done. We do not recommend not doing the last two sections, but certainly, focus your efforts on the sections that are worth the most points!

3. **Gather your resources together.**
   - Will you be using the Internet or a modem to connect to the library computer to complete your search of the literature?
   - Will you need to go to the library in person?
   - Be sure to keep some type of card system that provides detailed notes of each source you plan to use.
   - Refer to your APA manual (or whatever format your school is using) to determine what is needed in the citations and references.
   - Most style manuals require that you at least keep track of the author(s), title, journal or publisher, and date published. The process of writing down this information will save you many hassles when you can't find a reference, or the year is illegible on your copy of the article, or the journal name is not listed on the article.
   - When you proofread your paper, you can double-check all of your references to see if they are accurate.

4. **If at all possible, do not reinvent the wheel.**
   - Use the same topic over and over.
   - We have had a few students use the same basic topic throughout an entire nursing program!
   - Just think what a relief it would be not to have to do a complete search of the literature for each paper. You may have to do a limited search, but think of the time you would save!

How is this possible? Think of a topic that you are really interested in. An example might be eating disorders. Ways that you could adapt this topic to several different courses include:

- Eating disorders in adolescence for *pediatric* nursing
- Eating disorders during pregnancy for *obstetrics*
- Drug treatment for eating disorders in *pharmacology*
- Nutrition and eating disorders for *nutrition* class
- Treatment of eating disorders for *psychiatric* nursing
- The relationship between eating disorders in young women and their participation in group sports for *research*

Think about the possibilities! And, you can think about using the same topic in courses other than nursing. It is possible to use the same topic the entire time! Of course, one drawback to this approach is that you will probably never want to read or write anything about the chosen topic again! So, be sure that when you choose a topic you *really* like it, or at least want to know a lot more about it!

Things to Consider When Choosing a Topic

- Be wary of choosing a topic that is one of the instructor's favorites or one that they have written a book about or have done research on; chances are your ideas will be scrutinized closely because of the topic.
- Don't choose controversial topics that the instructor might be emotionally involved in, unless it is a debate or pro and con paper.
- Be wary of topics that you cannot find any additional information about, unless you are doing some original research.
- Also, be wary of topics that have too much information available; you will never be able to find it all and you will have to wade through tons of material.
- Be selective in choosing a topic and narrow the focus.

Cheating

Invariably, there is one student who tries to beat the system and cheat on a paper. Or better yet, the student gets someone else to do it for him or her.

> *For those of you who think that downloading or purchasing ready-made papers off the Internet is a great way to write papers, think again. There is a fairly new Internet site, www.plagiarism.com, that checks submitted material against millions of online pages. This site will not only detect word-for-word copying of another's material, but it can also detect if a paper is composed of bits and pieces of familiar texts. Many schools have already contracted with the site to scan all submitted papers. Professors are also able to contract individually with the site. Once a faculty member receives a report from the site, it is still necessary to make a decision about whether or not*

a student plagiarized. For example, if a paper is lacking a citation in one area, the site may report to the faculty member that the content was plagiarized. However, most faculty members would be open to the idea that perhaps a student just neglected to include that one citation. Whether good or bad, this site is available, and a word to the wise—don't plagiarize.

Just a few words of wisdom:

- Do your own work!
- Do not plagiarize!
- Put everything in your own words!
- Document your work from accepted sources!
- Do not do someone else's work for him!

Unfortunately, student nurses tend to be "caretakers." They are often "helpers" and feel that they are "needed" when others seek them out for help with papers. There is nothing wrong with sharing information or resources, but when you are doing more work than the person you are helping, you are allowing yourself to be used! You are not doing the person a favor; you are hindering his or her learning!

Remember the story about waking up in the recovery room with the nurse who cheated on exams to take care of you (see Chapter 1)? Would you want a student who had relied on others to do his or her work taking care of you? Would you trust him or her with your life? You will trust that person with other lives! Believe us, at some point in your career, you will find yourself in the position of being asked to do for or help a fellow student. This can happen with paperwork and in clinical settings. Be sure that your help is really needed and that you are not doing someone else's work for him. Nurses who depend on others to always do for them will also cut corners in other ways. They may short-change a patient on their medications, or rely on others to chart for them. The possibilities are frightening! It is important for you to stop this kind of cheating.

Not everyone will enjoy writing papers, but most schools do require them. Remember to clarify the criteria and then follow it exactly.

Typists

For those of you who choose to have someone else type your paper, whether it is for time reasons or financial reasons, you will need to do some preplanning. Be sure that you find someone before you need him or her! Get to know them and tell them what you will need. It is not a bad idea to show them your syllabus with paper deadlines highlighted so that you can work out a potential time schedule. Be sure that the typist is familiar with the required paper format such as APA.

Most likely, you will need to give the typist a lot of lead time. Find out how far in advance the rough draft will be needed, and what the lag time is between turning in the draft and getting back a paper for review. You will also need to plan for time between the first review, making any corrections, turning it back into the typist, and receiving the final copy. Sometimes this process will take 2 to 3 weeks, so you really need to plan ahead! If you are a procrastinator, you will most likely run into some problems!

Proofread! Proofread! Proofread!

Once you have your paper back for review:

- Be certain that the typist followed the correct format for citations in the body of the text and in the references or bibliography.
- Check to see that the paper is paginated correctly.
- Be aware of any changes that were made to the original content.
- Be certain that any alterations in content did not change the intended meaning of the original paragraph.
- If you don't proofread well, find someone who does.

The proofreader does not have to be familiar with the content of the paper. There is no reason why someone majoring in another field cannot check your paper for you. You are not looking for someone to see if the paper is good, you are looking for errors in spelling, sentence structure, and grammar. If you cannot find anyone on your own, check with the English department to see if they have a senior or graduate student who is looking for some outside work. Pay them. If you do not invest in a proofreader, you may lose many hard-earned points because of mistakes.

Be wary of relying on relatives and friends who volunteer to type papers for you. Remember that your deadline is not always their deadline! It can be very difficult to tell your mother that she is not following the correct format for a paper. Or even worse, you may not get the paper until the day that it is due. You will not have had a chance to proofread it before you turn it in, or if you find errors, you will not have time to get them fixed. We had one student whose mother-in-law offered to type her papers. Her mother-in-law learned to write using the Turabian format. When the student turned in her paper, she did not realize that her mother-in-law had changed the paper from APA format to Turabian. Unfortunately, this was one of the student's senior papers and she did not realize the error until it was time to turn the paper in. This senior student lost several points for using the wrong paper format.

Checking a Paper

When checking a paper, be sure of the following:

- You have the correct paper. It has your name and the correct course information on it.
- It has the correct number of pages.
- The pages are in the correct order.
- The lettering is dark enough to read and consistently clear. Make sure that the ribbon or ink cartridge did not run out in the middle of your paper.
- There are no additional or unwanted lines, streaks, or other distracting marks from printers or copiers.
- The bibliography or reference page is attached to the paper.

Writing papers can be fun and challenging. As long as you recognize that computers require a certain amount of special handling, you should do fine. Always remember, backup all of your work, have someone proofread your papers, and check to be sure that all of the pages are in order before handing in your paper.

4

Computers

Computers

Be sure that you choose a word processing software program that is capable of doing all the work you will need throughout the nursing program. If the university uses a specific one, and you will be using their computers, be sure that the same software is available in all the places where you plan on working. There is nothing worse than being forced to use the library computers because the nursing department is closed, and finding out that the library uses an entirely different software program! Be sure that you familiarize yourself with the software program. We find it helpful to have a book about the program that you can use. Either the software book itself or books from the *Idiot's Guide* or *Dummy* series will be helpful. Most common programs have several books available for you to look through. Find one that you can live with. If you are not that adept at computers, find yourself a computer troubleshooter in case of emergencies. Trust us, emergencies do happen.

Computer Tips

1. Find out if you can connect to any or all of the university computers by modem.
   • Can you download data from other places?

35

- Be certain that your data is protected by a password and that you don't share it with others!

   We once had a student report that one of her *friends* had destroyed her paper because her *friend* was failing the class and wanted her to fail too. (These kinds of incidents do not often happen, but once is enough.)
2. Take advantage of any short computer courses that are offered on campus.
   - Most universities have free or reduced-fee sessions to help students learn a variety of software programs.
   - Most sessions last an evening or 1 or 2 days.
   - These sessions can help you get started and provide lots of information in the way of handouts and tips.
   - An added plus of taking a course is that you have contact with someone who may help you find the computer person you may need as a future resource.
3. Take a day or two to find out how the various computers on campus are used.
   - You need to check for signup sheets, busiest hours, and what software programs are available.
   - Jot down notes to keep with you so that you can refer back to them during the crisis times when your favorite computer is taken! One problem is that throughout the semester, students frequently end up with similar course deadlines. This can cause long lines at most campus computers.
   - Be sure that you prepare for a time when you will not be able to use the computer. Be flexible!
   - Allow for busy hours and downtime in your planning.

■ Troubleshooting Tips

Computers are a godsend for most of us, but they are not without their drawbacks. Mistakes can happen when you are first learning to use a computer to write papers. Even seasoned, computer-literate students can run into problems with campus computers. We wanted to share some of the problems that we have encountered during our years of teaching, as well as some possible solutions.

- **If you are planning to use a library or university computer, be sure that you check for viruses before loading any diskettes on to your own, or anyone else's, PC.** Multiple-use computers frequently carry viruses that are capable of destroying all of your information and stored data.
- **To access the university computers you may need to work at odd hours or on weekends.** Be certain that you allow enough time to complete papers so that one day of downtime will not disrupt your schedule. A number of

students have run into problems when a university computer was down or there was an unexpected power failure. A lot of students may have papers due around the same time. If you have to schedule times, make sure that you will be able to complete your work on time. Always remember to backup your work on a diskette before leaving the computer.

- **Be sure to save your work after every couple of paragraphs or, if your computer program has an AutoSave, set it for at least every page.** If you need to, consider setting a timer for every 20 to 30 minutes to help you get into the habit of saving your work; otherwise you could be wasting precious time. Be certain to backup your work at the middle and end of every work session. Even if you have saved your work on the hard drive, you still need to save it on a diskette. We would recommend a double backup such as two separate diskettes, a diskette and a tape, or a diskette and a Zip drive—anything to ensure that you have a copy in at least two places (Figure 4–1).

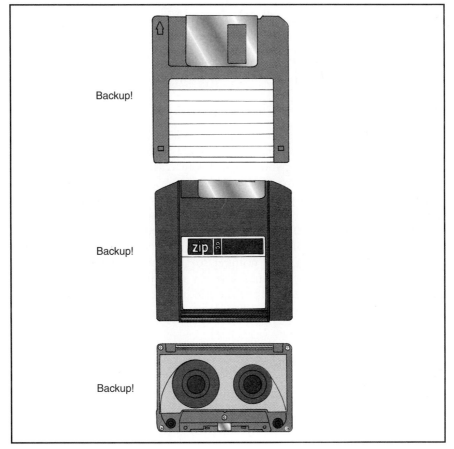

Figure 4–1. Back up all data several times.

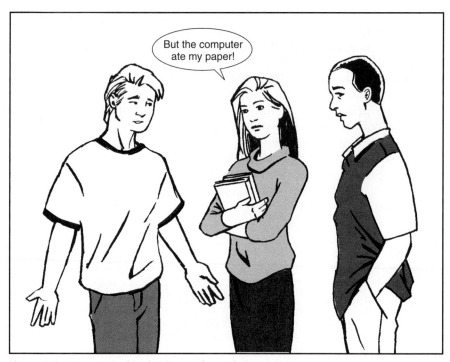

Figure 4–2. Be sure to make a hard copy of your drafts.

We recommend that you print a hard copy at the end of each work session. By having a hard copy, you can read your material and make any necessary changes before your next work session. There was once a student whose helpful husband decided to load some new software on the family computer the day before her research paper was due. Not only did he delete the word processing software program that her paper was saved on, but she was unable to retrieve information from her backup diskette. She came to class the next morning totally distraught with nothing to show for an entire semester of work (Figure 4–2). The school had a policy regarding point deductions for late papers so she lost some points. If she had had a hard copy to turn in, even if it wasn't a final copy, she may not have lost as many points.

5

Texts and Other Learning Resources

▮ Textbooks

Most students believe that information given in textbooks is always reliable. We have had students point out that information in a text sometimes conflicts with what we have said in class. It is for this reason that you should note the following points:

1. Texts are not infallible—many contain errors.
   - If your instructor says one thing and you read something else in your textbook, be sure to ask for clarification.
   - A good way to clarify a conflict is to ask your instructor, "If you ask a question on the test, which answer should I give?"
   - Be as specific as you can possibly be when asking a question.
2. Be wary of information in a text that contradicts common sense.
   - If you are studying dosages and calculations and you read that $4 \times 15 = 45$, or if you read that a major cause of heart disease is eating too many vegetables, you will know that there is an error.
   - If there is one major error, chances are there are several more.
   - Be sure to point out any errors you discover to your instructor.
   - Be careful! Many students overlook an obvious error because they inherently believe that textbooks are perfect.

3. Texts are often out of date.
   - New information is learned on a daily basis, and some areas of technology change minute to minute.
   - Texts are written over a period of a year or two, and in production for another year or more.
   - When reading about areas that are in constant flux such as AIDS, drug development, and others, you will need to rely on more up-to-date sources.
4. Texts reflect the beliefs and biases of the writer or writers.
   - Your instructor may or may not agree with the writer's experience and conclusions. Sometimes, the textbook will say "A." Your instructor will say, "I think B."
   - Be sure that you clarify which response is desired in a testing situation.

Journal Articles

Journal articles are usually more timely than textbooks, but information may still be 6 months to 1 year old or more at publication. Articles also contain errors. Be wary of articles or research that is supported by major companies with a vested interest in the information presented in the article. For example, we have read that eating a vegetarian diet can be detrimental to your health. Interestingly, a member of a beef producers' organization wrote this article. I have also read that drug A is better than drug B, but the pharmaceutical company that makes drug A paid for the research!

A majority of the information contained in texts and journals is accurate; however, you need to remain on alert. It is important to remember when you are reading texts and journals that some of the information presented may be quite old, and that not all information may be accurate.

Where Do I Find It?

In many nursing courses you will be looking for information that is not in your textbooks. Here is some basic information on reference sources that should help you locate that information with minimal frustration.

- **Librarian:** This individual can be of immense help. We highly recommend that you take a trip to the library and meet the reference staff. No, they will not do the work for you. They can, however, help you utilize your library time wisely!
- **Medical dictionary:** Although most of your textbooks have some medical terminology, we strongly recommend that your personal library contain a recent medical dictionary.

- **Cumulative Index to Nursing and Allied Health Literature (CINAHL):** One of the most frequently used multidisciplinary databases. It includes nursing literature as well as 15 to 20 allied health fields. You can access CINAHL by the hard copy version as well as by CD-ROM and online at the library.
- **Nursing journals:** There are over 100 American nursing journals. Contents vary from journals with a broad range of topics, such as the *American Journal of Nursing,* to those with a narrow focus such as the *Journal of Intravenous Nursing.* Once you have searched CINAHL, and have located an article, you may need to use interlibrary loan services to receive a hard copy. Remember, it may take 10 to 14 days for the article to arrive at your library, so plan ahead.
- **Morbidity and Mortality Weekly Report (MMWR):** The MMWR is an excellent source especially when you are searching for information focused on community and epidemiology issues. It is a weekly publication from the Centers for Disease Control and Prevention (CDC) that provides statistical information for a number of selected reportable diseases (e.g., mumps, tuberculosis, measles, and hepatitis). The information is provided for each state, as well as select cities. The MMWR also provides information on causes of deaths in 122 U.S. cities. Copies of MMWR are usually located in the documents area of the library. You may need to ask the librarian for help. The MMWR can also be accessed at: *http://www.cdc.gov/.*
- **Agency for Health Care Policy and Research (AHCPR):** This is an agency of the U.S. Public Health Service created in 1989 to enhance the quality, appropriateness, and effectiveness of health care services and access to these services. It sponsors a great deal of research and strives to provide the results of such studies to the public in an understandable form. Some of the many topics available from the AHCPR include cancer pain control, AIDS, pressure sores, incontinence, and recovery from a stroke. The agency's Web site is: *www.ahcpr.gov.*

You may also find the following resources helpful:

- OSHA—Occupational Safety and Health Administration
- JCAHO—Joint Committee on Accreditation of Healthcare Organizations
- CDC—Centers for Disease Control and Prevention
- FDA—Federal Drug Administration
- AHA—American Hospital Association

You are no doubt going to find that your main reference sources in school will be your textbooks. These have been selected by faculty who believe that the adopted book will do the best job of presenting the course material. However, there are still going to be information gaps in any text. This chapter has presented some basic references, which we believe will help you fill in the gaps.

RESOURCE WEB SITE

The Agency's Web address is: *http://ahcpr.gov*
For ordering information on AHCPR guidelines:

Call 1-800-358-9295
or write:
Government Printing Office
Superintendent of Documents
Washington, DC 20402

6

Faculty Variability

Faculty Variability

We think that the most important thing for you to realize about your faculty members is that they are people too. Each instructor is an individual with wants, desires, needs, and problems. Nurses become teachers for many reasons, but most of us do so because we want to instill something of ourselves in future generations of nurses to make the profession better. A majority of instructors are not teaching for financial gain.

It is important for you to know that the teachers are there to educate you and to guide you through your nursing program. They are not the enemy. They are not there to weed out a large number of students. They *are* there to help you graduate!

Faculty Members

We think it is important for you to know the following things about your faculty as people:

1. Give your faculty members some respect!
   - Treat them with respect and they will respect you as well.
   - Find out if the instructor has office hours, make an appointment, and keep it.

43

- If you cannot keep a scheduled appointment, cancel it.
- If an instructor asks you to do something, do it.
- If you are unable to do what is asked, explain why you can't do it.
- Don't be afraid to speak up and let your teacher know what you need to meet your goals.
- Remember that the faculty is there for you. They are rational human beings and they will try to understand your dilemma. For example, we recall a student who refused to go to a specific clinical agency during her maternal–child community rotation. The student was very angry with her instructor, and the faculty in general, because she was assigned to this agency. It wasn't until she sat down and explained her reasons (it was an abortion clinic and she was pro-life) that something could be done to rectify the situation (she was given an alternate assignment).

2. Remember, as human beings, your instructors will have good days and bad days.
   - Most of us have families, parents, spouses, and children.
   - Our parents get sick and die, our husbands and wives have their own set of problems, and our children go through adolescence and have extracurricular activities that we want to attend.
   - We get sick, have problems, and worry. We get anxious, depressed, and angry.
   - This is not to say that we have a right to take our moods and problems to the classroom, but rarely, this can happen.
   - If an instructor is having a bad day, and if you know and respect your instructor, you will probably be able to tell when it is a bad day. You might want to acknowledge it.

   For example, if you have a dreaded problem that you want to discuss with your instructor, instead of saying, "I have a problem and we need to talk." It might be better to say, "I have a problem that I would like to discuss with you, but this doesn't seem like a good time. When could I make an appointment to see you?" In this way, you acknowledge that now is not a good time, but that you still need to see him or her at his or her convenience.

3. It is also important to respect your instructor's privacy.
   - One of us used to arrive on campus at 6 A.M., long before classes would begin. It was made very clear to students that from 6 to 7 A.M. the instructor was busy working. Students were asked to address problems or questions between 7 to 8 A.M. prior to class and not to disturb the instructor prior to 7 A.M. Most students respected this private time. However, some were insistent that their question or problem could not wait 30 minutes. Because it was well known that 6 to 7 A.M. was private time, the instructor was less than pleased by interruptions. One student made the statement, "I can tell that you don't like me because you are always so cool to me." In response, she was told that she was well liked, but interruptions between 6 to 7 A.M., as stated earlier, were not welcomed.

- This is an example of a personal quirk. Everyone has quirks.
- Your instructor will try to work around your quirks. Please do the same for your instructor.

4. Your instructors will have a variety of personalities.
   - Some will appear to be very tough and demanding, while others will be laid back, and some might be overly friendly.
   - You will need to be flexible!
   - Most students will dislike tough and demanding faculty and complain that they expect too much (Figure 6–1).
   - In the long term, many students learn to respect these instructors. I have heard some students say that they learned the most from the tough ones.
   - Your teachers will let you know about things like how to address them (Dr., Mrs., Mr., Ms., etc). We expected students to call us by our title and last name until graduation, at which time they were free to call us by our first names. We believe that addressing someone by his or her last name is a sign of respect.
   - If a patient or instructor asks you to address her by her first name, then by all means feel free to do so.

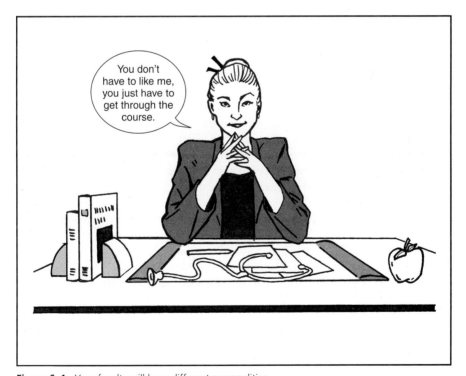

Figure 6–1. Your faculty will have different personalities.

Contrary to what some students believe, the faculty does not spend a lot of time talking about students. Students always want to know what faculty members discuss during course meetings. For the most part, meetings focus on topics such as curriculum, textbooks, exam planning, and exam results. Occasionally, a student problem is discussed as a means to assist the student.

For example, a particular student was having a great deal of difficulty in the clinical setting, but she was an "A student" in theory. Her difficulty was one of many issues discussed in a meeting to find ways to help her adjust to clinical work. As a result of our discussion, her instructor decided to spend more time with the student in the clinical work and "buddy" her with a more outgoing student for 2 weeks. At the end of the 2 weeks, the student was much more comfortable and confident.

Personality Conflicts

Sometimes students develop a personality conflict with a particular nursing instructor. There are a number of ways of dealing with this potential problem.

1. Can you identify what the conflict is with this particular instructor?
   - If so, is it something that you could discuss with the instructor?
   - Perhaps you think the instructor expects too much from you?
   - Perhaps you resent something the instructor said or did?
   - Perhaps you need more assistance than you think he or she is providing?
   - Remember that your instructor is a person too.
   - Take the time to discuss your mutual conflict. If this does not resolve the conflict, there are other options.
2. Is there another student or instructor to talk with about the conflict?
   - Perhaps this third person could assist you in dealing with the conflict.
   - Perhaps they can help you gain insight into the instructor's behavior, or into your own.
   - Remember it takes two to have a relationship. The instructor may have treated you poorly, but how have you treated the instructor?
3. Is there a way for you to avoid a conflict with this faculty member?
   - Are there other instructors who teach the same course?
   - Could you request a change in classes or clinical instruction to accommodate you?
   - Do you need to talk to someone else about the conflict?
   - One thing that is very important is for you to follow the chain of command. This means that you go up the ladder rung by rung without trying to jump ahead.

For example, if your problem is with a certain instructor who teaches the course with three other instructors, is there a course leader? After first speaking with the instructor, the next person in the chain of command is the course leader. After the course leader, there may be a team leader. Next in line is probably an assistant administrator, program director, department chair, and then an assistant dean or dean. Remember that it is important to make appointments with each person, and be courteous.

4. If the problem is still unresolved it might be time for you to file a grievance.
   - Most colleges and universities have a formal grievance procedure.
   - Get out your student handbook and read about students' rights.
   - There should be a detailed process to follow about filing a grievance.
   - Be sure that you follow it to the letter.

Ninety-nine percent of problems are handled long before a formal grievance. If you respect the person you have a problem with, and he or she respects you, most conflicts can be easily dealt with. In the majority of cases, all it requires is the courage to identify the conflict and then to be willing to sit down and discuss it with another individual.

A CASE IN POINT

We can recall hiring a new nursing instructor with very good credentials. Around her third month of teaching, the faculty members began to notice some small problems regarding tardiness and dress. By the sixth month, a couple of us began to wonder if she might have a problem with alcohol, but we had nothing to go on other than a few odd behaviors. By the ninth month, we realized that even with assistance, she would not be able to meet all of her required teaching duties. Unfortunately, we were still unable to discover exactly what her specific problem was. This particular instructor decided to move on to another job after only 10 months of teaching. Over a year later, a student remarked that this particular instructor used to drink vodka in her coffee during clinical hours. She stated that the instructor had also been drinking heavily after work and was rarely able to meet her students at the specified times. Several students were aware that the instructor had a drinking problem, but no one brought it to the faculty's attention. This instructor may have been able to be helped, but instead she moved on to another job, continued to drink heavily, and is no longer able to work. Her career has been ruined because people either did not recognize her problem or did not speak up if they knew about it.

A CASE IN POINT

A nurse at a clinical facility was abusing drugs. She was taking 1,500 mg of Demerol during an 8-hour shift. You might think this nurse was incapable of doing her job in the intensive care unit, but she was actually doing quite well. A problem developed when she started diverting, or using Demerol meant for her patients for herself. She would disappear into the bathroom and reappear some time later. A student finally came to one of the instructors to report the nurse's unusual behavior. It was found that the hospital was already gathering information to turn over to the peer-assistance program. This particular nurse entered treatment for her addiction, and is now in recovery and back at work. She is once again a valued employee. This student did her part in saving this nurse's life and keeping her patients out of harm's way.

Peer-Assistance Issues

Rarely during your nursing education, you might find an instructor, another student, or nurse in a clinical setting who has a major problem. By a major problem we mean a severe psychiatric illness or chemical addiction.

- State boards of nursing across the country are attempting to deal with these problems in a professional manner by assisting nurses and nursing students.
- Students and nurses with this type of problem are able to get help and remain in the profession.
- There are peer-assistance programs in most states and in some colleges and universities to help nurses and nursing students.
- Review your student handbook for specific information.
- If confronted with someone who you believe has a problem with severe mental illness or chemical addiction, remember, speak up, and report your observations! Protecting other nurses is only harming them, your patients, and you.

It is important to remember that in all areas of nursing you will be having contact with a variety of people. It does not matter whether you are a student or a practicing nurse. Part of learning to be a good nurse is learning to get along with many different people with a variety of personalities and cultural backgrounds.

7

Assertiveness

Assertiveness

Assertiveness is a trait that nurses need to develop. Being assertive means being positive, direct, and genuine. An assertive nurse will maintain eye contact and know when to say no. Assertiveness allows us to develop inner satisfaction, self-respect, and confidence in our new abilities. It allows us to be open and honest, and to maintain a sense of self-control and independence. In being assertive, we can choose how and when to respond; we can even choose to be nonassertive when the situation warrants it (Herman, 1978).

Nonassertive Behavior

People who are nonassertive may be viewed as being passive. Nonassertive nurses avoid conflict and rarely express feelings, which leads to increased resentment. Nonassertive nurses often feel helpless and powerless and may feel hurt or sorry for themselves. Many times, these nurses will spend more time complaining about how awful the work situation is because they are allowing themselves to be "used and abused" rather than speaking up for their personal rights. Often, these nurses are perceived as dependent or lacking in self-control and decision-making skills. They may feel angry and possess little self-respect.

49

A CASE IN POINT

Everyone loves working with Betsy. Betsy works hard and is more than willing to do her work and some of yours as well. Betsy never has a cross word for anyone but often complains about how the system "uses" her. She is the first person that the supervisor calls when another nurse calls in sick because the supervisor knows that Betsy cannot say no. Betsy will work overtime even when she has plans with her family. Betsy often feels helpless and gets depressed because she is always taking care of someone else. Unfortunately, our society in general and the nursing profession in particular may reward Betsy's nonassertive behavior by saying, "She'll do anything you ask her to," or "She is always so kind, you never hear her say a bad word about anybody" (Herman, 1978).

Aggressive Behavior

Aggressive nurses tend to be dominating, loud, and insensitive to others. Aggressive nurses want their way at all times, regardless of how others feel. They are frequently confrontive and leave other nurses feeling angry and belittled.

Passive–Aggressive Behavior

Another form of aggressive behavior is more indirect. Many nurses use this form of behavior. Rather than being assertive and directly asking for what they need, some nurses use indirect methods such as trickery, seduction, or manipulation. Often, women in our society are praised for learning these indirect behaviors.

Assertive Rights

All of us have the right to behave assertively. For some of us, the transition to assertiveness is easy; for others, it can be quite difficult. Only you can know for yourself. After reading this introduction, you probably have a good idea about whether you are assertive, nonassertive, or aggressive. Everyone can use all three types of behavior, but one tends to dominate. So, if you are aggressive or nonassertive, you might want to think about becoming more assertive.

A CASE IN POINT

> Katie is a terror at work. She used to work in the emergency department, but the other workers complained about her obnoxious behavior. She was transferred to same-day surgery. She makes fun of the other nurses and is rude to patients. When it is time for a break, Katie just leaves the unit. It doesn't matter if she is due to give a medication or receive a patient from surgery. The student nurses hide from her because she constantly reminds them that they don't know anything. Daily, a student leaves the unit in tears because Katie has been harassing him or her all day. Fortunately, overtly aggressive individuals do not usually find nursing, with its focus on caring and compassion, to be a profession that they would choose (Clark, 1978).

As we said earlier, we all have the right to be assertive. Nurses also have other basic human rights to which we ascribe (Table 7–1). Although nurses have these rights, there tends to be a "hierarchy" in the medical profession that gives more "value" to certain individuals. Many of us fall into the trap of thinking that doctors are higher on the value scale than nurses and therefore deserve *more* respect and have *more* rights. If we fall into this erroneous assumption, it would then follow that patients have the *least* rights of all! Is your dentist any more worthwhile than your plumber is? Is a male more worthwhile than a female? If you answered yes to these questions, then you believe that some people should have more rights than others. Is that valid? We believe that *all* people have the same value and rights and deserve the same treatment!

A CASE IN POINT

> Lois was angry with her supervisor for changing her schedule. The supervisor explained that another nurse was going to be absent for a week to attend a convention at the hospital's expense. Lois had already made plans to spend the weekend with her husband. Rather than telling her supervisor that she had made plans with her husband and would not be able to work that day, she waited and called in sick. Another example of passive–aggressive behavior would be giving a co-worker "the silent treatment" rather than coming out and saying what it is that you are angry or upset about (Clark, 1978).

TABLE 7–1. Nurses Bill of Rights

- The right to be respected—to be listened to
- The right to have and state thoughts, feelings, and opinions
- The right to question or challenge
- The right to understand and have in writing what is expected at work
- The right to say no
- The right to be an equal member of the health team
- The right to ask for changes in the system
- The right to a reasonable workload
- The right to make a mistake
- The right to make decisions regarding health or nursing care
- The right to do health teaching
- The right to choose not to assert oneself
- The right to be a patient advocate or to teach patients to speak for themselves
- The right to change one's mind

From: Herman, S. J. (1978). Becoming assertive: A guide for nurses *(p. 27). New York: D. Van Nostrand Co. Used with permission.*

How You Can Be More Assertive

1. Believe in yourself!
   - Believe that you have rights.
   - Build your confidence.
   - If you think positively about yourself you will build your self-esteem, which decreases your need for approval from others.
   - If you are not constantly seeking approval from others you are better able to make independent decisions and handle conflict more directly.
2. Make your needs a priority!
   - Frequently, nurses put everyone else's needs above their own.
   - You need to consider yourself a priority.
   - Do unto me, as I do unto others.
3. Think before you speak!
   - Are you into the "yes" habit?
   - Do not automatically say yes. Some of us are so ingrained with the yes-word that we will say yes before we know what the other person is asking.
   - Instead, say, "I need to think about it." Then you have time to decide whether you are doing something because you want to or because you feel obligated.

4. Learn to initiate conversations instead of waiting for someone else to speak first.
   - Say what you want to say, do not wait.
5. Use "I" statements rather than "you" statements.
   - If you say to another nurse, "I think we need to call Dr. Creed about this blood pressure, I don't want to wait until rounds," the message is clear that you have thought about the situation and have made a decision. If you say, "You had better call Dr. Creed about that blood pressure," the message is confusing and open to interpretation by the other nurse.
   - Many of us react negatively to someone else's telling us what to do.
   - In this situation, not only are you telling the other nurse what to do, but the other nurse can decide not to call, which is not what you want to have happen.
6. Do not offer explanations!
   - Do you feel the need to explain why you cannot do something?
   - For example, your supervisor asks you to stay late. Do you say, "No, I can't," or, "No, I'm so tired, and I promised my son I'd take him to his soccer game, and it's my fourth wedding anniversary, and my mother is ill."
   - All you need to say is no.
7. Be persistent!
   - For example, x-ray arrives to transport Patient A to a CT scan, even though Patient B is having the same scan and has been waiting 2 hours. You say, "Patient B has been waiting 2 hours and needs to go first." The x-ray transport worker responds, "I only do what I'm told." You reply, "I understand, and I'm telling you that Patient B needs to go first. Would you like me to call the department and tell them?" The x-ray transport worker says, "No, that's okay, I'll take Patient B down first."
8. Give and receive praise and criticism.
   - Are you able to tell someone that they have not done the job expected of them?
   - Can you tell someone they did a great job?
   - Can you accept someone telling you that your work is not up to par or that you handled a stressful situation extremely well?
   - Being able to give and receive praise and criticism is an important aspect of assertiveness.

How to Increase Assertiveness

So now you have a good idea of what constitutes assertive behavior. You may have also decided that you need to learn to be more assertive. For some individuals, group support can be very helpful when working on assertiveness skills.

It takes a lot of practice to change behavior. You may find that you need additional help. We would recommend finding a support group where you can practice your skills as you learn. Some business and professional groups offer assertiveness training classes as do colleges, counselors, and some churches. Check your local area for available classes. We have included some sample conversations to help you develop your assertive skills.

REFUSING REQUESTS

1. *Another student:* Can I see your careplan? I forgot to do mine again.
   You: No, I'm putting the final touches on mine and it is due in 15 minutes.
   Another student: But I don't have one to turn in.
   You: I think you should have thought about that before now.
2. *Colleague:* I'm going on break now, would you finish Mrs. T's bath for me?
   You: I can't, I haven't finished bathing my patients yet.
   Colleague: Okay, I'll find someone else who is already finished.

MAKING REQUESTS

1. *Student:* Dr. Moss, I've never done a Z-track injection before, but I read the procedure manual and I would like to go over the injection with you before I give it.
   Nursing instructor: That's good, I appreciate your honesty, now tell me step by step how you'll give the injection.
2. *Nurse:* I don't see any more fruit salad in the case.
   Cafeteria worker: Nope, me either.
   Nurse: Could you please check and see if there is any more available?

ASKING FOR A BEHAVIOR CHANGE

1. *Nurse:* Dr. Fulton, I've noticed that you often leave the unit without signing your telephone orders.
   Dr. Fulton: So what, I'm a very busy man and I'm in a hurry.
   Nurse: I understand that you are busy, but I must have all telephone orders signed within 24 hours, it is a hospital policy.
   Dr. Fulton: Oh, I didn't realize that. If someone would mark the charts that I need to sign, I'd be glad to sign them.
   Nurse: Thank you.

2. *Nursing instructor:* Miss Taylor, this is the second time that you have not followed the clinical dress code.

   Student: I'm sorry, my mother hasn't done the laundry again.

   Nursing instructor: I suggest that you learn to do your own laundry. You will not be allowed to return to clinical until you are properly dressed.

GIVING A COMPLIMENT

1. *Nurse:* I was very impressed by the way you handled that emergency. I noticed that you stayed calm and followed the procedure.

   Student: Thank you. I appreciate your saying that. I was really scared that maybe I wouldn't be able to handle an emergency situation, but now I know that I can.

ACCEPTING CRITICISM

1. *Colleague:* I can't believe that you stuck that baby four times! Now they are going to have to do a cut down!

   Nurse: You're right. The veins were too fragile. I should have called someone else. Next time I'll know better.

It is important for all of us to learn to use assertive behavior. Assertiveness can help you in a variety of settings. If we were all assertive, there would be a lot less game playing and a lot more honesty with our colleagues, patients, and ourselves.

8

Professional Possibilities

Professional Possibilities

The nursing profession is replete with job opportunities. There are some standard jobs, such as hospital or home health nursing, in which a large number of nurses work. However, there are also very unique job opportunities for nurses such as parish nursing and flight nursing. One of the things that most nurses love about our profession is that we can all find our own niche in a job that fits us as individuals (Figure 8–1).

The majority of nurses work in hospitals, clinics, home health, or extended care settings. These jobs can be extremely rewarding and often offer good benefits. As a student nurse, you will probably be exposed to all of these nursing opportunities in a variety of clinical areas. Since there is already a great deal of information available about these common types of nursing, we will not spend a lot of time addressing them. If you are interested in a particular type of nursing, contact a hospital, clinic, home health agency, or extended care agency at the location where you intend to begin working. All agencies will send you information about their facility, a job description, and an application.

Other Opportunities

Some of the other opportunities for nurses include:

- **Occupational health nursing:** Working for a large industrial company providing preventive and emergency care.

56

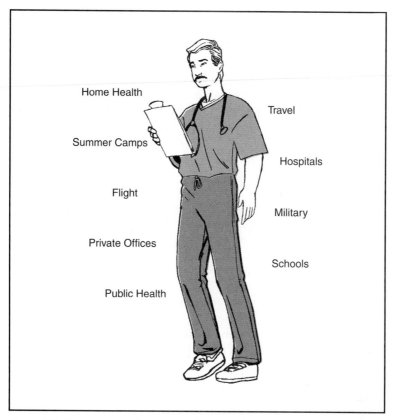

Figure 8–1. There are many job opportunities for nurses.

- **Private-duty nursing:** Working with an individual patient for an extended period of time. Most private-duty nurses work for an agency or for themselves.
- **Nursing education:** Teaching nursing at the vocational and practical level (requires at least a baccalaureate degree), the associate or baccalaureate level (requires at least a master's degree in nursing), or at the graduate level (requires a master's degree in nursing and usually a doctorate).
- **Physician offices or nurse-managed offices:** Working in an office for an advanced practice nurse or physician.
- **Student health or school nursing:** Working in a student health center at a university or in a school district.
- **Camp nursing:** Working at a camp (usually seasonal).
- **Short-term nursing assignments:** Working in areas where there is a shortage of nurses. Most assignments last 1 month or longer and lodging is provided.

- **Veterinarian or zoo nursing:** Working for a veterinarian or in a zoo providing care to animals under the direction of a veterinarian.
- **Parish nursing:** Working within a parish setting to provide preventive health care to parishioners.
- **Missionary nursing:** Working with a missionary group to provide health care in underdeveloped countries.
- **Military nursing:** Joining the Air Force, Navy, Marines, Army, or Coast Guard and serving as a nurse in a variety of settings. Offers many benefits and opportunities.
- **Public Health Service or Indian Health Service:** Joining one of these federal services to provide health care. Offers many benefits and opportunities.
- **Veterans nursing:** Providing nursing care at a veterans' hospital or clinic.
- **Flight nursing:** Providing emergency trauma care and transport, usually associated with a trauma center.
- **Travel nursing:** Escorting disabled or ill individuals who are traveling and need someone to accompany them.
- **Nurse entrepreneurs:** A variety of opportunities exist for nurses who wish to open their own business. Some examples are: home health agencies, medical equipment suppliers, infusion agencies, nurse-managed centers, consultation, private practice, providing workshops or seminars, creative apparel for newborns or the disabled, and holistic health care.

Other opportunities in nursing require advanced degrees (e.g., a master's degree with specific course requirements and certification exams).

Certification

After graduation, you may be interested in becoming certified in a specialty field. Certification is different from an advanced degree in a specialty area. Certification is available in nearly all specialties.

The American Nurses Credentialing Center (ANCC) at 1-800-284-CERT or online at *www.nursingworld.org* currently offers exams to become certified as a generalist, nurse practitioner, clinical nurse specialist, and nursing administrator. Each certification has specific application criteria. However, the fundamental requirements are:

- Valid RN license in the United States or its territories
- A specified minimum number of hours of clinical practice in the area
- Passing a written exam in the chosen specialty area

- An Associate Degree Nurse (ADN)/Diploma is required for the following specialty areas:
  - Psychiatric and Mental Health Nurse
  - Medical–Surgical Nurse
  - Pediatric Nurse
  - Gerontological Nurse
  - Perinatal Nurse
- Associate Degree Nurse/Diploma nurses may also request certification in case management or ambulatory care if they are already certified in a co-specialty area.
- A baccalaureate degree is required for all other areas of certification, and a master's degree is often required for nurse practitioner and clinical nurse specialist certifications.

The American Nurses Association (ANA) provides the majority of certifications, although there are a number of specialty organizations that have their own certification available. For further information about other specialty certifications visit *www.springnet.com*. Other areas available for certification include:

RESOURCE WEB SITES

American Association of Critical Care Nurses	*www.certcorp.org*
American Board of Neuroscience Nursing	*www.aann.org*
American Board of Perianesthesia Nursing	*www.cpancapa.org*
American Holistic Nurses Association	*www.ahna.org*
American Board for Occupational Health Nurses	*www.abohn.org*
Board of Certification for Emergency Nursing	*www.ena.org*
Certification Board Perioperative Nursing	*www.certboard.org*
Certifying Board of Gastroenterology Nurses	*www.cbgna.org*
Intravenous Nurses Certification	*www.ins1.org*
Hospice and Palliative Nurses	*www.hpna.org*
Certification for School Nurses	*www.nbcsn.com*
Diabetes Nurse Educators	*www.ncbde.org*
Pediatric Nurses and Nurse Practitioners	*www.pnpcert.org*
Obstetric, Gynecologic, and Neonatal Nurses	*www.nccnet.org*
Ophthalmic Registered Nurses	*www.webeye.ophth. uiowa.edu/asorn/ certif.htm*

RESOURCE WEB SITES (Cont.)

Nephrology Nurses Certification Board	*www.annanurse.org*
Oncology Nursing Certification	*www.oncc.org*
Orthopedic Nurses Certification	*www.naon.inurse.com*
Plastic Surgical Nurses	*www.asprsn.inurse.com/psncb/default.htm*
Rehabilitation Nursing Certification	*www.rehabnurse.org*
Vascular Nursing Certification Board	*www.svnnet.org*
Wound Ostomy Continence Nursing Certification	*www.wocncb.org*

9

Legal/Ethical Concerns

■ Legal/Ethical Concerns

This chapter was designed to assist you in avoiding legal problems while practicing as a nursing student, registered nurse, or licensed practical nurse. One of the most important legal concepts for you to grasp is standard of care. All professions have standards of care, or minimal levels of expertise, that must be delivered to the patient. Nurses are responsible for both *external standards* (those set on the national level) and *internal standards* (those set by the role of nursing). You are responsible for all standards of care as they pertain to the profession of nursing. You are required to maintain competence and skills by reading professional journals and attending continuing education and in-service programs.

If you are ever summoned to appear in a court of law, you will be judged by the standards of care in your community. You are responsible for delivering care that at the very least meets the standards in your community or exceeds them. By adhering to care standards, your patients will receive competent, high-quality nursing care.

According to Guido (2001), you should familiarize yourself with standards of care through the following:

- Your state nurse practice act
- Standards published by the American Nurses Association (ANA)
- Standards published by any applicable specialty organization, such as American Association of Critical Care Nurses (AACN) if you work in a criti-

cal care area or American Psychiatric Nurses Association (APNA) if you work in psychiatric nursing

- Federal agency guidelines and regulations such as those designated by the Occupational and Safety Health Administration (OSHA)
- Employment policy and procedure manual
- Your job description

Nursing Students

Nursing students are required to demonstrate the identical standard of care as a registered nurse or licensed vocational nurse, depending on the type of program. Nursing students have the ultimate responsibility for their own actions and may be liable for their own negligence. Students who are underage and not considered by state law to be adults may still be held liable for their actions.

Clinical Performance Requirements for Students

The role of the nursing student is one that requires the same competent care as that provided by a registered nurse (RN). This requirement places a great deal of accountability on you, the student. Students are legally responsible to inform their instructor if they are unprepared or require any special assistance. Students are accountable for their skills and their knowledge. Nursing faculty members or staff nurses may be accountable for a student's lack of preparedness or competence.

- Be certain that you know the policies and procedures of the clinical facility.
- Be adequately prepared for the clinical experience. Know your patient's treatments, interventions, and any medications.
- Be sure to inform the instructor if you are unprepared for the clinical experience. (If you don't know your patient, the treatments, surgery, medication, etc., you are unprepared!)
- If you are asked to perform a procedure or give a medication that you are not familiar with, say **no!**
- If you have practiced a skill, procedure, or medication administration, but are unsure of yourself, ask for help from your instructor. If your instructor is unavailable, ask the nursing staff to complete the task for you.
- Know what treatments, procedures, and skills students are allowed to perform in each institution. (They are not all the same.) If asked to perform something that is not allowed, **refuse!** Offer to assist the staff nurse in some other way.

- If you are working in an institution as an employee, clarify what skills, if any, are allowed for employees that you are not allowed to complete as a student.
- Be certain that you follow policy and procedure at *all* times. We have been appalled when students told us that they were allowed to start and give intravenous (IV) medication as nursing assistants when the skill was not listed under the job description of a nursing assistant. You must be aware of your own accountability and liability. No one else will be as careful as you will be!
- Most schools require that all of their students purchase liability insurance before clinical experience. If your school doesn't require liability insurance, consider purchasing it on your own. Liability insurance is available through a number of insurance companies. Most schools of nursing have brochures that will provide information about liability insurance carriers.

(Guido, 2001)

Avoiding Legal Problems

- Treat patients and family members honestly, respectfully, and openly.
- Be compassionate and professional.
- Make your patient aware of all facets of treatment, and of their prognosis when appropriate.
- Know the law and incorporate it into your practice.
- Know your competence level and work to improve it through continuing education (Figure 9–1).
- Be active in your professional organizations.
- Be aware of patients who are prone to sue. (Refer to List A in this section.)
- Be aware of nurses' personality traits that trigger lawsuits. (Refer to List B in this section.)

(Guido, 2001)

Vincent, Young, and Phillips (1994) found four main themes when examining why patients and their families take legal action. These four themes are:

1. **Accountability:** Wishing to see staff disciplined and called to account.
2. **Explanation:** A combination of wanting an explanation and feeling ignored or neglected after the incident.
3. **Standards of care:** Wishing to ensure that a similar incident did not happen again.
4. **Compensation:** Wanting compensation and an admission of negligence.

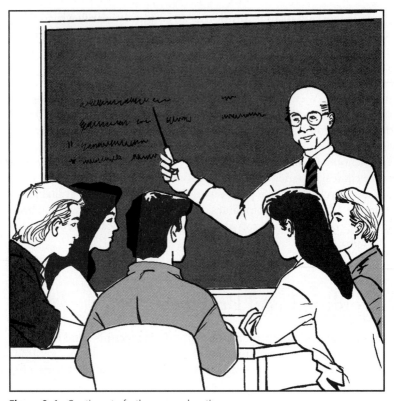

Figure 9–1. Continue to further your education.

List A: Patients Who Are Prone to Sue

There seems to be a profile of patients who tend to sue health care providers. The following are traits to be aware of:

- Overly dependent
- Hostile
- Uncooperative
- Noncompliant
- Blame others
- Insecure

(Guido, 2001)

If your patient reacts in this manner, it is important that you know how to deal with him or her. Rather than react negatively, which will increase resentment and the possibility of a lawsuit, choose to be empathetic and responsive. These patients tend to experience a lot of anxiety so it helps to provide as much information as possible, and to do so repeatedly. If the patient shows any efforts at cooperation, praise these efforts. Although there is no guarantee that you will avoid a lawsuit, it helps to recognize the type of patient who might sue.

List B: Traits of Nurses Who Trigger Lawsuits

The following is a profile of nurses' traits that trigger lawsuits:

- Have difficulty developing close relationships
- Insecure
- Tend to shift blame to others
- Insensitive to patient complaints
- Fail to take patient complaints seriously
- Aloof
- More concerned with technology and machines than the patient (Figure 9–2)
- Delegates to others to avoid patient contact

(Guido, 2001)

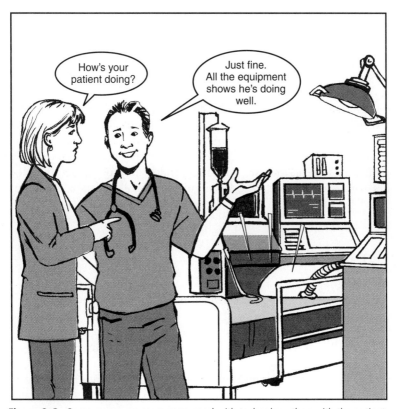

Figure 9–2. Some nurses are more concerned with technology than with the patient.

All nurses need to be cognizant of legal issues both at school and at work. It is important for you to learn how to protect yourself and your employer from litigation. Remember that it is important to treat others as you or a member of your family would want to be treated.

Delegation

As a student, you are not in a position to delegate nursing activities to unlicensed assistive personnel (UAP), individuals who participate in direct patient care but are not licensed. An older term for this group was *nursing assistants;* another common term is *PCA (patient care assistant)*. However, a few words regarding delegation seem prudent.

Many students work in a UAP position while in school. When doing this, it is *crucial* that you keep your student role and work role *separate*. As a student, the nursing board's rules and regulations permit you, under faculty supervision, to perform those activities legally allowed only for an RN. When you are working as an UAP/PCA, these rules and regulation **do not apply.** You are an employee and not a student. However, nurses frequently mix your roles and may delegate activities to you that your state regulating board says a UAP/PCA may *not* do. So, carrying out the assignment will put *both* you and the delegating nurse in legal jeopardy. Therefore, clarifying your role and capabilities is essential.

As a graduate, you will be on the delegating side. Therefore, you will want to know the rules and regulations of your state about delegation. You will have classes on this topic; pay attention. Should an issue arise that concerns a delegation assignment, you will not be able to use ignorance of your state's rules and regulations as an excuse. Although there may be some differences in specifics between the states, the basic guidelines are the same. A summary of these guidelines by Guido (2001) is seen in Figure 9–3.

Ethics

Very often, you hear the phrase *ethical–legal* used as if the terms are interchangeable. They are not. In health care, you may be faced with situations in which only one of these concepts is involved or both concepts are involved. Let's separate the concepts by looking at some basic definitions.

- **Law** has to do with rules and regulations established by a society to govern the behavior of its members. Laws can be classified into several categories

Actions that may be delegated include those that have:
1. A low potential for harm.
2. Minimum complexity of nursing activity.
3. Minimum required problem solving and innovation.
4. High predictability of outcome.
5. Ample opportunity for patient interaction with the staff nurse.
6. Adequate RN ability to supervise the delegated activity and its outcome.

The nurse who delegates the action is responsible for:
1. Using a thoughtful decision-making process in deciding to delegate.
2. Providing clear and specific directions.
3. Individualizing the plan of care to meet the patient's unique needs.
4. Communicating the method of performance, expected outcomes, and parameters.
5. Supervising performance of the task.
6. Evaluating the patient outcome.

The person receiving the delegation is responsible for:
1. Demonstrating competence to perform the specific task.
2. Asking questions if directions are not understood.
3. Following directions from the RN.
4. Following established protocols and guidelines.
5. Reporting observations and activities to the delegating staff member.

The employer, nurse-manager, or supervisor is responsible for:
1. Providing adequate staffing and other resources needed for safe and effective patient care.
2. Following up on every report of concern for safe staffing or concern for safe practice and taking steps to correct situations which prevent safe or effective care.
3. Providing education and orientation to all employees, including education on delegation (Minnesota Nurses Association, 1997).

Figure 9–3. Guidelines: Delegation. From: Minnesota Nurses Association, 1997. In: Guido, G. W. (2001). Legal and ethical issues in nursing (3rd ed.). *Upper Saddle River, NJ: Prentice Hall Health.*

such as constitutional law, statutory law, and administrative law. Statutory laws are of major interest to nurses. These laws create standards as a means of protecting the public from harm. For example, statutory laws establish the criteria that only licensed electricians are allowed to work on public buildings. And statutory laws set the standards that city water supplies must meet to ensure the safety of public drinking water. Although there are many divisions of laws, there are two of importance to health care providers.

- **Civil law:** Civil laws of paramount interest to nurses are the licensure laws enacted by each state. These are the rules and regulations that protect the public by setting the criteria that must be met before an individual can practice nursing in any given state. Also under civil law are a great many other issues that concern the health care giver such as invasion of privacy, slander, libel, negligence, and false imprisonment. By and large, civil laws concern actions that are seen as offensive to an individual rather than society, and when they are settled, the result is monetary compensation to one of the parties involved. This division of the law is the one that is involved when nurses find themselves in court regarding nursing interventions and adverse client responses.
- **Criminal law:** Criminal laws concern behaviors that are considered offensive to society rather than the individual. Violation of these laws results in a criminal trial, with punishment ranging from fines to jail to execution. Nurses seldom are involved in a criminal law situation as a result of their work. However, nurses occasionally have been charged with murder of clients under their care. How sad.
- **Ethics** has to do with the more fluid areas of values, morals, personal beliefs, and philosophy used in determining *right* from *wrong* behavior. You are, no doubt, acutely aware of situations in which the issues are not about the law but about hard-to-make choices. Some recent examples have to do with our new knowledge regarding genes and genetic disorders, genetic counseling and an unborn fetus, and the issues surrounding a 90-year-old who needs an amputation to save his or her life but refuses surgery. Another example is parents' refusing, on religious grounds, permission for a blood transfusion for their child. (These are situations that a policy, procedure, or protocol book cannot handle.) Because of different values in such circumstances, no one solution is acceptable to everyone concerned, thus the term *dilemma,* a situation in which all possible choices to a resolution are unfavorable/unacceptable to at least one side of the situation. When such dilemmas arise in health care settings, resolution requires *ethical decision making,* a process that utilizes one or more ethical principles. A few of the more frequently used principles are:
  - **Autonomy**—the belief that a competent individual has the freedom to make and act on choices, even when the health care provider does not agree with the choice. This principle is often referred to as the right to self-determination.
  - **Beneficence**—the belief that the caregiver has a moral duty to help an individual; doing what is good for the patient
  - **Fidelity**—the action of honoring promises, being faithful to commitments
  - **Veracity**—the action of truth telling; not deceiving or misleading
  - **Confidentiality**—the act of respecting patient's information/privacy

A CASE IN POINT

A 78-year-old patient, who resides in a long-term care facility, has the following health problems: mild right sided paralysis from a stroke 3 months ago with no apparent cognitive damage; diabetes with poor lower extremity circulation and stasis ulcers; hypertension; and congestive heart failure. The patient is very frail and becomes short of breath with only minimal activity. He is refusing to take any of his medications, stating that he is tired of his quality of life and wants to die. However, the physician, the nursing staff, and the patient's children do not agree with this decision. They all believe that the patient should be made to take the medications, even if it means disguising them in food or fluids.

- **Nonmaleficence**—the belief that the individual has the right to be protected from harm; sometimes seen as the companion principle to beneficence

There are times, however, when the dilemma is such that one of the parties, the patient or the heath care system, is unwilling to accept the decision. In this situation, the issue is taken to court for resolution. Now legal and ethical issues are gnarled. In these situations, the court utilizes both ethical and legal principles to reach a conclusion. Resolution by means of the court, however, does not mean that all parties believe that the resolution is "right."

Nurses are expected by the public to act in an ethical manner. Several ethical codes for nurses exist (see ANA Code of Ethics on the inside back cover of this text).

As you reflect on the case in point, can you identify where the principles of autonomy, beneficence, and veracity are involved? Therefore, in order to resolve this situation, *many* questions need to be asked and answered. One central question is who has the right to make the decision about taking or not taking medications? On the surface, many would say that the health care providers' and family's perspective should prevail. They sincerely believe that it is in the patient's best interest to have the medications. If the patient were incompetent, this view would probably predominate. However, the question now arises of how has or will "competency" be determined? Such a determination, in fact, may require that a judge have a hearing and make a declaration of the patient's competency, which in turn leads to a whole new set of questions. Have you noticed that the patient's age and the fact that he resides in a long-term care facility are not the foundation for decision making? (However, they would be part of the information used to arrive at a resolution.) You can see that reaching an ethical decision in this relatively uncomplicated situation is not clear-cut. As you study ethics, you will learn about the use of various frameworks to aid in the analysis and resolution of ethical dilemmas.

RESOURCE WEB SITE

Bioethics Online Service: *www.mcw.edu/bioethics/index.html*

10

Risk Management

Risk Management

Risk management is a specialized field within the general realm of management. Risk management in health care is similar to risk management in business as it focuses on minimizing the financial effects of accidental loss. Some of the financial losses that risk management is concerned with include property loss by fire or flood; income loss due to decrease in census; personnel loss through injury, illness, or death; machinery breakdown; and being named as a defendant in a lawsuit.

Risk managers perform frequent analyses of losses that occur within a facility. Risk managers also deal with identifying and decreasing the potential liability of the facility. Managers keep databases that reflect all losses over time. Their primary job is to stop losses from occurring or to provide means (financial) for losses that are going to occur regardless of attempts to stop them from happening. For example, in our litigious society, chances are that a health care facility may be faced with a number of lawsuits on a yearly basis. The risk manager is responsible for seeing that a certain amount of financial cushioning is provided to handle these suits.

The risk manager also serves as an insurance liaison for the facility and is sometimes responsible for the automobile, property, general, professional, and workers' compensation insurance policies. The risk manager is also a legal contact for the hospital and provides information about advance directives, adoptions, questions regarding consent forms, contract reviews, and any correspondence or contact with attorneys. The risk manager is not just concerned about one aspect of the health care facility, but rather with the broad picture. The risk manager has a responsibility to employees, visitors, patients, physicians, and to hospital property.

What the Risk Manager Monitors

According to Cindy McClelland, risk manager, some of the things that a risk manager might be responsible for monitoring include:

- Safety
- Fire protection
- Employee health
- Incident reports
- Bomb threat procedures
- Americans with Disabilities Act (ADA) compliance
- Patient complaints
- Security
- Physician credentialing
- Damaged or lost equipment

Often, nurses are not clear about what exactly a risk manager does. As you can see, the risk manager is responsible for the day-to-day activities in the health care facility. Because of such a unique position, the risk manager can serve as a source of information about a number of things that nurses are interested in.

The Risk Management Plan

The risk manager is also responsible for developing a facility-wide plan of risk management. According to Sullivan and Decker (1992), the risk management plan might consist of some or all of the following:

- Identify potential risks by working with all departments and inspecting the facility.
- Review and monitor systems such as incident reports, audits, committee minutes, and patient complaints.
- Monitor laws and standards that relate to patient safety, consent, and care.
- Review and appraise new programs such as managed care, home health, rehabilitation, and infusion therapy.
- Eliminate or reduce a specific risk through education, policy, or insurance financing.

- Analyze trends and causes of incidents by their frequency and severity.
- Identify educational needs—staff education needs about new equipment, policies and procedures, and patient needs on admission and discharge.
- Evaluate the effectiveness of the risk management program.
- Provide reports and documentation of trends to the chief executive officer and respective committees.

Risk management is important to you for a number of reasons.

- If the facility continually loses money, you may be out of a job.
- Theft can cause the employer to stop providing necessary supplies.
- Injury and illness on the job are important to your well-being.
- The risk management program can support and provide you with information on ways to make your nursing care better and your job safer.

Areas of High Risk for Nurses

Nurses tend to be involved in the areas of risk management given in the following list. It would behoove you to pay special attention to these areas, as well as finding out for yourself which problems occur most frequently in the area in which you work.

- Medication errors
- Complications from diagnostic or treatment procedures
- Falls
- Patient or family dissatisfaction with care
- Refusal of treatment or to sign a consent form

What the Risk Manager Can Tell You

- The risk manager can provide you with data about these high-risk areas for nurses.
- The risk manager can also give you specific information about the area in which you work.
- Does your area have more falls than others do? If so, why?
- What are other areas doing that your area is not?
- How can you fix the problem?
- The risk manager can help you with all of these questions and make your area safer for you, patients, and visitors.

Tips From a Risk Manager

1. **Communicate!** Let those individuals who need to know, know what is going on.
2. **Document!** Remember, "If you didn't chart it, you didn't do it."
3. **Follow!** The chain of command is there for a reason!
   - If you need help, ask your immediate supervisor.
   - If you are not satisfied with the results, ask your supervisor's immediate supervisor.
   - Do not skip steps and go directly to the chief executive officer.
4. **Maintain confidentiality!**
   - Keep hospital and patient information confidential.
   - Do not gossip.
5. **Incident reports!**
   - Always ask, and if you are still in doubt, fill one out.
   - The incident report form is a means of protecting you and the facility.
6. **Communication!**
   - Be honest but careful.
   - Remember, what you say can be used against you.
7. **Education!**
   - Stay up to date in your field.
   - You can *never* know too much.

RESOURCE WEB SITES

If you are interested in more information about risk management, visit the following Web sites at *www.riskweb.com.*

Risk Management Overview: *www.sei.cmu.edu/programs/sepm/ risk/risk.mgmt.overview.html*
Risk Management Internet Services: *www.rmis.com*
Global Risk Management Network: *www.grmn.com*
Risk Management Foundation: *www.rmf.harvard.edu*

Functioning
in Clinical Settings

11

Communication

Communication

Communication is an essential part of our lives. We communicate with each other constantly. As a student nurse, you will be learning to communicate therapeutically with patients. Most nursing schools do a good job of teaching therapeutic communication. Unfortunately, some students have difficulty grasping this concept.

You have been living in the real world for some time now. You have already witnessed millions of ways of communicating from one person to another. You will have developed methods of communication that feel comfortable to you. We tend to develop communication patterns that we use over and over again with the various people in our lives. We communicate one way with our parents, another way with the grocery store clerk, and now you are in the process of developing ways to communicate with patients. Some of the communication patterns that you use will be new; others will be old.

You will find that some nurses treat patients as objects or things. These nurses tend to be condescending, derogatory, unconcerned, and lacking in warmth. It is essential that you treat patients and others with respect. Remember that patients are people too. They are not just the disease that they represent. A patient is Mrs. Williams, who happens to be in room 107 and happens to have abdominal pain. She is not room 107 or abdominal pain. There are also many nurses who are compassionate, respectful, understanding, and caring. What kind of nurse will you be? You do have a choice! Remember the old adage: Treat people as you want to be treated. Treat your patient as you would want your loved one to be treated (your mother, father, sister, brother, spouse, or child). Many times, nurses are so busy doing various tasks that they forget that all of those various tasks have a purpose. The purpose is to provide high-quality care to our patients.

Let's look at two different scenarios regarding your decision to purchase a pair of athletic shoes for the first time.

Scenario 1: You go to a local sporting goods store and as you enter the shoe department you see three salespeople in store uniforms milling around. You walk past them and head toward the shoe department. Not one of the three employees gives you a second glance. As you approach the athletic shoes, you find that there are at least 100 different kinds—running, cross-training, walking, basketball, and tennis—as well as several different brands. Feeling totally overwhelmed, you start searching for some assistance. You finally locate an employee and request help with the selection process. The salesperson says, "Yeah, I'll be there in a minute." You wander back to the shoes and sit down to wait. After 5 minutes, you start hunting another salesperson. You locate another employee who is busy sharing details of the latest movie with other salespeople. By now, you are getting annoyed because no one will help you. You once again ask an employee for help. The salesperson reluctantly follows you to the athletic shoes. You explain that you need help choosing a shoe for aerobic dancing in a 9 narrow. The salesperson proceeds to pull out five pairs of 9 narrow shoes from the stacks. When you ask what the differences are in the shoes the employee says, "I don't know, what difference does it make, just find one that fits," and walks away. You feel as though no one is making an effort to help you and that the salesperson could not care less whether you are satisfied with the service or not. The employee obviously has more important things to do than to pay attention to you!

Scenario 2: You decide to try a different store. You find the shoe department and when you walk in a salesperson comes over to you and asks, "How may I help you?" You tell her that you are trying to find a shoe for aerobic dancing in 9 narrow. As she walks you toward the end of the aisle, she explains that you are bypassing tennis, walking, and other shoes that will not provide enough support for aerobics. At the end of the aisle, she points out the aerobic shoes and explains the cushioning and asks whether you have any problems with your feet. You explain that you tend to wear down the outside of your shoes very quickly. She chooses a pair of shoes for you to try and tells you that they provide a lot of lateral support. As she guides you to your selection, she smiles frequently and is extremely attentive to your facial expressions. You feel as though she is really focused on you and will stay with you and help you find the correct pair of shoes that are the best suited for you.

The next time that you go shopping for a pair of shoes, where will you go?

Communication and Nursing

Patients are consumers too. They want to be treated well. If they are mistreated, they will take their business elsewhere. Many hospitals have started giving patients report cards so they can grade their hospital stay. Part of our job is to keep our patients happy. Mark Twain said, "Kindness is a language which the deaf ear can hear and the blind can see." In business, there is a slogan, "The customer is always right." In other words, you should do everything in your power to keep the customer happy so they will return.

Nurses who are disrespectful and who treat patients badly can cause patients to go elsewhere for care. Remember this and learn to respect patients! Remember another old adage, "It is not always what you say, but how you say it"? That nonverbal message will come across loud and clear.

Communicating Nonverbal Messages

- **Communicate that you care.** How do you know when someone cares about you? He or she gets down on your level (sit down if your patient is sitting, or pull up a chair if the patient is lying in bed). You might reach out and hold a hand or touch a shoulder. Nod your head to let the patient know you are listening.
- **Communicate that you are empathetic.** Use eye contact to indicate that you are listening and that you understand. Nod your head and smile as you listen to what the patient is saying. Again, touch is important here.
- **Communicate that you want what is best for your patient.** If you have demonstrated that you care and are empathetic, your patient will know that you can be trusted and that you want to help. Your patients will be grateful, and your employer will be pleased.

However, some nurses have a tendency to have more difficulty communicating with other members of the health care team than with their patients. As technology improves, more specialties develop, leaving nurses responsible for communicating with more people on a daily basis. To streamline communication for the benefit of patients, it is important for us to know which member of the health care team needs what information.

Guidelines for Communicating with Team Members

PATIENT

- Perhaps the most important team member is the patient.
- Unfortunately, many specialists want to "do for" or "do to" the patient without allowing the patient's active participation.

- As changes occur in the health care system, patients are becoming more and more knowledgeable and are demanding to be included in all aspects of their health care.
- Patients have a right and a responsibility to participate in their own health care.
- It is necessary that all members of the health care team keep patients informed so that they will be sufficiently informed to make decisions about their own health care.

PHYSICIAN

- The physician is responsible for diagnosing, treating, and preventing disease.
- Typically, the doctor will use medications and/or surgery to treat patients.
- The physician used to be considered the "captain" of the health care team and was responsible for directing all aspects of care.
- Today, the doctor is considered a member of the health care team and needs to collaborate with other team members to provide patients with the best possible care.
- The physician needs to be informed about all aspects of the patient's care.
- It is important that you discuss with the physician any changes in health status or any changes in therapy provided by any other health team member.

PHYSICAL THERAPIST (PT)

- The PT focuses on problems of a musculoskeletal nature.
- The PT uses exercises and therapies to increase muscle strength and decrease loss of function.
- The PT needs to know about problems with musculoskeletal function, mobility aids, and anything else that has an impact on the patient's ability to participate in physical therapy.

OCCUPATIONAL THERAPIST (OT)

- The OT focuses on the patient's ability to maintain his or her independence in activities of daily living.
- The OT assists patients in adapting their home and/or using special equipment to continue to take care of their home or personal activities.
- The OT needs to be aware of any physical, mental, or emotional limitations the patient might have, or any problems the patient is having with activities of daily living or home maintenance.

SOCIAL WORKER

- The social worker attempts to better the patient's life outside of the hospital through referrals to community agencies, counseling, or finding alternative placement.
- The social worker helps organize care for the patient at home or in short-term or long-term living facilities.
- Social workers need to be informed about the patient's physical, emotional, and mental limitations.

DIETITIAN

- The dietitian is responsible for providing nutrition counseling and therapy.
- The dietitian helps develop an individual nutrition plan that takes into account things such as the patient's culture, ethnicity, financial status, and health status.
- The dietitian needs to know the patient's typical diet, what type of diet the physician has ordered, and any other information that pertains to the patient's nutrition status.

RESPIRATORY THERAPIST (RT)

- The RT focuses on the patient's respiratory function and treats any problems of a respiratory nature.
- In some facilities, the RT and the nurse work together to provide treatment.
- The RT needs to know about changes in respiratory function or any problems the patient is experiencing related to their respiratory treatment.

As a nurse, you will be responsible for communicating with all of these different specialists and may be responsible for coordinating information between and among them. To assist you with coordination of care, it is important that you recall two aspects of professional behavior that may impact your teamwork: advocacy and accountability.

Aspects of Professional Behavior

ADVOCACY

- To protect your patient's interests, you may need to be a **patient advocate.**
- Occasionally, you will find that a particular patient's needs are not being met, or the patient may actually be in jeopardy of having rights violated.
- It is your responsibility in either of these situations to speak on behalf of your patient.

- Technically, all health care team members share in this responsibility, but nurses tend to be in a better position to act as a patient advocate.
- This is one of the reasons that it is so important that you spend time getting to know your patient and your patient's wishes.

ACCOUNTABILITY

- As a member of the health care team, you are **accountable** for your own actions.
- You are responsible for informing your team members about any changes in the patient's status or about any information that the patient shares with you that is pertinent to the team.
- You are not only accountable to the patient, you are also accountable to other team members and the team as a whole.

As stated earlier, it is important that you respect your patients and treat them the way that you would want your loved ones to be treated. It is just as important that you treat other members of the health care team with respect. By fostering mutual respect among team members, you enhance the development of a collegial relationship.

Since there are a number of members on each patient's health care team, roles sometimes become confused. You may already have run into this situation where you are given conflicting orders. It is vital that team members delineate their roles in the care of patients. You can help facilitate this by encouraging group meetings to discuss patient care. You may find that you will need to further develop your ability to be assertive (see Chapter 7).

Communication can be a daunting task. However, communication patterns can be changed. You can learn new and better ways of communicating with your patient and others. Remember to respect yourself and others, to treat everyone with kindness, and to be genuine.

12

Documentation

Documentation of patient records is key to all areas of nursing practice. It is vital that nurses address individual patients' needs, problems, limitations, and progress. Unfortunately, documentation is often viewed as a chore more often than a challenge. It is important to know that documenting is a challenge because it is most likely the one issue that ends up winning or losing most lawsuits.

Documentation Facts

You need to be certain that in documenting you follow the policy and procedure manual of your institution and your state's nurse practice act. The following guidelines should also help with documentation.

- Documentation should focus on continuity of care, interventions used, and patient responses.
- If there is no change in the patient, that should also be noted at least once per shift or per visit.
- Documentation should also be concise, clear, timely, and complete.
- A complete nursing assessment should be included in the patient's record as well.

Documentation and Nursing

There are several types of documentation, but this chapter will address taped reports and charting (narrative, computer-generated flowcharts, and charting-by-exception).

Taped Reports

Some facilities tape the end-of-shift report that provides oncoming shift personnel with current information on all patients assigned to a particular nurse or group of nurses. A taped report can be a good way of transferring information from one group of nurses to another. Each facility will require different patient information during report depending on the focus of patient care. For example, a home health agency nurse will require much different information about his or her patients than a nurse on a hospital obstetrical unit.

Be careful about what you say during taping. We have heard many a value judgment about patients (e.g., "That one is just a crock"). We have also heard nurses laughing and joking about recent events on the floor. Remember, the report tape can be confiscated and used against you. We often wish that patients could be present at taped report to hear what is said about them. After all, the focus of report is to enhance exchange of information to provide better care to our patients. So, if your facility tapes reports, follow the guidelines of what to include so that others will be aware of the patient's condition, and leave out the extraneous comments.

Charting

Charting may include a handwritten record, a flow sheet, and/or a computer record. Whether a record is handwritten or entered into a computer, the same principles apply. It is imperative that you remember that patient records are admissible in court; therefore, you must be extremely careful in what you document.

We will never forget when one of us was called to appear in court to testify in a case where an infant had died in a neonatal intensive care unit (NICU). Although some of the events surrounding the infant's death were able to be recalled, it had been 5 long years since we had actually worked with the infant. The only way to refresh your memory about certain events that occurred in the past is to read nurses' notes. Luckily, this particular charting was descriptive enough to fill in any gaps in memory. However, being notified to appear in court can be a very scary experience.

If you ever find yourself in a courtroom situation, you will probably find that your mouth is dry and your knees are knocking! If you can imagine being scared, stressed out, or a bit on the defensive with someone standing there pointing out to you any errors that you have made in charting, it might encourage you to chart more accurately. We highly recommend that you participate in a mock trial if you ever get the opportunity to. If you know any lawyers and if your student organization or school is interested, you might want to consider setting one up. Mock trials can be quite fun as well as a valuable learning experience.

TYPES OF CHARTING

There are seven types of charting discussed here, and they are as follows:

1. Narrative (Figure 12–1)
2. SOAP (subjective, objective, assessment, and plan)
3. SOAPIER (subjective, objective, assessment, planning, implementation, evaluation, and rationale)
4. PIE (problem, intervention, and evaluation)
5. Focus charting (flowsheets, checklists)
6. Charting-by-exception
7. Computer-assisted charting

Regardless of what type of charting is used in your facility, certain basic principles apply. As part of your clinical orientation as a student, you should be taught about the charting used in each facility that you rotate through. Remember that you can always look in the policy and procedure manual and consult with your instructor before making chart entries.

7:30 A.M. Forty-six-year-old white female admitted to 4SA for evaluation. Pt transferred from ER after commenting that she "Is tired of it all and would be better off dead." Dr. Creed visited pt and completed pt history. Pt oriented to unit and introduced to staff. Pt is coherent, communicates her needs, and is cooperative. Pt is dressed appropriately and is wearing appropriate makeup.
8:00 A.M. Pt served breakfast on the unit. She ate 75%. Pt has not made any suicidal statements.
9:00 A.M. Pt attended music therapy and interacted with other patients. She smiled during group and participated by choosing a song to sing.
10:00 A.M. Pt attended education group. She openly discussed her medications and how she adheres to a dosing schedule. Pt helped others see the need for continuing therapy even when feeling well.
11:00 A.M. Pt discussed current depressive episode with RN. Stated that she felt "overwhelmed by a teenage son and daughter and an unfaithful husband." Pt also stated that "My mother died a month ago and I don't think I'm handling it very well."

Figure 12–1. Narrative charting example.

Charting Hints

- **Make an entry for every observation.** Remember the slogan, if you didn't chart it, you didn't do it. Some of the newer forms of charting, most notably charting-by-exception, encourage gaps in charting information. Even with charting-by-exception, you are expected to document any abnormal or significant changes that veer from accepted standards or clinical pathology.
- **Follow up as needed.** Even if your charting is accurate and timely, you must also make and document efforts to notify others about changes in a patient's condition.
- **Read notes before giving care or charting.** As students, you are encouraged to read the chart, including the nurses' notes. As nurses, we often complain about lack of time, or we consider report as a sufficient exchange of information. However, reading the nurses' notes can provide an overall picture of how the patient is progressing or not progressing, and can also help identify any discrepancies in documentation.
- **Record entries must be timely.** As stated earlier, memories tend to fade over time and if you are going in a hundred different directions at one time, as most nurses do, you may not recall all of the pertinent details of what happened 3 hours ago. However, charting late is better than not charting at all. Be aware that if your late charting ends up in a courtroom, questions will be raised about documenting solely to prevent liability (Figure 12–2). In other words, the attorney will make it appear that you were only trying to cover up an error because something terrible happened to your patient (whether or not you did anything wrong, chances are you will appear to be guilty).
- **Chart only after the event.** Never chart prior to doing a treatment, giving medication, or anything else. More than one nurse has charted a medication prior to giving it, only to find the patient dead. Think about another of your patients going into respiratory arrest, a fire, or any number of other critical events occurring. If you charted that you gave your patient heart medication before you actually gave it, another nurse will think that it has been done, which can put your patient in jeopardy.
- **Use clear language.** If the patient is obviously bleeding, do not chart the patient "appears" to be bleeding. Rather, chart how much blood you observe. Do not chart the patient "ate well," chart how much the patient actually ate. Vague references will be attacked in court and your observation abilities will be called into question. Can you imagine charting that a patient "appeared" to be bleeding, and going to court because the patient hemorrhaged to death? How could you defend "appears" to be? The plaintiff's attorney will be asking you questions about your ability to identify when a patient is bleeding or not. This is neither a pretty picture, nor one that you would want to experience.

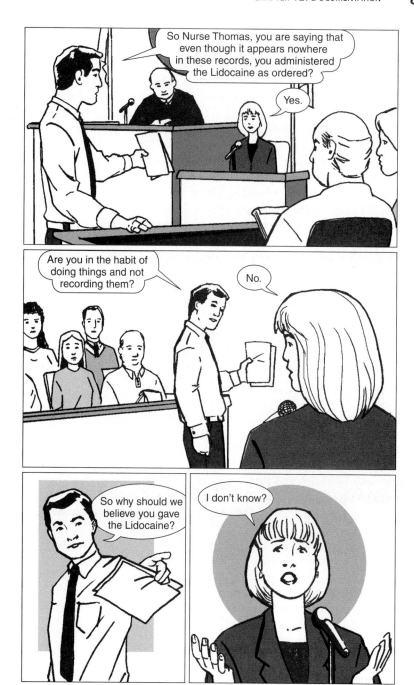

Figure 12–2. The opposing attorney will make you look like you did not know what you were doing.

- **Be realistic and factual.** It is important that you chart a true picture of your patient without personal comments. If a patient is noncompliant, chart, "Mr. Williams refused his 9:00 A.M. medication." Do not chart, "Mr. Williams does not seem to want to improve. He is very rude and doesn't want to get better." Patients who are noncompliant or those who are abusive or threatening may perceive that they have been treated unsuccessfully or unfairly. Patients who are not pleased with their hospital stay or treatment are more likely to sue you, the doctor, or the hospital.

- **Chart only what you observe.** When you chart for others, or chart in a patient chart other than your assigned patients, you can be called into court for questioning. If you are asked about the patient, even though you never cared for that patient, you may be unable to recall the specifics of the situation. So, if another nurse asks you to document an event, remember, it will be your license on the line. The same holds true when you accept information from others and document it. Some facilities still ask nurses to chart or cosign (sign your name after another person) for other staff members. When you do this, you are the one who is potentially liable for the care, observations, or any omissions that you chart. Be certain that you double-check all information before charting it yourself.

- **Chart errors.** Follow your institution policy and procedure manual regarding errors. Most facilities will ask that you draw a single line through the misspelled or wrong word and write the correct word above or to the right of it. You should also write your initials and the date and time above, or to the right of the new entry. Some facilities request that you write the word "error" or "mistaken entry"; others believe that using these reflects on the entire entry, not just a single word. To protect yourself, be certain that you follow your institution guidelines.

- **Identify yourself after every entry.** At the end of each entry you should write your full name and title, whether or not this information is given earlier in the chart. Some facilities have a space at the bottom or top of the page where you sign your name, title, and initials; your initials are used after each entry on the page.

- **All charting should be done in ink.** All entries should be legible and only standard institution-approved abbreviations should be used. Charting should be neat and organized (if your charting is sloppy and disorganized, a jury may conclude that you are sloppy and disorganized in your nursing care as well). Do not leave blank spaces or go back and try to chart between lines. Never leave a space for someone else to chart.

Flow Sheets or Checklists

Most institutions rely on some flow sheets or checklists to document routine care. Vital signs have been charted on flow sheets for many years (Figure 12–3).

F	C	04/08/98 Day: 1					04/09/98 Day: 2									
		03	07	11	15	19	03	07	11	15	19	03	07	11	15	19
104	40.0															
103	39.4															
102	38.9															
101	38.3															
100	37.7															
99	37.2															
98	36.6															
97	36.1															

	03	07	11	15	19	03	07	11	15	19	03	07	11	15	19
Temp		96 Orl		98 Orl		98 Orl	97 Orl								
Pulse		61		67		82	72								
Resp		20		18		20	20								
B/P		161/73		164/77		131/73	123/72								
*						*									

Wt Ht: 170lb

		NOCS	DAYS	EVES	TOTAL	NOCS	DAYS	EVES	TOTAL	NOCS	DAYS	EVES	TOTAL
I N T A K E	Oral												
	IV/Med Drips												
	TPN/Lipid												
	Tube Feed												
	Blood Product												
	Irrigants												
	TOTAL												
O U T P U T	Urine												
	Stool												
	Emesis												
	Drains												
	Blood/Drainage												
	EBL												
	TOTAL												
	NET												

Figure 12–3. Vital signs.

Today, flow sheets and checklists have been developed for most areas of nursing. Rather than having to write data over and over again, the flow sheet allows the nurse to enter only pertinent data (Figure 12–4). Although these sheets can be time saving, it is important to remember that they are also legal documents and admissible in court.

We have seen many charts in which the flow sheet says one thing and the nurse's notes say another. Be certain that you check the patient yourself and that the flow sheet is accurate! We cannot begin to count the number of times we have witnessed nurses continuing to check off the same columns as the previous shift. One time, the nurses were checking that the patient had ambulated four times a day for days, only to discover that the patient had a massive stroke and was bedridden. Of course, the nurses were aware that the patient was

Act	active	Frg	full ROM	Obc	obeys command	Sm	small
Alt	alert	Ics	incision	Orl	oral	Spn	spontaneous
Bld	bloody	Ita	intact	Per	person	Sta	stained
Brs	brisk	Liq	liquids	Plc	place	Tme	time
Clr	clear	Nds	nondistended	Plp	palpable	Unl	unlabored
Con	continent	Nor	normal	Pnk	pink	Wrm	warm
Dry	dry	Ntn	non-tender	Reg	regular	Yel	yellow
Evn	even	O3	orient(3)	Sft	soft		

Temp	04/08							
Graph	14:35	15:07	16:00	17:19	18:04	18:55	21:08	22:22
Vital Signs								
TEMP #1		94.3F Orl		98.2F Orl				
PULSE #1		67		74				
RESPIRATIONS		18		18				
BP #1		164/77		145/73				
Neurological								
Orientation/LOC			AltO3				AltO3	
Both pupils								
Pupil Reaction								
Motor Strength								
All extremities			Nor				Nor	
Open Eyes			Spn				Spn	
Best Motor Rsp			Obc				Obc	
Best Verbal Rsp			Clr				Clr	
Respiratory								
Resp Pattern			RegEvnUnl				RegEvnUnl	
Sound/Breathing			Nor				Nor	
Cardiovascular								
Heart Rate								
Pulses								
Radial			NorPlp				NorPlp	
Gastrointestinal								
Bowel Sounds								
all quads								
Swallows			Liq				Liq	
Abdomen			SftNtnNds				SftNtnNds	
Bowel Control			Con				Con	

Figure 12–4. Flow sheet charting report.

bedridden, but checklists are often completed while the nurse's mind is wandering or other events are occurring. Pay attention to what you are checking! Checklists and flow sheets are not mindless time-consuming tasks. Be sure that all of your data are reliable!

Charting-by-Exception

Charting-by-exception is a fairly new way of charting that encourages the nurse to only chart significant or abnormal findings rather than documenting normal findings over and over again.

- Document only significant or abnormal findings.
- Progress or lack of progress reflected in clinical pathways, nursing diagnosis–based standardized care plans and protocols, flow sheets, and checklists.
- Very streamlined and efficient.
- May leave major gaps when problems occur and the nurse is unable to thoroughly document all that was done for a patient.

For example, if you were working in a cardiac catheterization laboratory, you would use checklists for all data and document only significant problems. Since a hematoma is an "expected" complication of this procedure, it will most likely appear on a checklist. If the patient's hematoma is treated according to guidelines and the patient is discharged, but a thrombosis develops, what happens? What if you are called into court 3 years later and all you have to refer to is a checklist? Would you be able to remember who that particular patient was? Would you be able to defend your actions?

Computer-Assisted Charting

Computers have developed into a lifeline for most facilities. Computers can be used for everything including admission histories (Figure 12–5), nurses' notes, care plans (Figure 12–6), and many other types of data. Physicians can access patient records from their offices and transmit orders directly to the lab, pharmacy, and nurses.

- Nurses usually have access to a microcomputer through a video display terminal or a handheld portable terminal.
- Nurses are provided with computer training during orientation or other education program.
- Once a nurse is trained in the use of the computer, an access code is given.
- This access code is secured and is to be used only by the individual nurse who receives it.
- Allowing anyone else to use your access code number may result in termination of your employment.

Some computers have a keyboard to type in information; others use a penlight or other scanning device. Some of the newer computers have a bar-code reader that can scan a patient's ID bracelet prior to giving care or medications. If a medication is given in error, or at the wrong time, the nurse is notified immediately on a video screen.

COMPUTER CHARTING POSITIVES AND NEGATIVES
- Computer charting is our future. It not only streamlines our entries, it also generates typed, up-to-the-minute information.

```
                                                    04/09/00   10:13
                                                          Page: 1
                              Admission History
              From 04/07/00 07:00            To 04/09/00 07:00
              --------------------------------------------

        4068-A Name:_____ MD: _____
        Sex:___ Age: _____ Adm: 04/08/99 01:15  Patient Id:_____ Med Rec No: _____
```

Admission History

Religious Denominations
04/08 09:30   Religious Denomination: Episcopal. (CAL)

Admitted
04/08 09:30   Admitted ambulatory from admitting. Accompanied by: spouse/SO. Informant: patient/self. (CAL)
        09:30   ID bracelet on. (CAL)

Medications
04/08 09:30   Current med: Atenolol 50 mg q am Procardia XL 30 mg q HS. Last dose of this medication was taken: yesterday. Current med: Premarin po and 1.25 ng. Last dose of this medication was taken: yesterday. Current med: Synthroid 0.1 mg Tylenol Child. (CAL)
        09:30   Current med: Synthroid 0.1 mg q day. Last dose of this medication was taken: yesterday. (CAL)

Allergies/Adverse Reactions
04/08 09:30   Allergies/Adverse   Reactions: PCN,   Codeine—reaction—rash Dilaudid—reaction—spaced out. (CAL)

Reason for Admission
04/08 09:30   Reason for admission: (patient's understanding) patient to have surgery/procedure—bronchoscopy and cholecystectomy. (CAL)

Advanced Directives Information
04/08 09:30   Patient has not executed an Advance Directive. Information on Advance Directives: refused by patient. (CAL)

Previous Hospitalizations
04/08 09:30   Previous hospitalizations/out-patient treatments: year—1977. Reason: surgery—bladder suspension. Previous hospitalizations/outpatient treatments: year—1975. Reason: surgery—hernia repair—hiatal. (CAL)

Assistive Devices
04/08 09:30   Assistive devices: patient has none. (CAL)

Discharge Planning
04/08 09:30   Plans have been made for discharge. (CAL)
Care Provider: CAL

Figure 12–5. Admission history.

- Information tends to be more accurate and error free because the computer may prompt the nurse to fill in gaps or challenge conflicting information.
- Computer charting has the potential to cause problems with confidentiality.
- There is a possibility of a delay between giving a medication and when the computer permanently records the medication.

```
                                                    04/09/00  10:14
                                                         Page: 2
                          Cumulative Care Plan
         From 04/08/00 07:00              To 04/09/00 10:13
         ------------------------------------------


Name: _____  MD: _____
Sex:_____ Age: _____ Adm: _____ 01:15 Patient Id: _____ Med Rec No:_____

Cumulative Care Plan
Active          Inactive       Freq  NURSING DIAGNOSIS
04/08 (NH )                          1. Pain: Acute
                                     Defining Characteristics:
04/08 (NH )                            — c/o pain
                                     Related to
04/08 (NH )                            — surgical wound
                                     Secondary to
04/08 (NH )                            — cholecystitis
                                     Goals:
04/08 (NH )            PRN            — Verbalizes a reasonable level of comfort
                                     Interventions:
04/08 (NH )            PRN            — Administer pain medication per following
                                       plan, document response:
                                         instruct patient to request pain medication
                                         before pain becomes severe and adminis-
                                         ter medication before pain becomes se-
                                         vere.
                                     Assessments:
04/08                  PRN            — Assess effectiveness of pain control measures
Care Providers:
Nancy Hay, R.N.
```

Figure 12–6. Cumulative care plan.

Some of these problems are being addressed and new software is being developed to handle them.

Documentation is one of the most important things you will do as a nurse. The way you document can save you or hang you in a courtroom. Documentation can also be perceived as tedious, boring, and time consuming. It is a bit like any other repetitive task; it becomes what you make it. If you find charting boring, you will have a tendency to be sloppy and not pay much attention to it. If you look at it as a challenge, you will pay attention and do a good job. Think again about trying to organize a mock trial. Use some of your own charting or that of a colleague and look at it as a lawyer would. Are there any gaps? Are there any unapproved abbreviations? Make it an adventure!

13

Nursing Process, Case Management, and Clinical Pathways

Nursing Process, Case Management, and Clinical Pathways

The majority of complaints received from nursing students relate to the value of the nursing process. Students frequently want to know why nurses have to do all the paperwork or busy work. Often, the nursing process is seen as a waste of time until it is used in patient care. Unfortunately, some facilities reinforce this idea by requiring that careplans be up-to-date just prior to visits by the Joint Commission on Accreditation of Healthcare Organizations (JCAHO). In some situations, nurses are sitting at a desk filling in 3 weeks worth of nursing care plans on patients who have already been discharged because of a planned JCAHO site visit. It is unfortunate that the nursing process is not perceived in a more positive light.

The nursing process is a way of organizing data about patients. It also provides a blueprint, or map, for caring for the patient. When you decided to go to nursing school you were probably directed to an advisor. The advisor probably gave you a degree plan that provided you with information about what courses you had to take and when you needed to take them in order to graduate. It is similar to the nursing process for your patients. Imagine what would happen if colleges did not have degree plans. Trying to get a degree would be extremely confusing. Think about registration and picking courses that you thought might lead you to your goal without being sure. Attempting to reach your goal of graduation without a degree plan would be similar to trying to care for a patient without the nursing process or a care plan. Most educational and clinical facilities still use the nursing process, although some have chosen to use clinical pathways instead. The nursing process generally consists of a patient history and assessment and a nursing care plan. The history and assessment varies depending on many factors.

Factors That Influence the History and Assessment

No matter how varied history and assessments are, they are used to gather information about a patient and the patient's perceived need for health care. Your attitude and approach to the history and assessment can make a big difference in the ease with which you obtain important information. If you believe that the assessment is a big waste of time and its only purpose is to generate paperwork, then it is doubtful that you will have an easy time of gathering information. If, however, you view the assessment process as a way of getting to know your patient better and as a means of obtaining vital information, then you will probably see its value. Keep the following things in mind while taking a patient history or making an assessment:

- The nurse's objectives for completing the assessment (a hospital admissions assessment versus a reproductive clinic assessment)
- The type of care the patient needs or the amount of time available for completing an assessment (for example, emergency care versus home health care)
- The conceptual framework and mission of the institution (a Catholic university hospital may include different areas than a small, rural county hospital)

Generally, the nursing history and assessment is like a detective novel: You have to read the patient, fill in between the lines, and solve the puzzle. It can be a lot of fun!

The nursing care plan usually consists of four to six columns that help you organize assessment information and project some type of plan of care for your patient.

Nursing Care Plan Columns

Some examples of the information used in the nursing care plan are as follows:

1. **Assessment**
   - **Subjective data** (what the patient tells you)
   - **Objective data** (what you observe or read in the chart, lab values, vital signs, etc.)

- **Nursing diagnosis.** Some schools only allow students to use nursing diagnoses from an approved list such as North American Nursing Diagnosis Association (NANDA). Other schools encourage students to think independently and creatively to develop their own diagnoses in an accepted format. Since the original NANDA classification system started in 1973, NIC (Nursing Interventions Classification) and NOC (Nursing Outcome Classification) have been developed. These specific interventions and outcomes are associated with a specific NANDA diagnosis. If your school uses NANDA and/or the NIC and NOC guidelines, you will probably need a special book.

2. **Planning**
   - Goal or outcome. Stated as "The patient will . . ."
   - Short term—can usually be accomplished in less than 48 hours
   - Long term—sometimes not completed until discharge

3. **Strategies**
   - How the nurse is going to help the patient accomplish the goals
   - Some schools break down strategies into those that the nurse (student) can accomplish on their own and others in which the nurse is dependent on other caregivers (such as physical therapy).

4. **Rationale**
   - The nurse justifies why, or provides a rationale, for the strategies he or she chooses to use.
   - The rationale is the scientific evidence to support a specific strategy.
   - This is documented from a specific page in a text or nursing journal.
   - Some programs allow use of faculty lectures and/or common sense.

5. **Implementation**
   - What the nurse actually did for the patient

6. **Evaluation**
   - Evaluation and reevaluation of movement toward the original goals

A CASE IN POINT

Leslie is a 24-year-old female who was admitted to the acute psychiatric unit following a suicide attempt. Leslie is divorced and has one child. She appears to be sullen and sad. Both wrists are bandaged and the emergency room reports major lacerations with possible tendon damage. Leslie was admitted 5 years ago with a diagnosis of major depression, and her current medical diagnosis is major depression. You have been assigned to care for Leslie during your next clinical day and have been asked to develop a care plan for her (Figure 13–1).

Assessment	Planning	Strategies	Rationale	Implementation	Evaluation
Subj. Data "I don't have anything to live for. If only they hadn't found me when they did."	Short-Term Goal By the end of my shift the pt will state one thing worth living for.	1. Establish a therapeutic relationship.	1. Establishing trust allows the pt to share information in a confidential manner (Burgess, 1997, p. 175).	1. Had three 30 min one-on-one sessions with pt.	Goal met: Pt stated that her child was worth living for.
Obj. Data Sad affect Crying Bandaged wrists (each wrist required 20 stitches) Disheveled Poor hygiene	By the end of my shift the pt will comply with all suicide precautions. During my shift the patient will make no attempts to harm herself.	2. Provide close observation. 3. Encourage pt to sign a no-suicide contract.	2. Protecting patients from suicidal impulses is critical (p. 574). 3. A no-suicide contract is a time-limited verbal or written promise (p. 275).	2. Checked on pt every 15 min when not with her. 3. Pt signed a no-suicide contract.	Goal met: Pt was compliant with suicide precautions and signed a no-suicide contract.
Nurs. Diag. Self-directed violence related to feelings of hopelessness as evidenced by recent suicide attempt.	**Long-Term Goal** By discharge the pt will verbalize a desire to live and willingly attend outpatient therapy.	4. Use active listening techniques. 5. Provide an activity to release tension.	4. Nurses need to express concern and establish an alliance with the pt (p. 573. 5. Use positive interest and build mutual trust (p. 578.)	4. Used active listening. 5. Pt used the punching bag for 10 min and created a clay figure in OT.	Goal met: Pt did not try to harm herself.

Figure 13–1. Care plan for Leslie.

Nursing Students' House

Assessment	Diagnosis	Planning Short-Term Goal	Strategies	Implementation	Evaluation
Subjective: "I can't even see my floors. There are books everywhere!" *Objective:* 20 piles of unwashed clothes and 2 sinks full of unwashed dishes	Alteration in home maintenance related to nursing school attendance as evidenced by unwashed dishes and clothes, unmade beds.	1. The house will have no dishes in the sinks by 2 p.m. Wednesday. 2. The house will have clean floors by 9 a.m. Thursday. *Long-Term Goal:* The house will remain clean and free of clutter.	1. The student will wash one load of clothes daily for 3 weeks. 2. The student will purchase necessary cleaning supplies. 3. The student will wash dishes daily. 4. The student will wash one floor area daily. 5. The student will develop a plan to limit clutter.	1. I washed one load of clothes yesterday and today. 2. I went to the store and bought cleaning supplies. 3. I washed all of the dishes today. 4. I washed the kitchen floor. 5. I wrote down the places in the house that tend to collect clutter.	Goal 1 met 100%: All dishes are clean. Goal 2 partially met: Only one floor is clean.

Figure 13–2. Home "patient" care plan.

A humorous "nursing" care plan that most students can relate to can be found in Figure 13–2. The "patient" is the home of a nursing student.

Care Plan Pitfalls

There can be several pitfalls in any nursing care plan. Examples include:

- Getting bogged down in the paperwork part of the nursing process rather than following a logical step-by-step process.
- Difficulty focusing on one diagnosis and tending to want to incorporate all they have learned about a patient in one care plan. It is better for students to simplify the process by focusing on just one diagnosis at a time.
- Losing focus and wandering off to other problems during the process. For example, a nursing diagnosis might be anxiety, but halfway through the care plan, the student will develop strategies that deal with alterations in diet or incontinence, which would be better served by a separate nursing care plan.

Case Management and Critical Pathways

Case management is a way of organizing patient care to achieve a set of identified patient outcomes within a specific time frame. The individual who is responsible for coordinating this care is the case manager. **Case managers** are often nurses, but other health care workers also carry out case management functions.

Responsibilities of a Case Manager

In addition to acute care settings, case managers and pathways are being used in such diverse settings as home health, outpatient, rehabilitation, and long-term care. A case manager's responsibilities include:

- Coordinating and planning patient care
- Collaborating with other health care team members
- Monitoring the patient's progress
- Ensuring continuity of care
- Monitoring appropriate use of resources
- Controlling costs while maintaining quality of care

The guiding tool in case management is the **critical pathway** (i.e., care maps, interdisciplinary [action] plans, anticipated recovery plans). Regardless of the terminology, these pathways outline an anticipated progression for a patient with a specific condition. The pathways are used most successfully for patient conditions that have relatively predictable outcomes (Figures 13–3 and 13–4). Each pathway will "establish the sequence and timing of interdisciplinary interventions, and incorporate education, discharge planning, assessment, consultations, nutrition, medications, activities, diagnostics, therapeutics, and treatments" (Beyea, 1996, p. 3).

Although publications are now available with pathways for many patient conditions, several institutions develop pathways that are reflective of their specific patient populations. Both sources of pathways tend to have the following four features (Burrell, Gerlach, & Pless, 1997):

Date of Birth: _____   Time of Birth: _____

	0-6 Hours	7-12 Hours	13-18 Hours
Laboratory/ Diagnostic Tests	☐ Coombs ☐ Maternal Hep B status		
Treatments/ Procedures	☐ Stabilization ☐ Baby ID ☐ Vital signs as per patient standard ☐ Weight = _____ gm ☐ Bath	☐ Circumcision permit ☐ Hep B permit	
Medications/IVs	☐ Triple dye to cord ☐ Vitamin K ☐ Erythromycin ointment to eyes	☐ HBIG if mother Hep B positive or status unknown ☐ Hep B vaccine	
Consultations			
Activity	☐ Radiant warmer until stable temp	☐ Open crib	☐ Open crib
Nutrition	☐ Breastfeeding/or Glucose H2O	☐ Breastfeeding per policy / care plan or formula at least q 4hrs	
Assessments	☐ Apgar at 1 and 5 minutes ☐ Gestational age ☐ Nursing assessment for VS, feeding, voiding, bonding	☐ I + O ☐ Nursing assessment for VS, feeding, voiding, bonding	☐ I + O ☐ Assess circumcision site
Education/ Discharge Planning	☐ See mother pathway		
Home Care			
Variances			
Order			
Reason			
Order			
Reason			

RN Signature: _____   _____   _____
                 _____   _____   _____
                 _____   _____   _____

Target discharge status = Feeding well _____
                           Maintaining temperature _____
                           Voiding & stooling adequately _____
                           Bonding _____

Figure 13–3. Vaginal delivery critical pathway: infant. *(From Allen, C. V. [1997]. Nursing process in collaborative practice: A problem-solving approach [2nd ed.]. Stamford, CT: Appleton & Lange. Used with permission.)*

Target LOS= 24-48 Hours

	19-24 Hours	Within 2 Hours of Discharge	Home 24-48 Hrs. Post Discharge
Laboratory/ Diagnostic Tests	◄---------- PKU and bilirubin at age 24 hours ----------► Coombs results Maternal RPR status at delivery		PKU, if initial PKU done before 24 hrs Bilirubin if > 5 at age 24 hours or if baby jaundiced by home health nurse; report results to by pediatrician
Treatments/ Procedures	Circumcision care if circumcision done		
Medications/IVs			
Consultations			
Activity	Open crib	Open crib	
Nutrition	Breast–feeding/or formula at least q 4hrs	Breast–feeding/or formula	
Assessments	Physician assessment of body systems Nursing assessment for VS, feeding, voiding, stooling, bonding		HHC nurse assessment of physical environment and baby, including VS, feeding, voiding, stooling, bonding, jaundice
Education/ Discharge Planning		Instructions to parents	
Home Care			
Variances			
Order			
Reason			
Order			
Reason			

Confirmed by pediatrician:

_____   _____
Signature   Date

Figure 13–3. *(Continued)*

1. They identify patient outcomes expected at various points along the pathway and at time of discharge.
2. The pathways have time lines and sequencing of interventions are indicated.
3. Pathways reflect interdisciplinary collaboration and intervention.
4. They track holistic aspects of care such as diagnostic test, nutrition, mobility, and patient education.

	Prenatal Record to L&D by 36 weeks	Labor, Delivery, Recovery	0-12 Hours
Laboratory/ Diagnostic Tests	H + H Type + Screen Rubella RPR HBSAG	CBC per order MS BOS per order RPR	H+H or CBC if ordered Determine Rhogam and Rubella status

Treatments/ Assessments		Receive medical record from MD's
		  office by 36 weeks
		Assessment, vital signs and EFM
		  per patient care standard
			Post partum assessment per
			  patient care standard
			Peri care
			Hygiene + comfort measures
			Anesthesia follow-up if indicated

Medications/IVs	Prenatal vitamins	Analgesia/Anesthesia per order Pitocin per order	IV discontinued Analgesics as needed for pain
Consultations	Social Work per guidelines		Lactation consult if breastfeeding Social Work PRN Pediatrician visit with mother ⋯▶
Activity		OOB unless contraindicated	OOB with assistance Shower Voiding without difficulty Rest
Nutrition	Appropriate weight gain	Clear liquids per order Ice	Regular diet

Education/ Discharge Planning	Childbirth preparation classes
	Parentcraft classes
	Breast–feeding class if BF
	Orient to discharge program tour
	Contraceptive planning
	Select pediatrician
	*Preparing for Your Baby's Birth
	  at Jefferson*
	"Baby Talk" video
		Comfort measures and
		  relaxation techniques
		Orient to EFM
		2nd stage pushing
		Initial breast–feeding instruction
		  if breast–feeding
		Breast–feeding
			Handwashing
			Orient to baby's crib
			Infant positioning, feeding,
			  changing

Home Care	Referral to home care		
Variances *Order* *Reason* *Order* *Reason* *Order* *Reason*			

Date of Birth: _____

RN Signature: _____   _____   _____
_____   _____   _____
_____   _____   _____

Target discharge status = Minimal vaginal bleeding _____
Demonstrates parenting skills _____
Minimal physical discomfort _____

Figure 13–4. Vaginal delivery critical pathway: mother. *From Allen, C. V. [1997]. Nursing process in collaborative practice: A problem-solving approach [2nd ed.]. Stamford, CT: Appleton & Lange. Used with permission.)*

However, regardless of which pathways are used (individual institution or a generic publication), some patients will not progress as anticipated. When this occurs, it is called a **variance.** Three reasons that a variance might occur are (Beyea, 1996):

1. **System variance.** In this case, the health care institution or community is unable to provide the needed care (e.g., the patient may need to travel 50 to 60 miles to have an MRI because the institution does not have one).

Target Post Delivery LOS = 24-48 Hours

Time of Birth: _____

	13-24 Hours	Within 2 hrs. of Discharge	Home
Laboratory/ Diagnostic Tests	☐ Rhogam if Rh negative and baby Rh positive ☐ RPR results ☐ Rubella if not immune		
Treatments/ Assessments	☐ Assess parenting skills ☐ Post partum assessment per patient care standard ☐ Peri care ☐ Hygiene + comfort measures ☐ Anesthesia follow-up if indicated		☐ Follow-up phone call at 3-5 days post discharge by maternity nurse to assess ☐ Assessment by HHC nurse
Medications/IVs	☐ Stool softener as ordered ☐ Analgesics as needed for pain		
Consultations	problem (per BF Care Plan and Supplementation Policy/Procedure) ┄┄┄┄┄┄┄┄┄➤		☐ Lactation consult if breast-feeding problem ☐ Social work consult if needed
Activity	☐ OOB with assistance ☐ Voiding without difficulty ☐ Rest	☐ Escort mother and baby to car	
Nutrition	☐ Regular diet	☐ Regular diet	
Education/ Discharge Planning	☐ Sitz bath ☐ Infant care class ☐ Discharge planning ☐ Infant safety ☐ S&S of dehydration and infection ☐ Circumcision care if baby circumcized ☐ Breast pump if needed	☐ Discharge instructions ☐ Gift pack ☐ Infant car seat requirement ☐ Smoke detector ☐ Follow-up appointments ☐ Educational needs summary	☐ Reinforce teaching of infant and self–care by HHC nurse
Home Care	☐ Notify home care of delivery	☐ Home care contact in hospital	☐ Scheduled home care visits 24-48 hours post discharge
Variances *Order* *Reason*	☐	☐	☐ Earlier home care if needed
Order *Reason*	☐		☐ 2nd home care visit if needed
Order *Reason*	☐	☐	

RN Signature: _____   _____   _____
   _____   _____   _____
   _____

Confirmed postdelivery by obstetrician:

Signature _____   Date _____

Source: Thomas Jefferson University Hospital; Women and Children Care; Philadelphia

Figure 13–4. *(Continued)*

2. **Provider/clinician variance.** In this case, the health care provider's actions affect the patient's outcomes (e.g., a nurse's poor handwashing practices leading to a nosocomial wound infection).

3. **Patient variance.** In this case, the patient factors affect outcomes (e.g., a patient may not be taking a prescribed medication).

The nursing process, clinical pathways, and case management that you are exposed to in the facility where you work may vary from what has been presented here. It is important to remember that as students, flexibility is key to your learning. You will most likely be exposed to many different interpretations of these three concepts. Be certain that you know what is expected of you in whatever facility you are in at any particular time. If you are in doubt, refer to the policy and procedure manual.

14

Critical Thinking

Critical Thinking

Critical thinking (CT) is a phrase that you will hear frequently. What does critical thinking mean? At present, there is little consensus as to the definition but because it is a central theme throughout nursing programs, it is essential that you have your faculty define and give examples of this concept for you.

Even though we do not know exactly how your faculty defines CT, let's explore highlights of the topic and see what you can expect. To start, you may want to know why this is such an important issue.

Why Critical Thinking Is So Important

There are three main reasons CT is so important:

- **It is required.** All programs that are accredited by the National League for Nursing Accrediting Commission (NLNAC) have to demonstrate that their graduates have CT skills.
- **CT is essential for successfully answering questions on the National Council Licensure Examination (NCLEX).** Passing this state exam results in obtaining your license.

- **Your success and survival as a practitioner will depend on your CT abilities.** Among other things, you will be required to keep your knowledge base current, make decisions in complex situations, evaluate nursing interventions and patient outcomes, and quickly identify priorities. The foundation for these activities is CT.

Now that you understand why CT is so important to your faculty, let's explore some specifics. The reason we said earlier that you must have your faculty define CT is that the NLNAC leaves the specific definition up to faculty in each nursing program. The NLNAC does indicate, however, that the definition should indicate how the faculty measures or evaluates your ability to reason, analyze, and make decisions.

Because any kind of thinking (daydreaming, reasoning, problem solving, etc.) cannot be observed directly, faculty will use various observable ways to evaluate your CT skills. One of the most frequently used evaluation tools is the nursing process or nursing care plan. How you complete nursing process assignments tells faculty a great deal about your CT skills. For example, your written care plans give insight into your CT ability in such areas as ability to identify and collect valid objective and subjective data, make logical conclusions based on data, and identify nursing interventions based on these conclusions. In other words, the nursing process is one form of CT that utilizes problem-solving abilities.

Consensus among faculty in many disciplines, however, is that CT involves more than problem solving. Let's look at a small sample of other expanded views of CT. Paul (1993) states CT involves the "intellectually disciplined process of actively and skillfully conceptualizing, applying, analyzing, synthesizing, or evaluating information gathered from, or generated by, observation, experience, reflection, reasoning, or communication, as a guide to belief and action" (p. 110). This definition probably requires that you reread it and devote some thought to grasp its full meaning. Table 14–1 contains additional information on characteristics of critical thinking and critical thinkers by four individuals that are considered experts in the field. Although Table 14–1 presents four separate views, do you see anything that the four views have in common? Notice that although critical thinking requires a knowledge base, the crucial part is how that knowledge is processed. Knowing facts is not enough; it is how you put those facts together that is important.

We can see from this very cursory overview that CT is a complex concept. You, no doubt, have some CT skills on which to build. How one expands this skill is not well established. One essential element in its development, however, is a sound knowledge base. Without this base, CT about a specific problem or situation is not possible. So, your CT skills will start with learning specific information. In early nursing courses, faculty will have exercises and exams that only require that you recall the knowledge. However, faculty will expect you to demonstrate your knowledge base in clinical situations, written assignments,

---

Table 14–1. Four Perspectives on Critical Thinking

Characteristics of a Critical Thinker[a]
- Being open to views that are new and to different viewpoints.
- Being able to express and present ideas in an organized manner.
- Having evidence and logical reasoning to support ideas and views.
- Listening to others but thinking for one's self.

View of a Critical Thinker[b]
- Separates relevant from irrelevant information.
- Spots inconsistencies in a line of reasoning.
- Identifies and challenges assumptions.
- Separates verifiable facts from value claims.
- Identifies doubtful or unclear claims and arguments.

Characteristics of a Critical Thinker[c]
- Recognizes and challenges statements or ideas accepted as true without supporting data (these unchallenged ideas are assumptions).
- Identifies and explores as many alternatives as possible when analyzing a situation.
- Utilizes logical reasoning skills.

Questions a Critical Thinker Asks[d]
- What is the purpose of my thinking?
- How well am I articulating the question I am trying to answer?
- What is my frame of reference?
- What am I taking for granted (what assumption am I making)?
- Once I have come to a conclusion, what are the implications?

[a] *From Chaffee, J. (1985).* Thinking critically. *Boston: Houghton Mifflin.*
[b] *From Beyer, B. K. (1987).* Practical strategies for the teaching of thinking. *Boston: Allyn & Bacon.*
[c] *From Brookfield, S. D. (1987).* Developing critical thinkers: Challenging adults to explore alternative ways of thinking and acting. *San Francisco: Jossey-Bass.*
[d] *From Paul, R. W. (1993).* Critical thinking: How to prepare your students for a rapidly changing role. *Santa Rosa, CA: Center for Critical Thinking.*

---

class discussions, and exams in more complex ways. For example, faculty in maternity nursing could have a multiple-choice question on the age at which the anterior fontanel normally closes. Such a question, however, only provides an indication of your ability to recall the information. A question aimed at evaluating your critical thinking skills would be far different. For example, faculty could provide you with the following data.

You are assessing a 25-month-old child. On assessment, you find a smiling child with a soft spot in the area of the anterior fontanel. Based on this information, faculty might:

- **Ask you to describe (written or oral) your actions in order of priority with your reason for each action.** Your responses provide faculty not only with information on your knowledge regarding the anterior fontanel, but also with information such as your ability to prioritize and your written or oral communication skills.
- **Provide you with multiple-choice options in which you have to pick the best action.** This means that all of the answers are correct but one response is better than the others for various valid reasons. This type of question requires that you know the significance of an open anterior fontanel and the normal age for closure of the anterior fontanel, and can discriminate between the options and identify the one action that has priority.

This type of question is the type that you as a student may not like. You may feel that it is unfair since all the responses are essentially correct. However, the focus of this type of question is reflective of CT. Be prepared for this type of question in school and on the NCLEX.

Here is another example.

You are a school nurse. It is January and the weather has been cold. On Thursday, one of the 11th grade girls comes to your office. She states that she has been feeling sick to her stomach in the mornings, with dizziness and headaches. By the time her second class is over she feels better. She asks you to help her over this morning sickness since it is interfering with her early classes.

Based on this information, faculty may ask you to describe your actions. The depth of your response will help faculty evaluate how well you are able to use your knowledge base. Early in your studies you may only be expected to ask this student about her menstrual cycles. If this situation were presented in your last nursing class, however, faculty would expect much more, such as:

- In addition to the student's complaints, are you concerned with any other data in the situation? If so what and why?
- Are you curious why the symptoms seem to clear during her second class?
- Do you display in any of your responses consideration of ethical and legal issues associated with the role of a school nurse?

In place of a written or verbal response to this situation, faculty might instead have the following item on a test.

It is January and the weather is cold. A student comes to the school nurse with complaints of feeling sick to her stomach, dizziness, and headaches that lasts about halfway through her second class. She has had these symptoms for several days now. In addition to assessments regarding this student's menstrual cycle, what information is essential for the nurse to obtain at this time?

a. overall nutrition status
*b. health of family members
c. vital signs
d. date of last menstrual cycle

The answer is (b), for the following reason. Although the student's complaints are often signs of early pregnancy, they are also manifestations of carbon monoxide poisoning. (Note the major piece of information about the weather.) If this family has gas heat and if other family members have similar complaints, there may be a leak in the heating system. Responses (a) and (c) may be part of the assessment but there are no data to indicate that they are essential at this time. Response (d) is included in the stem of the question.

Note that in both the version in which you are asked to describe your actions with rationale and in the test item, you are pulling together information from more than one source or data bank. This is typical of critical thinking. Remember that if you can go to a page in a text and find the answer, it is not CT; it is basic recall of information.

Thus, CT is gaining prominence in schools of nursing as an essential skill for today's graduate. The amount of formal class time and content devoted to the topic is currently limited. You might want to expand your mind on the topic by reading some of the sources listed at the end of this chapter.

Books and Articles to Consider Adding to Your Personal Library

Kennison, M., & Brace, J. (1997). Digging deeper for creative solutions. *Nursing 97, 27*(9), 52–54.

Metheny, N. (1997). Focusing on the dangers of D_5W. *Nursing 97, 27*(10), 55–59.

Sloane, P. (1994). *Test your lateral thinking IQ.* New York: Sterling Publishing.

VonOech, R. (1990). *A whack on the side of the head.* New York: Warner Books.

Wilkinson, J. M. (2001). *Nursing process and critical thinking* (3rd ed.). Upper Saddle River, NJ: Prentice Hall Health.

15

Stress

Living with Stress

All human beings experience stress. Without stress we wouldn't be alive! Unfortunately, most of us experience more stress than we need! The growth of technology has changed our lives forever. Many of us rely on cellular phones, pagers, and faxes to keep in touch with our place of work. Some of us maintain 24-hour contact with our jobs. Stress has contributed to the development of many of the diseases experienced in our society. Some of the major diseases that have been linked to stress are asthma, coronary artery disease, hypertension, strokes, tension headaches, backaches, irritable bowel syndrome, colitis, arthritis, and diabetes.

To deal with stress we use ego-defense mechanisms. Our defense mechanisms help us to defend against threats to our psychological well-being. Coping behaviors (one of which is the use of defense mechanisms) help us to adapt to stressors. Over time, we tend to use those defense mechanisms and coping behaviors that have worked for us in the past. This continued use of the same defense mechanisms and coping behaviors develops into a habitual pattern. There are a number of ways of coping with stress. Various mental strategies to handle stress are listed in Table 15–1. Some coping behaviors are positive, others are negative.

For example, starting nursing school is a stressful event for most students. Student A copes by trying to get as much information as possible about each class, organizing a calendar, and thinking positively. Student B copes by drinking heavily on weekends and complaining about the amount of work expected

TABLE 15–1. Various Thought Strategies to Handle Stress and Their Rationale

Mental Response	Definition and Rationale
Use of knowledge	Learn causes of stress and ways to prevent or manage situation. Know personal limits. If problem is beyond your control and cannot be changed now, accept the situation until it can be changed.
Objectivity (reality orientation)	Sort out, compare, and validate events, ideas, and emotions to gain a total perspective and better understanding on basis of facts, not just feelings; maintain realistic perception.
Analysis	Study logically and systematically the component parts of a situation to arrive at realistic explanations and answers; manage part if not all of situation.
Concentration (mental self-control)	Deliberately set aside thoughts and feelings unrelated to the situation to master tension, save energy, find answers, and make necessary decisions for the task at hand.
Planning	Think through situation before acting to release tension, promote problem solving, and avoid unnecessary use of energy, error, and consequent frustration. Avoid too many deadlines. Decide on what drudgery chore you want to complete and do it as quickly as possible so it does not become a focus. Make a list of tasks and check off as they are accomplished.
Reconstruction	Review recent stressful event, writing ways it could have been better and ways it could have been worse. Write what could have been done to make it better, thus improving sense of challenge and control.
Fantasize (daydream)	Visualize release of tension and successful achievement rather than dwelling on fear of failure to plan strategy, ensure goal-directed action, cope with stressors, and relieve tension.

TABLE 15–1. Varous Thought Strategies to Handle Stress and Their Rationale (Continued)	
Mental Response	**Definition and Rationale**
Rehearsal	Fantasize or anticipate event or another's response before stressful event to practice coping mentally or behaviorally and to gain confidence in ability to manage.
Substitution of thoughts and emotions	State ideas and feelings that are different than real ones to avoid adding to stressful situation or to meet demands of the situation. Focus on one good thing that happened during the day.
Suppression	Hold thoughts and emotions in abeyance or momentarily forget to wait until it is more timely to change behavior, attack a problem, or implement a solution. Deliberately push all stress-producing thoughts aside for 60 seconds.
Valuing	Establish or reaffirm religious or sociocultural values to foster sense of balance and relaxation in face of stressors. Value and believe in yourself. Take an hour each day for yourself.
Empathy	Imagine how others in the situation are feeling so that behavior can take these feelings into account.
Humor	Point out inconsistencies in situation, laugh at self, and use past feelings, ideas, and behavior to be playful, keep objective distance from a problem, reduce anxiety, maintain self-identity, enrich solution, and add enjoyment to life.
Tolerance of ambiguity	Function in a way that lays the basis for eventual effective solutions when the situation is so complex that it cannot be fully understood or clear choices cannot be made now.

Source: Murray, R. B., Zentner, J. P. (1997). Health assessment & promotion strategies through the life span *(6th ed., p. 841). Reprinted by permission of Pearson Education, Inc. Upper Saddle River, NJ 07458.*

to anyone who will listen. Student A is attempting to problem solve, which is positive. Student B is reducing tension, which is not as healthy. Both students are coping with stress, although Student A is coping more positively.

Sample Coping Mechanisms

- Overuse of alcohol and drugs
- Overeating
- Humor
- Swearing
- Crying
- Self-pity
- Exercising
- Sharing with others
- Smoking

Some of us tend to deal with stress better than others. It is possible for an individual to develop stress resistance (an increased ability to tolerate stress) (Figure 15–1). Some of the things that help to increase our resistance to stress are under our control and others are not. For example, we can alter our lifestyle, but we cannot alter our genetic structure. Genetics may make us

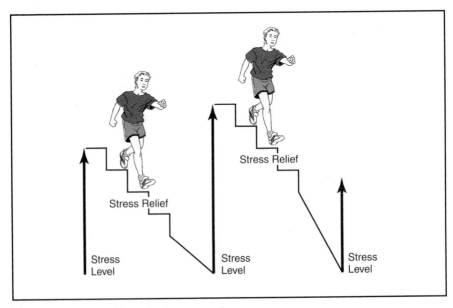

Figure 15–1. It is possible to develop stress resistance.

more vulnerable to stress. For example, if we are born with a heart valve defect, the defect cannot be altered to increase our stress resistance. If, on the other hand, we smoke, we can increase stress resistance by stopping smoking.

Factors That Increase Stress Resistance

1. Healthy lifestyle
   - Balanced diet
   - Regular exercise
   - Regular sleep
   - Avoidance of alcohol
   - Avoidance of tobacco and drugs
   - Keeping a routine of balanced activities
2. Sense of humor
   - Laughing at ourselves and others
   - Not taking life too seriously
3. Self-confidence
   - Feeling good about ourselves
   - Feeling good about our abilities
   - Feeling good about our relationships with others
4. Safety and security
   - Feeling safe at home and in our communities
5. Adequate social and material resources
   - Having enough money, food, shelter, clothing
   - Having help from others

(Berger & Williams, 1999)

Stress Management

Obviously, we can learn to increase our stress resistance by focusing on those areas that we can control such as lifestyle, sense of humor, safety and security, self-confidence, and adequate social and material resources. We can do this for ourselves and for patients.

STEPS TO STRESS MANAGEMENT

Unfortunately, we do not always have control over the stressful events in our lives, but we do have control over how we respond to them. Focusing on the benefits of an experience is not always easy, but it can be done, it just takes practice!

1. **Assess major life stressors.** There are a number of instruments that are available to measure stress. Most facilities have at least one instrument to measure stress, or you can find one in most psychiatric nursing textbooks.

2. **Help the patient understand the physical and psychological manifestations of stress.**
   - Increased heart rate
   - Increased blood pressure
   - Increased glucose
   - Hyperventilation
   - Delayed healing
   - Increased hostility
   - Increased sadness
   - Increased reliance on alcohol or drugs
3. **Determine if the patient has adequate support systems and how the patient usually copes with stressful situations.**
   - Help patients to focus on a balance in daily activities including diet, exercise, and rest (Figure 15–2).
   - Help patients to reframe negative thoughts about stress to positive ones.

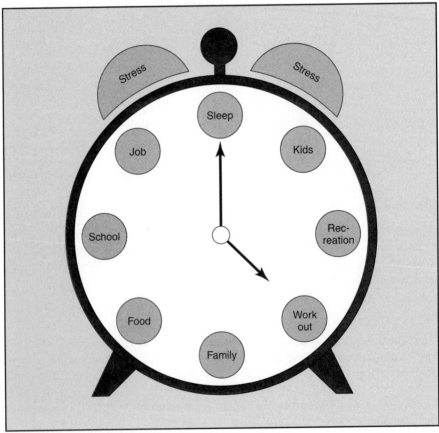

Figure 15–2. Help your patient learn how to balance daily activities.

Being admitted for alcohol treatment can be perceived as embarrassing, horrible, financially draining, and devastating. But, it could also be perceived as a second chance, a way to improve life, and make things right with family and friends. The second of these perceptions is much more positive than the first, and will be perceived as less threatening to the psychological well-being of the patient.

Nursing and Stress

Nurses are often much better at giving patients information to follow than following it themselves. How many times have you seen an obese health care provider telling an obese patient that the patient needs to lose weight? How many times have you stressed the need for a good diet to a patient and headed for the vending machine on your next break?

Nursing tends to be a very stressful profession, and nurses need to heed their own advice. A lot of times, nurses are working under conditions that produce stress including shift work, long hours, inadequate staffing, and dealing with people who are needy and suffering. The fact that we confront death and disease on a daily basis tends to threaten our sense of safety and security. Some patients will die; hence, we must confront the fact that we will die too. Nurses are accountable for their patients' lives and for vast amounts of technological information. After paperwork and other responsibilities, many nurses are dissatisfied with the amount of quality time that is left to spend with patients. New graduates also experience reality shock as they make the transition from school to work.

Burnout Hints

You have probably already heard the term *burnout*. Burnout occurs frequently in the nursing profession.

- It is easier to recognize burnout in others than it is to recognize it in oneself.
- Burned-out nurses are apathetic and uncaring and may also experience a number of stress-related symptoms.
- Burnout, once recognized, can be reversed with time and stress-reduction techniques.

Some nurses find that a change in job is beneficial. Perhaps a move from an intensive care unit to a clinic or home health agency might help. Nurses are lucky that there is such diversity in the profession. There are any number of job possibilities and most of us can find a place where we can be happy and where burnout is less likely. If you find yourself in a job where you are not happy, keep looking! Sooner or later, you will find a job that is right for you.

Some Ways for Nurses to Beat Stress

1. **Live in the moment!**
   - Most of us try to do five things at once and feel stressed as a result.
   - Concentrating on one thing can help decrease anxious feelings.
2. **Balance your life!**
   - Give some of you to work, some of you to your personal life, and some of you to your spiritual life.
   - This does not mean 80% work, 10% family, and 10% spiritual, it means balanced.
3. **Don't sweat the small stuff!**
   - Does it really matter if there are no tickets available to the movie that you want to see? Could you see a different one? Could you go see it next week? Does it really matter if the copier ran out of paper? Does it really matter that your co-worker has to leave 10 minutes early? Does it really matter that you have to wait in line 5 minutes at the grocery store?
   - Think about the long-term scheme of things.
   - These minor hassles can cause major stress if you let them.
   - Learn which things are of value to you—focus on those and forget the rest.
4. **Focus on things that are important to you!**
   - The things that are important are your health, family, friends, work, and home.
   - Avoid the things that are not important.
5. **Try meditation!**
   - Meditation can help you relax and feel ready to face the world again.
   - It does not have to last 30 minutes or an hour to be helpful.
   - Ten minutes of controlled breathing are enough to slow your pulse rate, your breathing, and even lower your blood pressure.
   - Meditation can also help clear your mind of thoughts and worries.
6. **Keep a journal!**
   - Write down the things that bother you—get it all out—even if you have to burn it when you're finished.
7. **Laugh!**
   - Laughter can reduce stress, so take time to see that new comedy.
   - Find a funny friend, call the joke hotline, or do whatever you need to do to have a chuckle.

Nursing Students and Stress

Nursing students are often under a great deal of stress. Stressors that are common to students can be the result of outside stressors (family, friends, finances, etc.) or school stressors (grades, coursework, clinical, faculty, etc.).

Family

Family stressors can be the result of poor planning, or they can be unexpected. Nursing school is extremely demanding and families need to be prepared for what is ahead (Figure 15–1). Spouses need to realize that the student will be gone (at odd hours) for long periods of time. They need to know that studying is a priority and that things like laundry are not. You will need to keep channels of communication open and be flexible, so will your spouse! Talk things out and take time for each other. The divorce rate among student nurses and graduates is high. If your marriage was good prior to school, it will most likely survive. If you and your spouse were having problems, they will most likely intensify. Seek help early! We have seen some students lose a marriage and flunk out in the same semester.

Children also need to know that school is demanding. Young children often feel abandoned when a parent is in nursing school. When not at school the parent is usually busy studying or trying to fit too much into too little time. Remember that your children will be there long after you finish nursing school. They are more important than school and they need you to keep that in perspective. Sure you are trying to provide them with a better life, but if they do not feel loved, they will resent the time that school requires. Do fun things with your children. Be there when they need you. Help them to understand when school takes priority.

Friends

Your friends will either lend their support or complain that you no longer have time for them. You will need the supportive ones. Set aside times for your friends. You are not entering a monastery or being confined to jail. There is a life outside of nursing school and you need to cultivate it to decrease your stress.

Finances

All colleges offer financial assistance through grants, scholarships, and loans. If you need financial assistance, find the financial aid office and go there. You are not seeking a handout. Colleges are required to give a certain amount of financial aid each year. If you don't ask for it, someone else will get it anyway. Talk to your department head or faculty. Ask questions! For your own good, go check it out.

Grades

School stressors are discussed in Chapter 1. One stressor that seems to stand out above all others is grades. Not everyone in class will get all A's. Some students are not satisfied unless they get an A; not making an A will become a significant source of stress for these students. We have had students fall apart because they got a 95% grade on an exam. We have had students who wanted to rewrite a paper because they only received a 97%. You are not your grade. Whether you make a C or an A, you will still graduate and receive the same diploma. If settling for a lower grade means that your marriage might survive nursing school and that your kids will remember who you are, it is worth it to give up the A. Would you rather be a nurse with straight-A grades or one who has a life? Some students can have both, but most have to give up one or the other. Which one is worth more to you?

Stress is something that we all have to deal with. It is important to control and decrease our stress levels whenever possible. Nursing and nursing school are both very stressful. Learning how to control your stress is essential to your livelihood. Controlling stress will also help you and your family lead a healthier and happier life.

16

Pain

Pain

Pain is a phenomenon that you will encounter in almost all clinical environments, and is one of the most studied human experiences. Even if as a graduate you manage to work in a setting with healthy individuals who have no pain episodes, you will be exposed to pain away from work: pain experienced by yourself, by relatives, and by friends. Perhaps it is because pain is such an omnipresent occurrence that providing effective interventions is often a great nursing challenge. Starting in 2001, the JCAHO (Joint Commission on Accreditation of Healthcare Organizations) will have documentation of pain assessment as a required standard. Pain is now being considered the "fifth vital sign."

The consequences of unrelieved pain are many. Some of the common ones are rather obvious, such as irritability, restlessness, and anorexia. At the opposite end of the continuum is suicide. And the fear of uncontrollable pain is one of the major factors in the current national debate on physician-assisted suicide and euthanasia (see Chapter 23).

Pain can be analyzed from many perspectives, including duration (acute or chronic), location, etiology, and severity. Pain is often the single most common symptom that causes a patient to seek help. In one respect, nature is kind to us in relation to pain. At the time the pain is experienced, we are miserable. However, after the pain is gone, we remember only how miserable we were. Although the remembering may be distressing for some individuals, the actual pain itself is not reexperienced. Pain is also the one human sensation for which there is such a wide variety of vastly different intervention techniques for relief.

Three Basic Components of Pain

1. **Reception at the site of origin to the brain.** Nociceptors are the nerve fibers that carry the pain impulse to the spinal column. You can expect to see this term in all current literature and research on pain.
2. **Perception of the pain.** This occurs at two levels:
   - Physiological perception: Brain reception and interpretation of the pain impulse (dull, sharp, aching, etc.)
   - Psychological perception: The individual's mental interpretation of the pain based on such factors as past experiences with pain, current situation, anxiety, culture, gender, and age
3. **Response to the pain perception.** This also has two basic levels:
   - Physiologic response: Changes in body physiology such as pulse rate, concentration, and blood pressure
   - Behavioral response: The objective indicators of the pain including pacing, gritting the teeth, crying, irritability, groaning, inability to keep still, and distorted facial expressions

This list of objective indicators could be very lengthy because these behavioral responses will be individual and influenced by the psychological factors at the perception level. The list can also be very short because there are individuals who present very few objective indicators of pain.

Three Types of Pain Assessment

When dealing with patients who are experiencing pain, the first nursing action is to assess the pain.

1. Determine the pain's etiology.
   - Where is the pain?
   - When did it start?
   - What is it like?
   - Does anything make it better? Worse?
     On the surface, this may sound rather silly. After all, if a patient just had surgery, we expect him or her to have pain. Many a nurse, however, making such an assumption, has medicated a patient only to discover later that the pain was not related to the surgery. The patient, in fact, was developing a pulmonary emboli or having cardiac pain and, therefore, proper medical intervention was delayed.
2. Determine the severity of the pain experienced.
   - There are a number of pain assessment tools useful with adults and a few for young children. One of the more common tools used with adults is a

numerical rating scale based on zero (no pain) to 10 (maximum or severe pain). In addition to the various pain assessment tools that focus on pain intensity, a nurse, Fannie Gaston-Johansson, has developed a pain assessment tool called the "Painometer." This assessment tool assesses pain on four dimensions: intensity, quality, location, and duration. This tool is being used in major cancer centers in the United States and is widely used in hospitals and clinics throughout Sweden.

- A common scale for children is the Wong–Baker Faces Rating Scale (Figure 16–1). This scale is sometimes used with hearing-impaired patients or non–English-speaking patients. However, more research needs to be conducted on its validity in these groups.

The key to using any pain assessment tool is consistency. All individuals working with the patient should use the same pain-rating system. This helps to create uniformity in assessment and documentation of pain and the effectiveness of intervention. In actuality, as your nursing skills become more proficient, you will be blending these first two assessments of etiology and severity into one.

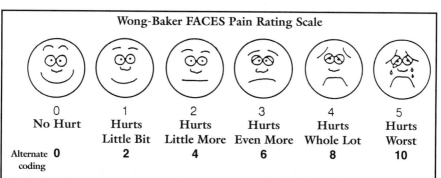

Wong-Baker FACES Pain Rating Scale

0	1	2	3	4	5
No Hurt	Hurts Little Bit	Hurts Little More	Hurts Even More	Hurts Whole Lot	Hurts Worst

Alternate coding:

0	2	4	6	8	10

Explain to the patient that each face is for a person who feels happy because he has no pain (hurt) or sad because has some or a lot of pain. Face 0 is very happy because he doesn't hurt at all. Face 1 hurts just a little bit. Face 2 hurts a little more. Face 3 hurts even more. Face 4 hurts a whole lot. Face 5 hurts as much as you can imagine, although you do not have to be crying to feel this bad. Ask the person to choose the face that best describes how he is feeling.

Rating scale is recommended for persons age 3 years and older.

Brief word instructions: Point to each face using the words to describe the pain intensity. Ask the child to choose face that best describes own pain and record the appropriate number

Figure 16–1. The Wong–Baker Faces rating scale. (*From Wong, D.L., Hockenberry-Eaton, M, Wilson, D, Winkelstein, ML, & Schwartz, P [2001]. Wong's essentials of pediatric nursing [6th ed., p. 1301]. St. Louis. Copyrighted by Mosby, Inc. Reprinted with permission.*)

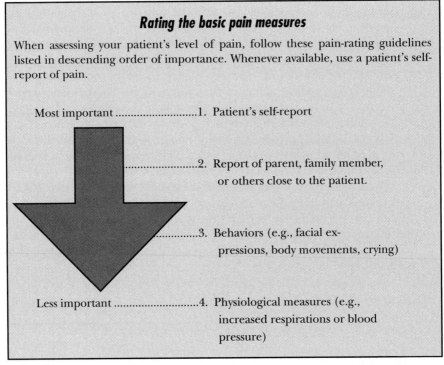

Rating the basic pain measures

When assessing your patient's level of pain, follow these pain-rating guidelines listed in descending order of importance. Whenever available, use a patient's self-report of pain.

Most important ....1. Patient's self-report

.......................2. Report of parent, family member, or others close to the patient.

...............3. Behaviors (e.g., facial expressions, body movements, crying)

Less important ....4. Physiological measures (e.g., increased respirations or blood pressure)

Figure 16–2. Pain-rating guidelines. *(From McCattery, M. Pain management handbook.* Nursing *97, 27 [4]: 42–45. Used with permission.)*

3. Determine the intervention's (e.g., medications, massage, distraction) effectiveness.
- This is done approximately 30 minutes after the intervention.
- One of the most common indicators of effectiveness is again a pain-rating scale.
- The scale used in the first assessment should be used to evaluate effectiveness. Figure 16–2 presents, in descending order of importance, pain-rating guidelines, which apply at all stages of pain management.

Up to this point, we have been considering pain in children and in adults. For many years, it was believed that neonates did not experience pain. Currently, however, there is almost complete agreement by health care providers that neonates do experience the sensation of pain. The belief is that any event that would cause pain in a child, would also cause pain in a newborn. To date, however, there is no valid assessment for pain in neonates.

One possible tool, however, is the Neonate Infant Pain Scale (NIPS) as illustrated in Table 16–1. Note that the scale requires a baseline assessment that includes several variables prior to a painful intervention. So far, little is known regarding the strengths and weaknesses of the scale and its use has been lim-

Table 16–1. Neonatal Infant Pain Scale (NIPS)

Facial Expression

0 = Relaxed muscles	• Restful face with neutral expression
1 = Grimace	• Tight facial muscles, furrowed brow, chin, and jaw (*Note:* At low gestational ages, infants may have no facial expression)

Cry

0 = No cry	• Quiet, not crying
1 = Whimper	• Mild moaning, intermittent
2 = Vigorous cry	• Loud screaming, rising, shrill, and continuous. (*Note:* Silent cry may be scored if the infant is intubated, as indicated by obvious mouth or facial movements)

Breathing Patterns

0 = Relaxed	• Usual breathing pattern is maintained
1 = Change in breathing	• Indrawing (retraction of chest), irregular, faster than usual, gagging, or holding breath

Arm Movements

0 = Relaxed/restrained (with soft restraints)	• No muscle rigidity, occasional random movements (not fighting the restraints)
1 = Flexed/extended	• Tense, straightened arms; rigidity; or rapid extension and flexion

Leg Movements

0 = Relaxed/restrained (with soft restraints)	• No muscle rigidity, occasional random movements (not fighting the restraints)
1 = Flexed/extended	• Tense, straightened legs; rigidity; or rapid extension and flexion

State of Arousal

0 = Sleeping/awake	• Quiet, peacefully sleeping; or alert and settled
1 = Fussy	• Alert and restless or thrashing

Adapted with permission from the Children's Hospital of Eastern Ontario.

ited to responses to heel sticks in infants over 28 weeks of gestation. However, further research by nurses and others will hopefully create a valid and reliable neonate pain assessment tool.

There are many phrases associated with pain. Two that send up a red flag are, "This patient has a low pain threshold," and its opposite, "This patient has a high pain threshold." Pain research has not identified what a *pain threshold* is; it is not a measurable concept. However, these terms, and others like them, are heard in health care settings with regularity. The first phrase is basically a euphemism for "This patient sure asks for pain medication a lot; he or she is probably addicted." This is a red flag that the health care team does not have the latest information about pain management.

When a patient has what is commonly considered a painful condition and the opposite phrase, "This patient sure has a high pain threshold," is used, the second red flag goes up. Not seeing any of the anticipated behavioral pain indicators, the physician and/or nurse jump to the conclusion that

Table 16–2. Common Nonpharmacological Interventions

- External TENS units
- Distraction
- Relaxation
- Imagery
- Biofeedback
- Acupuncture
- Hypnosis
- Behavior modification
- Meditation

Table 16–3. Pharmacological Pain Interventions

- Nonopioids
  Acetaminophen
  Salicylates
  NSAIDs (nonsteroidal anti-inflammatory drugs)
  Supportive
    Anti-anxiety
    Antidepressants
    Corticosteroids
- Opioids

Table 16–4. Surgical Interventions

- Nerve blocks
- Percutaneous cordotomy
- Commissural myelotomy hypophysectomy
- Spinal cord stimulation (implanted TENS units)

Most surgical interventions occur after pharmacological and nonpharmacological techniques have not provided adequate pain control.

the patient experiences less pain than the "average" individual in a similar situation. In actuality, it is much more likely that this patient is experiencing pain but has had a poor pain assessment by the nurse and physician.

Unlike many other human experiences, there are a great variety of interventions for pain relief. These interventions can be placed into three main categories: nonpharmacological (Table 16–2), pharmacological (Table 16–3), and surgical (Table 16–4). Each table contains only the most common interventions for each category. Note that the interventions in Table 16–4 are generally used after the nonsurgical methods have been tried and have not been successful. Also be aware that the trancutaneous electrical nerve stimulation (TENS) intervention can be implanted, a surgical intervention, or worn externally as a nonpharmacological intervention (Table 16–2). Just from personal experience you no doubt realize that the current interventions used most often for pain control are in the pharmacological category (Table 16–3). However, the use of interventions in the nonpharmacological areas are becoming more popular. And, some individuals with complex pain problems may be treated with a combination of all three techniques.

Pain medications are one of the major tools used with individuals who have pain associated with cancer. It is not unusual for these individuals to need frequent adjustment in their medication. Over time, their narcotic medication will be changed to another route of administration for the same medication, a different pain medication, or a different combination of medications. When the medication is changed from one route of administration to another, a calculation is required to obtain the correct dosage.

Here is an example. (Note that *breakthrough pain* is severe pain that occurs between the regular doses of an opioid.)

A patient has been on Dilaudid (hydromorphone), 16 mg (PO) every 4 hours, plus 3 breakthrough doses of 8 mg each in a 24-hour period. The physician is switching the patient to morphine via continuous intravenous administration. The order reads: "Change to IV morphine at 21 mg per hour IV." Is this correct?

1. Determine current use of PO Dilaudid per 24 hours.

$$\frac{24 \text{ (hours)}}{4 \text{ (frequency of dosing)}} = 6 \text{ regular doses of Dilaudid/24 h}$$

6 (regular doses) × 16 (mg/dose) = 96 mg of Dilaudid/24 h

3 (breakthrough doses) × 8 (mg/dose) = 24 mg Dilaudid

The patient receives 120 mg of Dilaudid in 24 hours.

2. Multiply the current dose by its conversion factor for the 24-hour dose. For Dilaudid the conversion factor to parenteral morphine is 6.7 (Table 16–5).

Table 16–5. Drug-to-Drug Conversion Guide[a]

Oral Conversion		Parenteral Conversion	
To Morphine From	**Conversion Factor**	**To Morphine From**	**Conversion Factor**
Methadone	1.5	Methadone	1
Hydromorphone	4	Hydromorphone	6.7
Meperidine	0.1	Meperidine	0.13
Levorphanol	7.5	Levorphanol	5
Codeine	0.15	Codeine	0.08
Oxycodone	1		

[a] Directions to convert from another narcotic to morphine.
1. Determine the amount of analgesic it takes in a 24-hour period to effectively control the patient's pain.
2. Multiply the 24-hour total by the conversion factor shown in the table.
3. Because there is often incomplete cross-tolerance from one opioid to another, a lower dose than that calculated may be needed to maintain efficacy. To account for this, divide the above result by 2 to arrive at a *starting* dose. *Note:* There is great individual variability here. Monitor the effect and be prepared to titrate the dose during the first 24 hours.
4. Divide the calculated 24-hour dose by the appropriate number of doses per day (e.g., six doses for regular [immediate release] oral morphine at 4-hour intervals or two doses for controlled-release morphine at 12-hour intervals).

Example: Mrs. Brown has been getting good pain control with hydromorphone by taking two 4-mg tablets orally every 3 hours. However, she complains about having to wake up several times during the night to take the medicine and keep her pain under control. The doctor decides to change to controlled-release morphine to simplify the program and allow for longer periods of sleep. To determine the appropriate equivalent dose of morphine, the following calculations are made:
1. 8 mg (two 4-mg tablets) × 8 doses per 24 hours = 64 mg
2. 64 mg × 4 (conversion factor) = 256 mg morphine
3. 256 mg divided by 2 (to allow for incomplete cross-tolerance) = 128 mg every 24 hours
4. 128 mg divided into 2 doses = 64 mg every 12 hours (The closest tablet size is 60 mg.)
5. Provide morphine sulfate 10–15 mg prn to titrate or treat breakthrough pain

Source: Thorpe, D. M. Pain. In Burrell, L., Gerlach, M., & Pless, B. (1997). Adult nursing: Acute and community care. (2nd ed.). Reprinted by permission of Pearson Education, Upper Saddle River, NJ 07458.

$$120 \text{ mg} \times 6.7 = 804$$

$$804 \div 2 = 402 \text{ mg of IV morphine per 24 hours or}$$
$$16.76 \text{ mg per hour}$$

The patient should, therefore, receive 16.75 mg of IV morphine per hour.

The nurse should check with the physician before proceeding with the ordered change from PO Dilaudid to IV morphine. The 21 mg per hour rate exceeds the calculated conversion rate.

Another conversion concerns changing from one narcotic to another. This conversion also requires calculation. Table 16–5 provides information needed to make such conversions and gives a typical example.

Three Concepts Associated with Pain

Three concepts that are central to pain control are addiction, drug tolerance, and physical dependence. Understanding the meaning of each provides a strong cornerstone for adequate pain control.

1. Addiction
   - A psychological dependence on a drug in the opioid group.
   - The drug is sought out at all costs by the individual only for its emotional and psychological effects.
   - The drug is not used for pain relief.
2. Drug tolerance
   - The body's physiological adjustment to an opioid so that greater amounts of the drug are required to produce the desired physiological response. (*Note:* Tolerance can also occur with nonopioid drugs.)
   - Tolerance occurs rather quickly with opioids.
   - Fearing the possibility of creating an addict, the physician seldom increases the dose. The rationale generally goes along the line of "After all, the patient is receiving the recommended dose."
   - For individuals with chronic, severe pain of any etiology, the markers for medication dose should be the patient's response—is the pain at a tolerable level and are adverse reactions acceptable—not the dose.
3. Physical dependence
   - The body's physiological adjustment to a drug that results in withdrawal symptoms if the drug is not received at regular intervals.
   - The time for physical dependency to develop varies.
   - It is not uncommon for it to occur in as little time as 1 week.
   - Dependency can develop for drugs other than opioids.

Addiction, drug tolerance, and physical dependency are terms associated with opioid use. Although often lumped together as if they were one, they are three distinct body responses. Note that most individuals who are on opioids for intractable, chronic pain will develop both a drug tolerance and physical dependency. Research has shown, however, that less than 1% will become addicted. (It is not unusual for individuals with cancer to develop tolerance and, over time, to require as much as 8,000 mg of morphine—or more—every 24 hours to achieve pain relief that was originally obtained at 60 mg every 24 hours. The 8,000 mg is not a misprint.) This individual also has a physical dependency and will experience withdrawal symptoms if their medication is suddenly stopped. However, this individual is not addicted or considered a junkie. The extremely high dose is required for adequate pain relief.

It is confusion over these physical responses and the fear of creating an addict that leads to patients being undermedicated for pain. In addition, in many states, physicians who have prescribed long-term use of opioids for individuals with chronic, intractable pain have found themselves before their state medical board facing disciplinary action. As research sheds more light on pain and treatment options, as medical and nursing schools include pain control in the curriculums, and as practitioners who have been in the field for a number of years become aware of pain treatment advances, undermedication of those in pain will hopefully decrease.

Table 16–6. Pain Patient's Bill of Rights

You have the right to:

- Have your pain prevented or controlled adequately.
- Have your pain and pain medication history taken.
- Have your pain questions answered freely.
- Develop a pain plan with your doctor.
- Know what medication, treatment, or anesthesia will be given.
- Know the risks, benefits, and side effects of treatment.
- Know what alternative pain treatments may be available.
- Sign a statement of informed consent before any treatment.
- Be believed when you say you have pain.
- Have your pain assessed on an individual basis.
- Have your pain assessed using the 0 = no pain, 10 = worst pain scale.
- Ask for changes in treatments if your pain persists.
- Receive compassionate and sympathetic care.
- Receive pain medication on a timely basis.
- Refuse treatment without prejudice from your doctor.
- Seek a second opinion or request a pain care specialist.
- Be given your records on request.
- Include your family in decision making.
- Remind those who care for you that your pain management is part of your diagnostic, medical, or surgical care.

Source: Adapted from Cowles, J. (1994). Pain relief! Portland, OR: Master Media.

At one time, medical literature contained little information on pain control. This, of course, is no longer true. In addition to professional publications, lay literature (books, newspapers, magazines, information on the Internet) contains a vast amount of information on the nature of pain, as well as pain control techniques. Cowles (1994) developed a pain patient's bill of rights (Table 16–6). This bill of rights has appeared in many magazines, including the article "Take Charge of Your Pain," which appeared in the January 1995 issue of *Modern Maturity* (the official publication of the American Association of Retired People). The article provided an analysis of the 19 rights that give nurses a good perspective of the expectations of their patients. In addition, this article, like so many magazine articles, gave the reader five sources for more information on pain, including the Agency for Health Care Policy and Research Publications (AHCRP). It is clear that patients are becoming very aware that pain is controllable and they are being educated to expect adequate treatment.

Difficult Aspects of Pain Management

1. **Not being judgmental.**
   - Pain is what the patient says it is.
   - Placebos should never be given as a way to prove or disprove the existence of pain.

     Many health care workers look for certain behavioral or outward responses to pain. If these responses are absent, the nurse or physician automatically jumps to the conclusion that the patient does not have "real" pain. There was a time when such a patient was given a placebo to prove he or she really did not have any pain. The current standard is for some nurses to be the *keeper of the keys* (i.e., having access to and control of pain medications), which creates a sense of power. If the pain medication order states it may be administered no sooner than every 4 hours, that is what the nurse does, despite evidence that the patient is not receiving adequate pain relief. Hopefully, the advent and increased use of patient-controlled analgesia (PCA) will help alleviate this nursing response.

2. **Helping the patient (and often his or her family) understand the following.**
   - Pain does not have to be tolerated. On the other hand, the patients with chronic pain may need help understanding that it may not be possible to be totally pain-free. Perhaps the goal is to reduce the pain level to a 1 or 2 on the 10-point rating scale.
   - Taking opioids for pain may lead to tolerance and dependency but not addiction.
   - There are many interventions for pain.

- Patients often need encouragement to try some of the nontraditional interventions.
- Pain intervention used should be initiated before the pain becomes severe.
- Some patients may need a referral to a local pain clinic.

3. **Around-the-clock (ATC) medicating.**
   - The patient may need to be awakened to receive a night dose.
   - Caregivers may need help realizing that waking the patient is more important to pain relief than uninterrupted sleep.

Before we leave the topic of pain, we will spend a few words on *phantom limb pain*. There are many theories regarding phantom limb pain, but to date this is a phenomenon that is not well understood. Most explanations found in textbooks agree that the nerves at the amputation site continue to send impulses to the spinal cord and then on to the brain where perception occurs. This does not, however, explain why or how some paraplegics with complete breaks of the spinal cord experience leg pain. Since the spinal cord damage prevents transmission of impulses to the brain, how do impulses get to the brain? So, although much progress has been made on the physiology of pain, phantom limb pain is an area with many questions.

Continuing research by Melzack (1998) has generated additional information to the experience of phantom pain. Melzack has studied individuals who were born without a limb. Approximately 20% of the group "reported feeling—often vividly—in an arm or leg they had never had or known" (p. 20). Although current theories may explain some aspects of phantom pain, the perceptions of some individuals born without a limb indicate that a great deal is still unknown.

And like the experience of phantom pain, pain in general remains a topic that requires further research. In addition to the work being done with neonates, other groups require research, such as the elderly, who often receive poor pain management. Mechanisms of pain, and techniques to manage it, will continue to be developed. Pain will be one of the topics that you will encounter throughout your nursing career.

Resource Listings

American Society of Pain Management Nurses (ASPMN)
7794 Grove Drive
Pensacola, FL 32514
E-mail: *ASPMN@aol.com*

American Cancer Society
1-800-ACS-2345

American Chronic Pain Association
PO Box 850
Rocklin, CA 95677-0850
(916) 632-0922

American Pain Society
4700 W. Lake Ave.
Glenview, IL 60025
www.ampainsoc.org/

Agency for Health Care Policy and Research (AHCRP)
PO Box 8547
Silver Spring, MD 20907
1-800-358-9295
www.ahcpr.gov/

The publications from the AHCRP on pain include:

Acute Pain Management in Adults
Acute Pain Management in Infants
Pain Control After Surgery (including a consumer guide)
Management of Cancer Pain (including a consumer guide)

American Academy of Pain Medicine
4700 W. Lake Ave.
Glenview, IL 60025-1485
(847) 375-4731
www.painmed.org/

American Society for Pain Relief, Research, and Education
www.cris.com/

17

Rehabilitation

Rehabilitation

Rehabilitation is essential to many areas of nursing practice. As the aging population continues to grow, the number of individuals with chronic illnesses will increase. A number of chronic illnesses lead to altered functional ability and as a result, altered lifestyles. ***Rehabilitation nursing*** uses a problem-solving approach to diagnose and treat the responses of individuals with actual or potential health problems that occur as a result of the changes brought on by chronic illness or injury (Habel, 1997).

The Role of the Rehabilitation Nurse

- Focus on the patient's physical and mental status as well as their emotional responses to pain, disability, and alterations in self-concept.
- Assess self-care abilities and work with both the patient and the family to assess their ability to cope with changes.
- Understand the value of preventing complications and teach the individual and the family prevention techniques.

Frequently, nurses find that patients can be less than cooperative; therefore, they need to recognize when patients and their families are having a natural reaction to an illness or injury versus a true problem. It is important for nurses to prevent complications and deformities, start rehabilitation activities early, teach patients and family, and refer to other professions and agencies as necessary.

The nature of the term *chronic illness* should remind us that we are dealing with an illness or injury that is most likely incurable and that will last more than just a few months. Individuals with chronic illness or injuries are forced to deal with many lifestyle changes.

Lifestyle Changes of Chronically Ill Patients

All of these changes cause additional stress, frustration, and often, fatigue:

- Health status
- Body image
- Loss of self-esteem
- Relationships and roles
- Activities and leisure pursuits
- Sexual functioning
- Loss of income or financial stressors
- Multiple doctor or hospital visits
- Multiple laboratory tests and medication trials
- Exacerbation of the illness

Patient responses to injury depend on the following:

- Patient's personality
- How quickly the changes occur (e.g., spinal cord injury versus arthritis)
- How significant the changes are to that individual

It is important for the nurse to remember that our society emphasizes wholeness, youth, and beauty. Your patient is trying to deal with changes and put the new "self" into some perspective. The new self will also need to be accepted by the patient and society, and be deemed worthwhile. Some patients never make the adjustments necessary to adapt and accept the new person. Patients with chronic illness or injuries may experience reactions similar to patients who are grieving a loss. They may initially feel shock, but it soon becomes apparent that a change has occurred and they may feel angry, depressed, anxious, and hopeless. Often, the anger and hostility these patients feel toward themselves for becoming ill is projected onto others. Patients may also respond with anger and hostility as a result of their loss of power to make choices. In this situation, the nurse must offer choices in areas in which patients can make them.

Nurses need to recognize that patients will experience a variety of feelings that are not easy to deal with. Following an injury or diagnosis, the patient may cope (with an unconscious defense mechanism) by using denial. There are different levels of denial and its use can be healthy or unhealthy. Initially, the use of denial is considered healthy as the individual retreats into himself or herself to reduce the threat of what has occurred to his or her self-concept. Over time the individual is usually able to recognize that a change has occurred but may continue to use denial. You may hear a patient say, "I know that I'll never be able to snow ski again, but that isn't so bad. I can live with that." Other patients might ignore the problem by saying, "I know the doctor said I have high blood pressure, but these pills are for my kidneys." Unhealthy denial occurs when a patient continues to verbally deny that which is obvious.

For example, we had a young male patient who suffered a spinal cord injury as a result of a diving accident. He was only 28 years old when he became a C5 quadriplegic. He kept telling everyone who came into his room, "I can feel my legs. Watch, I'll move them for you." This young man was in complete denial. He was psychologically unable to adapt to the changes in his life, and unable to move forward as a result. He required a great deal of support and was eventually able to come to terms with his multiple losses.

When a patient is in extreme denial, it is very important to get the patient to share how he or she views the illness or injury. Some patients may need more information about the present changes or those that will occur. It is unfortunate that denial occurs at a time when most patients are experiencing a number of physical assaults. The physical becomes the priority of most health care professionals, leaving the patient to deal with the psychological changes on their own. As the patient's physical condition improves, health care professionals often move on to the next patient whose physical care is a priority. Patients need care at all stages of recovery, both physical and psychological!

Eventually, the individual is able to progress through the denial and acknowledge that in order to survive, certain changes will have to occur. At this time, individuals require a great deal of support as they learn to focus on the reality of their situation. The person must analyze who they were before, who they are now, and who they will become in the future. This entire process can be extremely traumatic.

Finally, the individual is able to reconstruct a new life, incorporating the changes brought on by the chronic illness or injury. For example, we know a young man, Sam, who became a paraplegic as a result of a horseback riding accident. An athletic man prior to his accident, he decided to take up paraskiing (Figure 17–1) as a sport following a period of rehabilitation. Although Sam

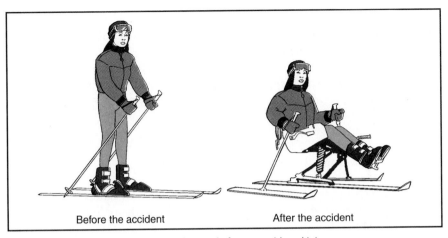

Figure 17–1. Participation in sports before and after an accidental injury.

was excited and pleased to be accomplishing new things, he still regretted the fact that he could no longer ski on his own two legs. These conflicting emotions (pleasure and regret) force the individual to confront an ambivalence that often leaves them confused, vulnerable, and frustrated. Having trusted people to share these feelings with is a necessity. The individual will be highly sensitive to how others treat them. If you or someone else regards the patient with pity or disgust, the patient will know it and you or others will be unable to help the patient through this change process. The individual needs to know that the changed them is a worthwhile person. They also need to know that they will develop other social relationships, formulate a redeveloped self-esteem, and create a new social identity.

◼ Mobility

One of the priorities of rehabilitation is to get the patient to become as mobile as possible. As a nurse, you should remember that there are positives and negatives involved when helping a patient become more mobile.

1. **Responsibilities of the nurse**
   - Reinforcing correct techniques
   - Offering encouragement
   - Assisting with exercises
2. **Mobility positives**
   - Be physically active
   - Become physically fit

- Build self-esteem
- Contribute to developing an activity and rest schedule that will allow for continued improvement

It is important to note here that some patients with deteriorating neuromuscular diseases such as amyotrophic lateral sclerosis (ALS), multiple sclerosis (MS), and muscular dystrophy (MD) may not experience improvement despite physical activity.

3. **Mobility negatives**
   - Decreased mobility and physical activity can lead to increased stress
   - Withdrawal and apathy will delay recovery
   - Decreased social contact
   - Decreased chance to control their interactions with others

   For example, for a patient who is bedridden, the only people the patient sees are ones that come to see the patient. The patient has no control over getting out and initiating contact with others. His or her world shrinks to just a few individuals. Imagine seeing the same people over and over only when they want to see you!

Nurses need to be attuned to changes in a patient's mobility status. It is important for you to have a mobility baseline assessment. Once the baseline is established, it will be easier for you to determine whether or not the patient is making progress. Remember, however, that some patients will not experience much progress. Patients with certain neuromuscular disorders may become more debilitated over time regardless of intervention. It is important to remember that any progress (no matter how infinitesimal) is positive. Whether your patient was formerly an Olympic athlete or sedentary, each individual will progress at different rates. For the former Olympic athlete who is now a quadriplegic, moving a finger may be a giant step. Adjusting your expectations to small steps is essential to your ability to become satisfied with rehabilitation nursing. You may see the occasional giant step, but they usually come slowly (Figure 17–2).

Mobility History Assessment

One way for you to establish a mobility baseline is through a mobility history and assessment. A number of good tools are available to help you gather this information. The basic areas of assessment include:

1. **Vocational:** Type of work, how much physical effort is required
2. **Home and family:** Relationships, ability to perform home maintenance, cooking, cleaning, and other daily activities
3. **Social:** Leisure activities (past and present); how the illness has changed these
4. **Sexual:** Satisfaction with relationships; how the illness has affected sexual functioning

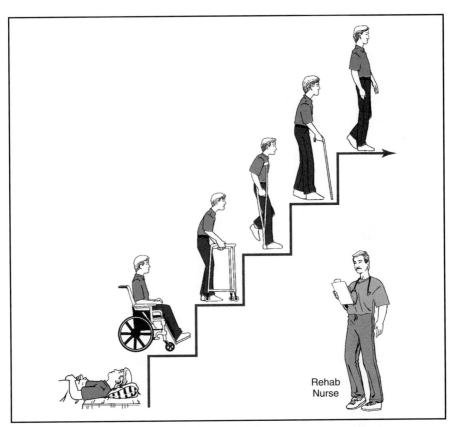

Figure 17–2. Changes may come slowly during rehabilitation.

5. **Activities of daily living**
   - Exercise—how much, what kind, how illness has affected methods of exercise choices
   - Sleep—how much, any problems
   - Nutrition—eating habits; how has the illness affected them, intake of beverages, tobacco use
   - Medications—what is used regularly, prescription, and over-the-counter; any affect on mobility
6. **Psychological:** Any concerns, method of dealing with problems, effectiveness of coping strategies; changes in the way patient feels about self

The actual physical mobility assessment focuses on assessing and evaluating integumentary, pulmonary, cardiovascular, musculoskeletal, neurological, and psychological functioning. Detailed information is obtained and incorporated into the mobility history to formulate a baseline assessment.

Once the baseline is established, nothing should be done for the patient that he or she can do for himself or herself. Every activity, no matter how small, contributes to strengthening. If you do everything for the patient, it will reinforce feelings of helplessness and hopelessness.

You have probably already studied the effects of immobility during a nursing fundamentals course. Prior to working with a patient who requires rehabilitation, we would recommend that you review the hazards such as osteoporosis, muscle wasting, contractures, and pulmonary embolism associated with immobility.

Sexuality

Changes in mobility have the potential to alter sexual satisfaction. The sexual changes that occur may be a result of fatigue, loss of independence, or inability to adapt to illness or bodily changes. During the time a patient is hospitalized, sexual satisfaction is often overlooked. If a patient requires extended rehabilitation, sexual outlets need to be provided. Caring staff members can provide for necessary privacy.

CHANGES IN SELF-CONCEPT

Patients and their partners frequently experience conflict as a result of added tensions listed below.

- Feeling that they are no longer desirable
- Fearing the reactions of their partner
- Fear may lead to a decrease in sex drive
- Possible withdrawal due to a fear of rejection

It is important for you to inform both the patient and the partner that this conflict is not abnormal. Your compassion and knowledge can help them both overcome the tension. Patients may also need information about how to make sexual activity a part of their new lives. Simple changes in positioning may be all that is needed for the patient to continue to have satisfying sexual relations. The patient may also need to know about ways of anchoring or removing catheters prior to intercourse. Sometimes, the timing of prescription medication (for spasticity, etc.) or taking a warm bath can enhance ability to perform. Your patients will have many questions about their changed sexuality, whether or not they ask. Your job is to provide opportunities for discussions about sexuality and to help the patient learn new ways of experiencing sexual satisfaction. Most rehabilitation facilities provide a resource person who can help guide you in your discussions with the patient, or there may be a sex therapist that can give your patient information directly.

Motivating for Change

Rehabilitation involves significant changes in almost every area of life. Motivation is the key to successful rehabilitation. Individuals who have been extremely independent and believe that they are in control of their lives tend to participate more readily in the rehabilitation process. However, all patients will require external reinforcement and support, especially during the early stages of rehabilitation.

ENHANCE MOTIVATION

1. **Listen.**
   - Be sure that you listen intently to both the verbal and nonverbal cues that the patient gives you.
   - Active listening will help you gain an understanding of exactly what might motivate the patient.
   - Remember that we are all different. I might be motivated by an ice cream sundae, whereas someone else might be motivated by some quiet time alone (Figure 17–3).

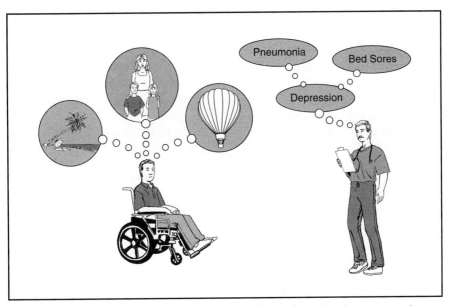

Figure 17–3. What motivates the patient may be very different from what the nurse perceives as motivating factors.

- It is up to you to figure out what the patient's motivating factors are.
- Remember you do not know what the patient is going through. Do you have the same disability? Do you think/feel/believe the same?
- Do not presume to know what the patient is experiencing.

2. **Active participation.**
   - The patient needs to participate in goal setting.
   - Work on establishing a goal that has meaning for the patient. For example, if the patient was an accomplished horsewoman, then perhaps a goal of getting back on horseback will have the most meaning.
   - Do not make the assumption that accomplishing any goal is impossible for the patient. There are numerous hippotherapy centers (therapeutic riding) across the country.
   - Plastering the room with pictures of horses may help reinforce this goal for the patient.
   - Often, if a person has a strong enough desire to accomplish a goal, nothing will stand in his or her way.
   - We have seen numerous patients who were told that they would never walk again, walk, and even complete a marathon.

3. **Choices.**
   - Allow the patient to make personal choices.
   - This will give the patient an increased sense of control.
   - Even small choices or forced choices are still choices, for example, "Lucy, would you prefer to bathe in the morning or in the afternoon?" or, "Would you prefer to wear your green shirt or the blue one?" or, "Would you rather have cake or ice cream for dessert?"
   - These choices might seem insignificant to you, but they can help your patient regain some semblance of control.

4. **Contract.**
   - A written or verbal contract can help the patient to work toward specific goals.
   - Keeping a diary can also help the patient to see progress when it is difficult to notice. For example, a patient might make a contract to walk one length of the parallel bars by the end of 1 month.
   - Each step is significant. Each pick-up, put-down of a foot. If the patient notes that, "I took one step today," "four today," "six today," they can look back and see progress.
   - Sometimes, the change is so small that it is difficult for the patient to see any improvement.
   - With a diary, the patient has no doubt that progress is being made.

5. **Work together.**
   - Work with other team members.
   - A group effort with everyone focusing on the same outcomes is best for the patient.

Complications

Often in chronic illness, complications cause more problems than the original disability. It is vital that you work hard to prevent, or at least recognize early, any potential complications. Not only do complications cause problems, but they also can cause more financial expenditure, increased discomfort, and potentially, death.

Some examples of problems that can be prevented with good nursing care include:

- Dehydration
- Distended or full bladder
- Rectal impaction
- Incontinence of bladder or bowels
- Decubiti (bed sores)
- Deformities from disuse
- Emotional distress

You also need to keep an eye out for depression, isolation, and fatigue. You provide nursing care to the patient, but the patient decides whether to accept or refuse it. Let the patient and family know why you are doing what you are doing, and why it is essential. Explain about decreased mobility and physical changes that occur as a result such as contractures, what they are, and how they are preventable.

Rehabilitation is a challenging endeavor in both chronic illness and injury. In order to succeed in rehabilitation nursing, a nurse must be patient, creative, and caring. You will need to develop an understanding of the rehabilitation experience from the patient's standpoint and be empathetic and genuine. The patient in need of rehabilitation will be extremely sensitive to rejection and will need your reassurance.

Books to Consider Adding to Your Personal Library

Backstrom, G. (1994). *The resource guide for the disabled*. Dallas, TX: Taylor Publishing.

Hawking, S. (1994). *Computer resources for people with disabilities*. Alameda, CA: Hunter House.

Maddox, S. (1993). *Spinal network*. Boulder, CO: Spinal Network.

RESOURCE WEB SITES

If computers are available to your patient, there are a number of disability-oriented Web sites that can provide information and support. Four of the best Web sites for people with disabilities are:

1. Disability Net: *www.disabilitynet.co.uk*
2. The Boulevard: *www.blvd.com*
3. Ability Online: *www.ablelink.org*
4. New Mobility: *www.newmobility.com*

18

Ageism

It is no secret that the population of older adults is increasing. Currently in the United States, there are approximately 35 million older adults. By 2020, it is estimated that this number will increase to 59 million, including approximately 266,000 individuals who will be 100 years old or older. You should, therefore, realize that a high percentage of patients in the near future will be older adults.

We begin by exploring the meaning of old—elderly—aged—senior citizen. The first, most obvious observation is that "old" is a relative term. To the 3-year-old child, anyone who is 5 years old is old; and this view tends to continue through the ages. Old only applies to those who are ahead of us in birthdays. The second observation is that many terms and phrases are used to refer to basically the same group of individuals.

What Is Old?

There are two objective ways to describe old.

1. **Chronological:** Selects an age as "old" and compares an individual's age to this number as a standard. Since the 1965 amendment to the Social Security Act, 65 has been the standard definition of old age. In addition, 65 was established as the minimum age for Medicare health care benefits, while the Age Discrimination in Employment Act establishes 70 as mandatory retirement age. Many commercial establishments also use chronological age to offer certain customers special benefits such as discounts on purchases. For example, 50, 55, and 60 are common ages business have selected as the number that fits a customer into the "senior

citizen discount" group. So, chronological age tells us when to have a birthday party, the age that makes us eligible to vote, the number we put on a form that has a space for "age," and when we can ride the bus free. Although chronologic age offers quick and convenient ways to determine who is "old," it does not give any indication of the individual's functioning or performance skills and abilities.

2. **Functional age:** Also referred to by some as *biological age.* This approach requires individual assessment on several levels rather than a number. It is not an easy concept to measure or define in a few words.

In an attempt to create more uniformity, there is a trend in **gerontology** (the study of aging) to use a single set of terms as reference points for definitions of old (Table 18–1). However, these definitions are not universal.

Another term worth exploring is *ageism.* Ageism is defined by Stanley (1995, p. 52) as:

> *a systemic stereotyping of and discrimination against people because they are old, just as racism and sexism accomplish this with skin color and gender, old people are categorized as senile, rigid in thought and manner, old-fashioned in morality and skill. . . . Ageism allows the younger generation to see older people as different from themselves; thus they subtly cease to identify with their elders as human beings.*

You have, no doubt, identified ageism in others. How about in yourself? No? Good! However, remember this the next time you have an older patient and you groan ever so softly: "Oh no. Not another old lady!" You too are expressing ageism!!!

Ageism is a complex subject that is easier to define than it is to understand. Stereotyping of the elderly—ageism assumptions—can lead to inferior medical and nursing care. All too often, the elderly patient's problems are seen as a direct result of the aging process and thus assumed by some health care workers to be inevitable and untreatable. In one way, ageism might be seen as an "occupational hazard" for health care workers since so many older patients are ill, frail, confused, and hospitalized, or in long-term care facilities. We fall into the generalization trap and do not separate facts from myths. A major myth is that all older adults are like those we see in our daily practice. Additional myths (Farrell, 1990) are listed in Table 18–2.

Table 18–1. Various Definitions of Age

Age (years)	Category	Definition
65–74	Early old age	Young–old
75–84	Middle old age	Middle–old
85+	Late old age	Old–old, frail elderly

Table 18–2. Common Myths About Aging

- Old age is a disease.
- Old age begins at 65.
- Senility is part of aging.
- Old people are all alike.
- Older people are usually unhappy.
- Older people are set in their ways and unable to change.
- Older people have no power.
- Older people are sexless.
- Most old people are poor.
- People become more religious as they age.
- In general, older people are lonely and socially isolated.
- Most older workers cannot work as effectively as younger workers.

Research has demonstrated some disturbing information regarding the elderly and health care, including the fact that elderly patients are less successful than younger patients are in capturing the attention of health professionals. The elderly are seldom successful in having their concerns addressed. However, this long-standing situation is changing. One reason for the evolving change is that although mainstream advertisements of all forms (TV, paper, radio, magazines) are aimed at the young, the focus of many ads now target older adults. A second reason is the explosion of information aimed at the elderly. Books, TV programs, special segments of news broadcasts, popular magazine articles, specialty magazines, organizations, and the Internet are readily accessed by the older generation. These sources provide the elderly with vast amounts of information on such topics as pain control, dietary needs, activity, sexuality, end-of-life decisions, what to expect (and sometimes demand) from health care providers. The list goes on. The point is, the elderly population is growing in number and, at the same time, becoming more active participants in many aspects of their lives. They are not willing to quietly accept less than that received by the "younger" generation.

Prominent Theories of Why We Age

For all cultures, and through the millennia, the process of aging has been of great interest. Currently, there are at least seven prominent theories of why we age (Table 18–3). We will look at the basic premise of each. Remember that each theory is complex and has various amounts of research to support it.

Table 18–3. Common Theories of Aging

- Immunity and autoimmunity
- Cross-linkage
- Free radicals
- Wear and tear
- Nutritional restriction
- Error
- Biological programming

1. Immunity and autoimmunity
   - Explains aging on basis that the immune system begins to develop antibodies to destroy older cells
   - Decline of the immune system contributes to the development of age-related diseases
2. Cross-linkage
   - Based on chemical reactions creating damage to DNA
   - If DNA strand is unable to repair itself, cell death will occur or abnormal cells will be produced
3. Free radicals
   - Thought that environmental pollutants cause molecules to break off cells
   - Believed that these free-floating electrons will then damage various cell structures
4. Wear and tear
   - Proposes that the body has a time schedule and wears out as its time winds down
   - Stress and damage play a role in this theory
5. Nutritional restrictions
   - Based on research that shows that laboratory animals maintained on restricted diets outlive their regular-diet counterparts
6. Error
   - Thought to be due to cells receiving wrong messages from the cell nucleus resulting in cell mutations
7. Biologic programming
   - Claims that life expectancy is governed by heredity
   - Humans have a preset biologic clock that determines the onset of aging and life span

The fact that there are so many theories of aging, each with its own research base, tells us that there are apparently many factors involved in aging and that eternal youth is not possible. Aging just occurs! If nothing else, there are three accepted characteristics of aging according to Matteson, McConnell, & Linton (1997):

1. Aging is common to all members of a given species
2. Aging is aggressive
3. Aging is deleterious, ultimately leading to death

In addition to theories that attempt to explain why humans experience specific physiologic changes with aging, various theories exist that describe developmental changes that occur at various stages of life. A few of the more prominent developmental theories are by Erikson, Peck, Havighurst, Ebersole, and Butler.

If aging is inevitable, what about ways to affect longevity? Like the many theories of aging, there are many theories about how to affect longevity including diet, exercise, vitamins, antioxidants, and antiaging therapies. As Hayflick (1994) points out, "no one has ever shown unequivocally that, in humans, any medical intervention, lifestyle change, nutritional factor, or other substance will slow, stop, or reverse the fundamental aging process or the determinants of life span" (p. 313). Hayflick notes, "we still do not know how to slow the aging process in humans, but we do know how to increase our life expansion by eliminating or reducing causes of death" (p. 341).

To study aging in a systematic, scientific manner requires time. Hayflick (1994) presents a great deal of information gleaned from one such long-term study known as the Baltimore Longitudinal Study of Aging (BLSA), which started in 1958. About 2,200 volunteers were followed for an average of 13 years. Many participants were elderly when they joined the study and have since died, while a number of volunteers who were less than 50 when they joined are just now reaching advanced age. So far, this study has provided data on both the physiologic and psychological dimensions of aging. One major factor is apparent—"older humans show a greater range of individual variation in many physiological and psychological measurements than do younger adults" (Hayflick, 1994, p. 140). The notion that all old people are essentially the same is a myth!

Nonetheless, from the BLSA and other research, we are learning a great deal about the aging process. Some of the findings support long-held beliefs, while a great deal of the new findings are shattering many others. (Thus, for some, the study has come to be called the "myth buster.")

A small sample of current information on aging from the BLSA follows.

- Predominant characteristics of old age are:
  1. A reduced capacity to adapt
  2. Reduced speed of performance
  3. An increased susceptibility to disease
- Maximum heart rate diminishes with age—this is not a health problem.
- When disease free, the heart of an older person pumps just about as well as a young healthy heart.

- Short-term memory declines with age.
- Vocabulary scores do not change with age.
- In the absence of disease, personality traits remain essentially the same throughout life.
- The common belief that as people age they become crankier or mellower is a myth.
- Lifestyle habits, such as low-cholesterol diets and not smoking, can influence the development or progression of some age-associated diseases, but there is no evidence of a direct effect on the fundamental aging process.
- Relative frequency of sexual activity does not change with age.
- The ability to identify odors declines earlier and more rapidly in men than in women.

The BLSA, and other research on aging, is providing data that distinguish between age-related normal changes and age-related illnesses. Table 18–4 lists some examples. Again, although there are many age-related conditions, they are not a part of the normal aging process. Hayflick (1994) points out this distinction between normal age changes and age-related illnesses. He writes that "physiological loses characteristics of aging eventually occur in the cells, tissues, and organs of all older members of a species, while changes due to disease occur only in some members" (p. 48). Note that although many of the normal age-related changes increase the older adult's risk to specific diseases, normal aging and age-related disease are not the same thing! Thus, the difference between two terms that are often incorrectly interchanged, geriatrics and gerontology. *Geriatrics* is the study and practice of dealing with elderly patients who have an age-related illness or condition, whereas *gerontology* is the term to indicate the study and practice of normal, age-related problems and changes. Although they are two distinct areas, it is possible to be dealing with both areas in the same patient.

Table 18–4. Normal Changes with Aging Versus Age-Related Illness

Age-Related Normal Changes	Age-Related Illnesses
• Loss of strength and stamina	• Cancer
• New hair growth in ears and nose	• Heart disease
• Decline in short-term memory	• Alzheimer's disease
• Balding	• Strokes
• Loss of bone mass	• Dementia
• Decrease in height	• Arthritis
• Hearing decline	• Parkinson's disease
• Reduction in visual acuity	
• Renal blood flow and glomerular filtration rate (GFR)	
• Liver spots on skin	

At times, a common difficulty for caregivers of the older adult is deciding if the patient is experiencing manifestations of illness. A good benchmark is the occurrence of "deterioration of functional independence in active, previously unimpaired elders is an early, subtle sign of untreated illness characterized by the absence of typical symptoms and signs of disease" (Besdine, 1990, p. 3). In other words, when an older adult suddenly demonstrates problems with mobility, cognition, continence, or nutrition, there is cause for an assessment and problem-oriented approach to identify the etiology. For many older individuals, loss of functional ability may not manifest itself until the individual is under stress, either physical or emotional. In addition, "most older persons have a most-vulnerable function" (Fretwell, 1990, p. 170). Examples are cognition, memory, and ability to remain continent or walk. Loss of one specific function (especially suddenly), is often the red flag of illness. So, for an individual who is 80 years old, well-oriented, and continent, sudden incontinence may be the initial symptoms of pneumonia. Remember that in older people, there is usually a poor correlation between the type and severity of problem (functional ability) they present and the etiology.

Two Common Assessments Specific to the Elderly

As with many distinct patient populations, there are a number of assessments specific to the elderly. Two of the most common and initially most useful ones are ADL and IADL assessments.

1. **Activities of daily living (ADLs):** Activities necessary for self-care such as bathing, toileting, dressing, and transferring.
   - There are a number of ADL assessment tools.
   - One well-known ADL tool is the **Katz Index.** This tool assesses the patient's actual performance on ADLs versus what they do that requires help provided in controlled settings.
   - Another tool used to measure ADLs is the **Barthel Index.** This tool assigns numbers to various activities based on the patient's degree of independence.
2. **Instrumental activities of daily living (IADLs):** A must for the elderly patient living in the community.
   - This is an expansion of ADLs.
   - Assesses items such as ability to carry out various household activities such as shopping or taking medications.

There are multiple issues associated with the older adult. In the following sections we will explore several specific ones: urinary incontinence, abuse, restraints, sexuality, and dementia.

Urinary Incontinence

Urinary incontinence (UI) is considered the involuntary escape of urine to such a degree that it causes a problem. Nurses usually think of urinary incontinence only as something that occurs in elderly, nonambulatory, institutionalized patients. Research has revealed, however, that in addition to the 1.5 million incontinent nursing home residents, UI occurs in 15 to 30% of noninstitutionalized individuals over age 60. For all of these individuals, UI has mental, physical, social, and economic consequences.

Like so many other situations, successful interventions for UI depend on identifying its etiology. For too long, this etiology was considered the individual's old age. However, UI is no longer considered a natural part of aging. Rather, at least 10 causes for UI have been identified (Table 18–5). UI can also be placed into a *type*. Each type provides a description of the circumstances when the incontinence occurs.

Four Basic Types of Urinary Incontinence

1. Urge incontinence
   - Involuntary incontinence that occurs as soon as a strong need to void is identified
   - Frequently associated with involuntary detrusor contractions
   - These individuals cannot get to the bathroom fast enough
2. Stress incontinence
   - Involuntary incontinence that occurs with increased intra-abdominal pressure without detrusor muscle contraction
   - Such examples are coughing, sneezing, laughing, assuming an upright position, and physical exertion

Table 18–5. Etiologies of Urinary Incontinence

• Urinary tract infections	• Weak bladder sphincters
• Vaginal infections and irritation	• Neurologic disorders
• Constipation	• Immobility
• Medications	• Benign prostatic hypertrophy
• Weak bladder muscles	• Impaired cognition

3. Overflow incontinence
   - Incontinence occurs when the bladder is not completely emptied
4. Functional incontinence
   - Involuntary incontinence that occurs in individuals with normal bladder functioning
   - Seen in patients with cognitive disorders

If you look at the table of etiologies you will see that the types of UI are associated with specific etiologies. For example, benign prostatic hypertrophy (BPH) can contribute to overflow incontinence, detrusor hyperreflexia from a stroke can create urge incontinence, and a severe head injury may lead to functional incontinence. Therefore, UI can be caused by pathologic, anatomic, or physiologic factors and at times, more than one factor may be operating.

Because the etiologies for each type of UI vary, so will interventions. One of the greater challenges for the nurse is to convince the patient that they do not have to tolerate UI. Urinary incontinence is not considered normal or an accepted part of aging. Once individuals accept this fact, they need to discuss their situation with their physician and determine the etiology. The problem, however, is that there are reports that many physicians do not respond when informed of the incontinence. If this happens, it means that you need to help the patient educate their physician or find another one (preferably a urologist or gerontologist). Once the patient has an understanding physician, the diagnostic process will start with a history and physical exam with special emphasis on the urinary system. Based on the history and physical, any number of specific urologic tests may be conducted from the simple to the complex.

Identification of the type of UI and the specific etiology is the foundation for treatment choice, which again, will range from simple to complex. The most common treatment modalities of UI are listed in Table 18–6.

Table 18–6. Treatment Options for Urinary Incontinence

- Medications
- Surgery
- Bladder training
- Pelvic muscle (Kegel) exercises
- Biofeedback
- Catheterization
    - Intermittent
    - Indwelling
- External collection devices
- Absorbent products

Abuse

Elder abuse (which is also referred to as *elder mistreatment*) is a very serious and prevalent problem that can occur at several levels. Like child abuse, the most obvious form is physical abuse such as slapping, hitting, and pushing. *Physical abuse* can also include neglect such as lack of physical care, inappropriate physical care, and inadequate nutrition. Physical abuse provides objective evidence. However, other less obvious forms of abuse include verbal abuse, exploitation, financial and psychological abuse, and sexual abuse. Although more literature is appearing on elder abuse, it remains a topic with little research. We do not know much about such topics as the nature of the problem, its causes, characteristics of the abuser and the elder, and aspects of prevention. Table 18–7 identifies factors for both the elder and the abuser that increase the possibility of elder abuse.

Since nurses have such frequent contact with elderly patients, they are often the first ones to suspect some form of abuse. With few exceptions, almost every state requires that anyone who is aware of elder mistreatment, or has strong reason to suspect it, is required by law to report it to proper authorities. In most states this authority has the title of Adult Protective Services (APS) and its number appears in local papers, government listings in telephone books, and can also be located through the telephone information operator. Once notified, it is up to the authorities to investigate and take appropriate action. If, however, you have reported a situation and continue to see or suspect that the mistreatment is continuing, report it again! History has shown us that problems are not always corrected in a timely manner.

The dynamics of elder abuse are complex. One factor, however, that seems to be related to mistreatment is caregiver stress. Some research has shown a correlation between the two. If the nurse identifies caregiver stress and pro-

Table 18–7. Risk Factors for Elder Abuse

Risk Factor	Victim	Abuser
• History of mental illness	●	●
• Shared living arrangements	●	●
• Family history of violence	●	●
• Isolation	●	
• Stressful events		●
• Poor health	●	
• Cognitive impairment	●	
• Substance abuse		●
• Dependency	●	●
• Lack of financial resources	●	●

Source: Lynch, S. H. (1997). Elder abuse: What to look for, how to intervene. AJN, 97 (1): 29.

vides interventions to relieve that stress, abuse may be avoided. In addition, some neglect problems may be corrected with caregiver teaching. Table 18–8 illustrates other intervention strategies.

If it appears as if elder abuse occurs only in the home, there is adequate research and anecdotal evidence to attest to the fact that it also occurs in long-term care facilities, as well as acute care facilities. In addition, it is not always someone else who carries out the mistreatment. There is a form of mistreatment classified as self-neglect. The individual does not seek out medical care, refuses care, is noncompliant, has poor nutrition, and lives in a dirty environment. All these actions are a result of the individual's choice. These situations

Table 18–8. Strategies for Intervention(s) with Elder Abuse

Patient Refuses Treatment

- Allow patient to make choice of refusal.
- Remain nonjudgmental.
- Educate regarding available services and incidence and severity of abuse increasing over time.
- Provide emergency contact numbers.
- Contact Adult Protective Services (APS) in accordance with state law.

Patient Lacks Mental Capacity

- Contact APS.
- Arrange for provisions to be made regarding guardianship, financial assistance, foster care, and court proceedings.

Patient Accepts Intervention

- Examine positive and negative aspects of change.
- Discuss safety options, such as hospitalization, changing living arrangements, obtaining orders of protection, changing locks, and pressing charges.
- As appropriate, refer to hospital social services, home health care, respite care, education, chaplains, and supportive counseling.
- Refer to APS for assistance contacting appropriate resources, such as case workers, counselors, and legal services.
- Allow patient to express feelings and fears.

For Abusers

- Remove victim from danger, relieving abuser of caregiving responsibility and stress.
- Provide support services, such as counseling, education, and rehabilitation for drug or alcohol abuse.

Source: Lynch, S. H. (1997). Elder abuse: What to look for, how to intervene. AJN, 97(1): 29.

often create more challenges than those situations in which another person causes the mistreatment. Until declared legally incompetent, the older person has the right to accept or reject care, including help with nutrition, medication, and living conditions. Many ethical factors need to be considered before making the decision to seek legal intervention. Nurses, as well as families, struggle with issues of self-neglect. There is no one or easy answer to the problem of elder abuse in any form.

Restraints

Over the years, nursing's answer to the elderly who were cognitively impaired and had behaviors that were considered potentially or actually detrimental to the individual (falling, wandering away, pulling at various tubes, etc.) was to use restraints. Restraint devices include such things as special restraint vests, sheets, belts, side rails, wrist restraints, and gerichairs. Most of the time, the devices were utilized solely at the nurse's discretion. (If the nurse was not satisfied with the effectiveness of the restraints, she would often ask and receive from the physician an order for some sort of chemical restraint such as sedatives and tranquilizers.) Despite their use, however, the problems that restraints were supposed to cure have remained! Eventually, some nurses began to doubt the wisdom of restraints and research to explore the consequences of restraints began. It soon became apparent that the use of restraints created as many, or more, problems as they were intended to prevent. As nurses began to doubt the wisdom of restraints, so did society. Many individuals and groups became involved in issues regarding the elderly. One of the most recent and influential developments was the Omnibus Reconciliation Act, commonly known as OBRA, passed by Congress in 1987. This legislation addressed many issues regarding quality of care in long-term care facilities, including residents' rights. Paramount among these rights is the right to be free of restraint (physical and chemical).

When the legislation regarding restraints became law, most nurses in long-term care facilities threw up their hands and said it could not be done, that the elderly "need restraints for their own good." It has not been an easy road, but time has proven those nurses wrong. With very few exceptions, safe, competent nursing care does not have to include the use of restraints.

One of the most striking changes with OBRA has been that the use of restraints now requires a physician's written order. The corresponding charting regarding use of restraints is extensive. For example, the charting must indicate not only the reason for the restraints (specific behavior) but indicate what alternative interventions were tried prior to the restraints. (Note that "lack of staff" to watch the patient is not an acceptable reason for restraints.) The documentation must also include such data as the times the patient was monitored, the patient's response to the restraints, care given during the restrained period, and reasons for prolonged use.

Today there are some long-term care facilities that are almost totally restraint free. Although OBRA addressed care in long-term care facilities, its influence has spread to other areas such as acute care facilities, adult day care, and home care. These areas of care, including various levels of intensive care units, are realizing that alternative actions to restraints are desirable and possible.

Sexuality

Although definitions of sexuality vary, they all convey the idea that there are more than physical activities associated with sex. It "encompasses the manner in which individuals use their own roles, relationships, values, customs, and maleness or femaleness" (O'Toole, 1997, p. 1473). Figure 18–1 indicates major fac-

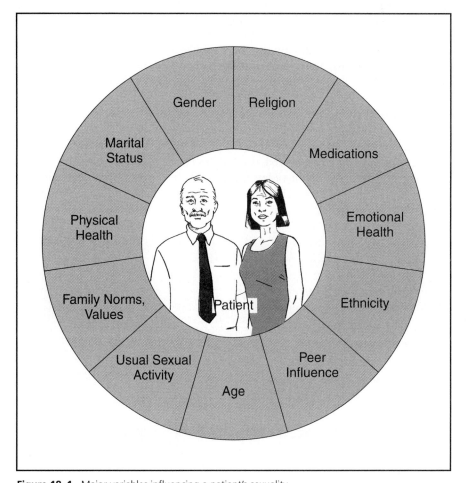

Figure 18–1. Major variables influencing a patient's sexuality.

tors that influence sexuality. For many individuals born in the first half of the twentieth century, sexuality was associated only with the sexual act. They were raised to believe that sex was an activity for married couples only; after the child-bearing years, sex was generally considered unnecessary or impossible. When it was discovered that an older man or woman wanted to or actually participated in sexual activities, he or she was labeled as a "dirty old man" or a "dirty old woman." This generation of individuals is today's patients who are in the age range of about 55 years and older. One of the major mistakes nurses make with this group is assuming that because of the patients' backgrounds, issues of sexuality and sexual activity can be deleted from their care. This is an erroneous assumption! Although many patients in this age group may in fact "be done" with sexual intercourse, they may have many concerns regarding their sexuality (Table 18–9).

Needless to say, during the second half of this century, society's attitudes toward sex have changed. Sex before, outside of, and without marriage for a large portion of society, is now more acceptable. In addition, many types of sexual activities between and among men and women, if not accepted, are tol-erated. The oncoming generation of older patients will not be the stereotypical heterosexual.

Despite this change in society, many health care workers ignore, neglect, or refuse to acknowledge sexuality issues. If you find yourself in this group, you are not providing optimal care to your patients. For example, assessment and care for two serious problems, acquired immune dificiency syndrome (AIDS) and sexually transmitted diseases (STDs), may not be carried out. Both are health problems in older adults. You are encouraged, therefore, to take steps to improve care. This may involve expanding your reading on the subject, attending workshops, or discussing the topic with colleagues who are well versed on the subject.

Table 18–9. Common Sexuality Issues of Older Adults

- Vaginal dryness
- Decreased sexual arousal
- Sex and heart problems
- Effects of medication on libido
- Being hugged and touched less by others
- Altered physical appearance
- Impotence
- Fear of revealing that they are not heterosexual

Table 18–10. Conditions That Can Create Manifestations of Dementia

- Alzheimer's disease
- Trauma
- Huntington's disease
- HIV-related dementia
- Brain tumors
- Multi-infarct dementia

Dementia and Delirium

One of the major frustrations for family and caregivers of the elderly is senile behavior. **Senile** is a nonspecific term used by the public to indicate mental disorders associated with aging. In today's medical and nursing publications the term is seldom used. Rather, we see the terms *dementia* and *delirium*.

True dementia is an irreversible form of impaired cognition with progressive deterioration in mental capacity. Table 18–10 lists some of the common conditions that can create the clinical manifestations of dementia. Table 18–11 differentiates between dementia and delirium. It is important to distinguish between the two because delirium has etiologies that can be treated and the impaired cognition, if not completely reversed, can be improved. Understanding the differences in the two conditions will help you in counseling family members and in developing appropriate nursing interventions.

Table 18–11. Character of Dementia and Delirium

Characteristic	Dementia	Delirium
Other names	• Organic brain syndrome • Often called by the etiology • Old terminology—senility	• Acute confessional state
Common etiologies	• Senile dementia of the Alzheimer type (SDAT) • Multicerebral infarcts • Long-term alcoholism	• Metabolic imbalances • Medication • Massive infection • Prolonged, high fever • Alcohol intoxication and alcohol withdrawal

Table 18–11. Character of Dementia and Delirium (Continued)

Characteristic	Dementia	Delirium
Onset	• Gradual, insidious; often not noticed until clinical manifestations are severe	• Fast; recognition that individual is not acting normal is readily apparent
Course	• Progressive; almost always irreversible • Aphasia • Anomia	• Reversible with prompt identification and treatment of etiology; "finding words" • Usually rapid speech

As discussed in the beginning of this chapter, the elderly will be a large portion of all patients in the health care system in the near future. This chapter has presented a few of the major issues associated with gerontological nursing.

Resource Listings

American Association of Retired Persons (AARP)
601 E Street, NW
Washington, DC 20049
(202) 434-2277
www.aarp.org/

This group has a *vast* amount of literature available on issues of concern to the older adult. A copy of their current catalog might be very useful in your personal library.

American Society on Aging
833 Market Street, Suite 511
San Francisco, CA 94103-1824
(415) 974-9600

Gray Panthers
PO Box 21477
Washington, DC 20009-9477
(202) 466-3132

National Council on the Aging
409 Third Street, SW, Suite 200
Washington, DC 20024
(202) 479-1200

Gerontological Society of America
1K Street NW, Suite 350
Washington, DC 20005
(202) 842-1275
www.geron.org/

Alzheimer's Association
919 North Michigan Avenue, Suite #1000
Chicago, IL 60611-1676
(800) 272-3900

Respite Programs for Caregivers of Alzheimer's Disease Patients
Hotline: (800) 648-COPE (648-2673)

National Council of Senior Citizens
1331 F Street NW
Washington, DC 20004-1171
(202) 374-8800

Children of Aging Parents
Woodbourne Office Campus, Suite 302A
1609 Woodbourne Drive
Levittown, PA 19057-1511
(215) 945-6900

19

Sexuality

We often wonder why it is that nurses can easily ask patients questions about their most intimate bodily functions but they are unwilling to ask questions of a sexual nature. If we consider such human needs as breathing, eating, and sleeping important, then why isn't sexual functioning (a primary physiological need) of equal importance? All of us are sexual beings. All of us wonder how changes in our health status might impact our sexual functioning. Unfortunately, some patients are afraid to ask questions about their sexual health, and as a rule, if the patient doesn't ask, chances are the nurse is not about to bring up the subject. It is equally bothersome to us that many nursing faculties avoid teaching students about sexuality. They may teach the pathophysiology, or even discuss coping with bodily changes, but few require their students to ask patients in-depth questions about sexuality in clinical settings. Is sexuality so taboo a subject that most health care providers refuse to discuss it? Is it more embarrassing than bowel movements and catheters (Figure 19–1)? What exactly is the problem?

■ Importance of Sexuality

We believe that human sexuality must be incorporated into high-quality health care. Perhaps you are thinking that nurses do discuss sexual health. We did a short, unscientific poll of our colleagues. Seven had had hysterectomies within the last 5 years. Not one of them had been told *anything* about sexual functioning! They had been told about estrogen therapy, staple and suture removal, and activity level. Not one was told when to resume sexual relations, how sensations might be different, or that lubricants might be needed for vaginal dryness. We find this to be an example of just how poorly informed patients often are about the sexual consequences of their treatment or surgery.

Sexuality is a vital part of our everyday lives. It is important to our relationships, self-esteem, and concept of our maleness or femaleness. Childbearing is also important to the psychological and social identity of many women. How can we ignore such an important part of the lives of our patients?

158

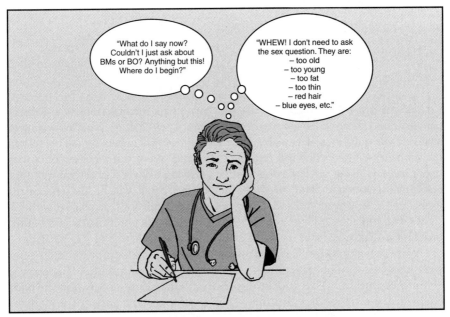

Figure 19–1. Students can be embarrassed to ask questions about sexuality.

Your Sexual Concerns

It is quite common for nurses to feel uncomfortable counseling patients with sexual issues. Some concerns include:

- Believing that you do not have the knowledge base or the skills that you need to respond to patients with sexual concerns.
- Feeling uncomfortable with your own sexuality and being afraid that you will not be able to handle the concerns of your patient.
- Believing that sex is something that you do not openly discuss with anyone.

All of these concerns can be dealt with. You need to be willing to work on opening yourself to learning more about sexuality.

Guiding Patients

To guide our patients, we have to ask questions. Don't be afraid to ask questions that relate to sexuality. If you don't ask, you will never know whether your patient has sexual concerns or not.

- Ask patients whether or not they have any sexual concerns.
- Ask how their illness has affected their sexuality.
- Ask if any of their medications are interfering with sexual performance.
- Ask if they have any questions or any concerns regarding changes in their sexuality.

To help patients with sexual concerns, you have to ask the questions. Many times, patients can read nurses' nonverbal behavior and know that they are *not* willing to answer their questions about sex. They sometimes test nurses by asking related questions to see how they will respond. They may point out a person on a soap opera and say, "That guy is having trouble satisfying his wife," and then wait for a response. If you say, "So," or, "That's too bad," that will be the end of the exchange. If, however, you say, "That must be difficult for him to deal with," it shows that you acknowledge the difficulty as well as the emotional aspects of the problem. Your patient may go on to discuss a problem that he or she is having.

We will never forget a student nurse who was watching a television show with her patient. The patient welcomed the student and said, "This show is about prostitution." The student responded, "Oh, I don't know how anybody could degrade themselves like that." She overlooked the patient's underlying message—the patient happened to have been a prostitute at one time. The relationship with the student was over. The patient would never ask the student another question because the student was obviously judgmental. Be careful about what you say, how you say it, and what your body says that you are not saying out loud.

Now you know that you need to be willing to ask questions and also examine your own beliefs about sexuality. To feel more comfortable about asking questions, you will need to develop a sexual knowledge base and also formulate a sexual history.

Developing a Knowledge Base

Most nursing schools will incorporate sexual information into nursing courses. For example, you might learn about taking a sexual history during your family (obstetrics–pediatrics) nursing course. You might learn about breast self-exam during a class on women and cancer. Some nursing schools will offer a nursing elective in sexuality.

Whether sexuality is a separate course or whether it is integrated into your other courses doesn't matter. It is essential that you learn the basics of sexual functioning so that you can provide accurate information to your patients. To determine what information your patient needs, you will need to formulate a sexual assessment. Before you begin a sexual assessment, it helps to know some of the things that will facilitate your accomplishing this goal. There are some

Table 19-1. Interviewing to Obtain Sexual Information—Some Do's and Don'ts	
Do	**Don't**
1. Obtain information about all needed areas.	1. Focus only on sexuality.
2. Provide privacy.	2. Obtain information when others are present or take copious notes.
3. Strive for an unhurried atmosphere.	3. Check your watch, tap your foot.
4. Maintain an attitude that is frank, open, warm, objective, empathetic.	4. Project discomfort, become defensive.
5. Use nondirective techniques when possible.	5. Ask many direct questions.
6. Have a prepared introduction to state purpose of interview.	6. Be vague about the purpose of the interview.
7. Use appropriate vocabulary.	7. Use street terms.
8. "Check out" words to ensure patient understands.	8. Assume the patient understands what you're saying.
9. Adjust the order of questions according to client's needs.	9. Follow a rigid format.
10. Give the client time to think and answer questions.	10. Answer questions for the patient.
11. Recognize signs of anxiety.	11. Focus on getting information without recognizing patient feeling.
12. Give permission not to do something.	12. Have preset expectations of the patient's sexual activity.
13. Listen in an interested but matter-of-fact way.	13. Overreact or underreact.
14. Identify your attitudes, values, beliefs, and feelings.	14. Project your concerns or problems onto the patient.
15. Identify significant others.	15. Assume that no one else is involved in the patient's sexual concerns.
16. Identify philosophic religious beliefs of patient.	16. Inflict your moral judgments on the patient.
17. Acknowledge when you don't have an answer to a question.	17. Pretend you know when you don't.

Source: Hogan, R. (1985). Human sexuality, a nursing perspective. *Reprinted by permission of Pearson Education, Inc. Upper Saddle River, NJ 07458.*

skills that you can develop that can help you get the most out of your assessment (Table 19–1). Typically, a nursing history will include information about sexuality. Some questions that you might want to include in a nursing history are found in Table 19–2. The information in this table will help you include basic sexual information during the nursing history. It is also important to include information that is specific to females and males (Table 19–3). There are

Table 19–2. Data to Be Collected by Nursing History for All Patients

Age	Identifies period in life cycle.	In what year were you born (month, day)?
Gender	Each gender may react differently to life events. Highlight gender identity problems.	[Usually is evident by dress, otherwise:] What sex do you consider yourself to be?
Education, occupation	Sexual practices may be related to education–socioeconomic class; change in occupation may contribute to role disturbances.	How far did you go in school? What do you do for a living? What change has there been in your ability to do your job?
Significant others	Other sources of support, stable or otherwise.	What persons do you consider most helpful right now? In what way? Are they available?
Quality of relationship with significant others	Relationship may be supportive, negative, or punitive, and these affect ability to cope with sexual problems.	Are there any differences in the way you get along with these people since you have been ill or hospitalized (or recently)?
Interests, hobbies	Indicates other support systems and avocational interest that contribute to self-esteem.	What do you do with your free time? What leisure and work activities are important to you? How are these being affected now?
Spiritual/ religious/ philosophical beliefs	Sexual practices may be related to beliefs. Guilt may occur if religious beliefs are compromised. Conflict and anxiety may be experienced by patient if different practices are suggested by nurse.	With what religious denomination are you affiliated? Can you describe any spiritual or other beliefs that are helpful to you now? Do you have or want the support of a clergyman (minister, priest, rabbi)?
Health problems, medical conditions, surgical procedures in past and anticipated in the future; medication therapy	Some medical problems, surgical treatment, or medications result in sexual dysfunction (physiologic changes). Anxiety over outcome or change in body image may lead to functional problems.	What illness and/or surgery have you had in the past? Did they affect your usual way of living or work? Did they affect sexual function? Do you expect this illness/hospitalization will have effects on your usual way of living or work? In what ways? What medications do you take?

Table 19–2. Data to Be Collected by Nursing History for All Patients (Continued)

Changes in role relationships and ability to carry out the usual sexual role	Change in ability to carry out what is perceived as the usual sexual role may cause anxiety, depression, and/or sexual dysfunction.	What difference has there been in your functioning in the family? Describe. Can you do your usual tasks or jobs? Describe. Have there been any changes in your relationship (with the way you get along) with others (male, female, significant others)?
Potential changes in ability to carry out usual sexual role	Expectations of problems may cause problems (self-fulfilling prophecy).	What changes do you expect after you get home (or in the future)?
Change in perception of self as male or female due to illness or life events	Anxiety and sexual dysfunction may result from threat to gender identify.	How do you expect this illness (or life event) to affect how you see yourself as a man/woman?
Existing or potential sexual dysfunction	Elicits problems (sexual dysfunction).	Has there been or do you expect to have any changes in sexual functioning (sex life) because of (illness, life events)? Describe.

Source: Hogan, R. (1985). Human sexuality, a nursing perspective. *Reprinted by permission of Pearson Education, Inc. Upper Saddle River, NJ 07458.*

a number of detailed sexual assessment forms that can be used for patients who are experiencing sexual dysfunction. However, individuals trained to deal with sexual problems generally use these assessment tools.

Normal Sexual Response

Following a sexual history, it is important for you to understand the basics of the normal sexual response. Although you will probably have learned about normal and abnormal male and female anatomy and physiology, sometimes little is offered about sexual functioning. According to Masters and Johnson (1966) there are four phases to the human sexual response cycle.

1. **Excitement:** When the individual becomes sexually excited by various stimuli. If for some reason the stimuli is withdrawn, then the cycle stops. If the stimulation continues, then the next phase is reached.

Table 19–3. Data to Be Collected About Sexual Function

Female	Male
1. Menstrual history: onset, duration, pain, number of pads, intermenstrual bleeding, discharge. Pregnancies: number of children, miscarriages, contraception, satisfaction with method.	1. Genitourinary problems: infections, penile discharge, pain with urination, difficulty initiating or nocturnal urination.
2. Sexual response: sufficient vaginal lubrication, pain with intercourse, frequency of coitus, achieve orgasm with intercourse or masturbation.	2. Sexual response: early morning erections, difficulty achieving or maintaining firm erection, change in sexual desire, volume of ejaculate.
3. Satisfaction with sexual response, partner's satisfaction.	3. Satisfaction with sexual response, partner's satisfaction.
4. Infections or venereal disease.	4. Infections or venereal disease.
5. Questions or problems they would like to discuss.	5. Questions or problems they would like to discuss.

Source: Hogan, R. (1985). Human sexuality, a nursing perspective. Reprinted by permission of Pearson Education, Inc. Upper Saddle River, NJ 07458.

2. **Plateau:** When sexual tension increases. This phase may be prolonged if the stimulation continues or shortened if the stimuli are withdrawn.
3. **Orgasm:** When sexual tension is released. It is important to note that this is entirely an involuntary response and is a total body reaction even though the most intense sensations are felt in the pelvic area in both males and females.
4. **Resolution:** Occurs following orgasm when the body returns to the pre-excitement state.

It is important to note that although males and females both experience the four phases of sexual arousal, they may experience them at different times (Figures 19–2 and 19–3). Note also that there is a refractory period in males. A female can immediately begin another sexual response cycle if adequately stimulated before sexual excitement totally resolves. However, the male requires a refractory period during which he cannot be restimulated. Usually, the length of the resolution period is similar to the length of the excitement phase. Also note that the female typically follows one of the three response cycles (A, B, or C in Figure 19–2). Males only have one (Masters & Johnson, 1966). In pattern A, the woman experiences multiple orgasms with a very short resolution period. In pattern B, the woman never reaches orgasm but has several peaks during the plateau stage and a prolonged resolution period. In pattern C, the woman experiences an interruption during the excitement phase with an intense orgasm and rapid resolution.

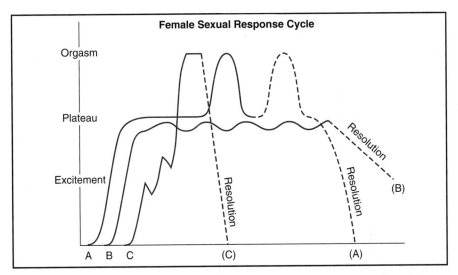

Figure 19–2. Female sexual response cycle. *(From Masters, W. H., & Johnson, V. E. [1966].* Human sexual response. *Boston, MA: Little Brown.)*

These differences in arousal can lead to sexual difficulty between partners if they are not understood. There have been cases of couples in counseling who were headed for divorce because they believed that if the man and woman do not have simultaneous orgasms, something is wrong with one or the other partner. Although simultaneous orgasms occasionally do occur, it is rare. Other couples have read that unless a woman experiences multiple orgasms,

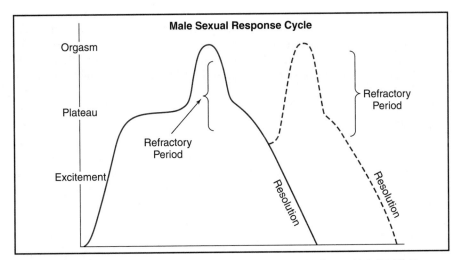

Figure 19–3. Male sexual response cycle. *(From Masters, W. H., & Johnson, V. E. [1966].* Human sexual response. *Boston, MA: Little Brown.)*

the man is not performing adequately. Although women are capable of having multiple orgasms, some do and some do not. These sexual concerns can lead to anxieties, anger, frustration, and eventually, termination of a relationship.

Illness and Sexuality

It is important for you to realize that there is a strong connection between illness and sexual functioning. Illness may cause a decline in the individual's physical abilities, a change in the individual's sense of maleness or femaleness, or a change in body image.

Many chronic illnesses have sexual repercussions. Some of the more common physical illnesses that cause sexual problems are:

1. **Diabetes:** Can cause impotence in males and frequent vaginal infections or orgasmic dysfunction in females.
2. **Arthritis:** The pain associated with arthritis can cause a decrease in desire for sex due to mobility problems or deformity.
3. **Spinal cord injuries:** The male will experience loss of sensation, but depending on the level of injury, he may still have an erection reflex. The female will experience a loss of sensation. Both males and females will find other areas of their bodies that cause sexual responses. Females may be able to get pregnant and carry a fetus to term. Males may benefit from various methods used to treat erectile dysfunction.
4. **Alcoholism:** Can lead to impotence and delayed ejaculation in males. Females can experience problems with sexual arousal and with decreased orgasmic frequency.
5. **Heart disease:** Can interfere with sexual functioning as a result of diminished blood flow, fatigue, or a decreased capacity for activity. Frequently, fear of another heart attack causes anxiety that can lead to sexual dysfunction.
6. **Cancer:** Can cause actual physical changes to sexual organs. Often causes changes in body image that can temporarily cause changes in sexual functioning.
7. **Gastrointestinal (GI) disorders:** Can result in an ostomy, which causes body image problems that cause temporary changes in sexual functioning.

Illnesses may cause specific physical changes, or they may cause a short-term lack of desire for sexual activity. At other times, the actual physical constraints forced on an individual by the environment may cause changes in sexuality. For example, hospitalization, diagnostic testing, and being separated from loved ones may all interfere with a person's normal sexual functioning.

For individuals who must be confined for long periods of time, day passes or other means of providing an outlet for sexual energy are suggested. Most long-term facilities can provide the time and privacy necessary for masturbation or sexual relations. We think that it is essential that we provide patients with an opportunity to maintain a sense of intimacy with their loved ones. Between illness and long-term confinement, we tend to strip all intimacy away. Intimacy is a basic need that we all share.

Caring for Patients with Sexual Concerns

You will have many patients who have sexual concerns. Some of these patients will approach you with questions, others will wait for you to question them. Please remember to include at least one question about sexuality in all of your assessments. This will help you to determine if you should follow up with other questions. As stated earlier, your willingness to address sexual issues will enable your patients to confide in you.

Nurses are in an excellent position to help most patients deal with sexual problems. Most sexual dysfunctions are the result of a lack of knowledge or inaccurate information. Consider how many of us learn about sexuality from our friends or the media. We are often too embarrassed to discuss sexuality with our parents, and some parents are too embarrassed to discuss sexuality with their children. As a result, many of us reach adulthood with little more than bits and pieces of information that we try to make sense of.

Many couples experience anxiety because they fear that they are "not normal." Sometimes, nurses can provide a small amount of seemingly obvious information about sexuality that can provide them with reassurance.

Medication Pointers

Nurses have an opportunity to provide patients with accurate information about medications and sexual functioning. For example, a patient once presented nine months pregnant even though she "was taking the pill daily." Upon further questioning, we discovered that the patient had inserted her birth control pills vaginally instead of orally. Many patients will be taking medications that interfere with sexual functioning. Again, the nurse is in a unique position to provide patients with information about medications and how they might cause problems.

- It is important for you to know about the effects of medications on sexuality. For example, over-the-counter antihistamines can cause vaginal dryness and subsequent pain during intercourse.
- Many medications cause decreased libido and erectile dysfunction. Some cause an increase in libido.
- If you are not sure of how a medication might effect sexual functioning, check your drug book or the *Physician's Desk Reference* (PDR) or check with a pharmacist.

- Let your patient know what to expect. All too often, a patient stops taking a medication and never informs the doctor of the real reason. How many patients do you know who are noncompliant with blood pressure medications because they cause impotence?
- Patients need to know that other medications are available that may not have the same side effects.

The following is a list of some medications that interfere with sexual functioning.

ANTICHOLINERGIC MEDICATIONS

Be aware that any medication that causes a dry mouth can cause sexual dysfunction. Most cause erectile failure and inhibit vaginal lubrication that can lead to dyspareunia (painful intercourse) and orgasmic dysfunction. Some of those medications include:

- Artane
- Atarax
- Atropine
- Antispas
- Anaspaz
- Benadryl
- Bentyl
- Cytospaz
- Kemedrin
- Norflex
- Pro-Banthine
- Procyclid
- Scopolamine
- THAM or THAM-e

ANTIHYPERTENSIVE MEDICATION

Antihypertensive drugs frequently cause sexual dysfunction. Most can cause decreased libido, delayed ejaculation or ejaculatory incompetence, and erectile failure. (Note that some patients will experience sexual dysfunction as a result of their hypertension.) All patients taking antihypertensive medications need to be questioned thoroughly about sexual side effects. One of the major problems with hypertension is noncompliance with medications. Although often unwilling to broach the subject, many patients discontinue use due to sexual side effects. If asked, patients will often admit to an inability to have satisfying sexual relations. The patient should be encouraged to speak with the doctor because there are many different medications available. The patient may experience fewer problems on a different drug. Antihypertensive drugs include:

- Aldactone
- Aldomet
- Catapres
- Dibensyline
- Inderal
- Ismelin
- Serpasil

NEUROLEPTICS

Most neuroleptic (antipsychotic) medications cause orgasmic dysfunction, ejaculatory incompetence, and erectile failure. Noncompliance with these drugs is common. If possible, patients need to be asked about sexual side effects and whether their noncompliance is due to these effects. Some of the newer medications (Clozaril, Respiradol) may not have the same sexual side effects but further study is needed. Neuroleptics include:

- Haldol
- Mellaril (frequently causes menstrual irregularities, gynecomastia, inhibited ejaculation, and vaginal dryness)
- Prolixin
- Serentil
- Teractin
- Thorazine

MOOD ACTIVE DRUGS

Lithium may cause erectile failure and ejaculatory incompetence.

Tricyclic antidepressants can cause erectile failure and ejaculatory incompetence. These drugs include:

- Anafranil (may cause spontaneous orgasm in women)
- Elavil
- Norpramin
- Pamelor
- Tofranil

Serotonin reuptake inhibitors (SSRIs) have fewer side effects and mild anticholinergic effects. These drugs include:

- Luvox
- Paxil
- Prozac
- Zoloft

Atypical antidepressants have fewer sexual side effects and include:

- Desyrel (can cause priapism [sustained erection], which is a medical emergency. If not treated immediately, it can result in irreversible impotence.)
- Effexor
- Serzone
- Wellbutrin

Monoamine oxidase inhibitors (MAOIs) cause impotence and ejaculatory difficulties as well as delayed orgasm in women. They include:

- Eutonyl
- Nardil
- Parnate

Tranquilizers affect the central nervous system (CNS). Changes in the CNS will cause changes in sexual functioning. Tranquilizers include:

- Alcohol (causes erectile failure)
- Librium (causes erectile failure and delayed ejaculation or ejaculatory failure)
- Valium (causes decreased libido)

OTHER DRUGS

There are many other drugs that can affect sexual functioning. Unfortunately, not many drug books mention sexual side effects. It is always important to assess patients' responses to medication, including any unwanted sexual side effects.

- Baclofen causes erectile failure.
- Clofibrate causes erectile failure.
- Pondiman causes erectile failure and loss of libido.
- Tagamet causes erectile failure that can progress to impotence, which can remain even after the drug is discontinued. Tagamet also causes a decrease in sperm count, which is important information for those concerned about fertility.

STREET DRUGS

Some street drugs, such as marijuana and heroin, can cause erectile failure.

Severe Sexual Problems

Occasionally, you will encounter a patient with problems with sexual functioning that needs to be referred for further assessment.

- If a patient discloses a problem that is long term or severe, referral should be made to a qualified sex therapist.

- Refer patients who may have a physiological sexual problem.
- Refer patients who are the victims of family violence.
- Refer patients who have long-standing problems related to incest or rape.
- Refer patients to someone else if you are unwilling, or unable, to deal with sexual issues.

Work on developing a comfort level in dealing with questions of a sexual nature. However, if your lack of ability is detrimental to the patient, find another nurse who is more comfortable in dealing with sexual concerns. Take the time to observe the other nurse and learn to handle sexual concerns on your own. Remember when you couldn't start an IV? Remember the fear and feelings of inadequacy? Learning to deal with sexual concerns is like learning any new skill. It all takes practice!

20

Culture

■ Cultural Challenges

Nursing in the twenty-first century will bring with it many challenges not faced by our earlier colleagues. One challenge that we currently must deal with is providing care to individuals from varied cultural backgrounds. The 1990 United States Census revealed that 32 million residents did not speak English as their primary language. Additionally, when we look at the 1994 data from the United States Immigration and Naturalization Service (INS), we find that in that year, the INS admitted 804,400 immigrants and 22,119,000 nonimmigrants. Therefore, in 1994 alone there were 22,923,400 new individuals in the United States with cultures different from the European–American culture. Add to this number individuals from other countries who are already permanent residents, and one can quickly determine that on a daily basis, nurses will be interacting with patients with varied cultural backgrounds. (And this phenomenon of multiple cultures is not unique to the United States. Countries around the globe are also finding their populations becoming more heterogeneous.) As the number of individuals with varied cultural backgrounds began to increase over the years, nurses realized that care for one cultural group was not always appropriate for another group. Thus the development of **transcultural nursing,** an area of nursing that focuses on how cultural values, beliefs, and attitudes influence an individual's health behaviors and, in turn, delivery of health care.

A major goal of health education programs is to have graduates who are **"culturally competent"** or who give **"culturally specific"** or **"culturally** congruent" care. What do these phrases mean? The commonality among the various definitions is that nursing interventions for health promotion, maintenance, restoration, and palliation are delivered in a manner that blends—are congruent with—the individual's cultural background. This requires not only learning culture differences, but also respecting the differences.

Initially, health care workers are interested in biological variations among cultural groups. These include body build and structure, skin color and texture, and enzymatic and genetic variations (Spector, 2001). In addition, different cultural groups are prone to varied specific health problems (Table 20–1).

Although health care workers tend to be aware of biological variations, they are only vaguely aware of the influence culture has on an individual's response to events along the health–wellness continuum. And in fact, "when there is conflict between the provider's and the client's belief systems, the provider typically is unable to understand the conflict and, hence, usually finds ways of minimizing it" (Spector, 2001, p. 4). A few of the most prominent areas in which culture is often the basis of behaviors include:

- Birth rites
- Death rites
- Dietary beliefs and practices
- Time orientation
- Attitudes toward the elderly
- Personal space
- Infant feeding beliefs and habits
- Gender roles
- Social roles

Religious and cultural beliefs are often the foundation for the values and practices displayed in many of these behavioral areas.

When considering culture, two terms come to mind:

1. **Acculturation:** The process of acquiring the behaviors, attitudes, and values of a different culture.
2. **Assimilation:** When an individual, over time, gives up the values, traditions, and traditional ways of his or her native culture and conforms to the standards and behaviors of the new culture.

Like the health–wellness continuum, you will have patients from foreign countries who will be at various points on the acculturation–assimilation continuum which is illustrated in Figure 20–1. Note how the two lines overlap. During this overlapping time, individuals are experiencing and living between two cultures.

When you observe a patient from another culture who now accepts practices such as eating common American foods and wearing the latest

Table 20–1. Examples of Biological Variations Among a Select Number of Ethnic Groups

African (Black) Americans	Asian/Pacific Islander Americans	American Indians, Aleuts, and Eskimos	Hispanic Americans	European (White) Origin Americans
Sickle-cell anemia	Hypertension	Accidents	Diabetes mellitus	Breast cancer
Hypertension	Liver cancer	Heart disease	Parasites	Heart disease
Cancer of the esophagus	Stomach cancer	Cirrhosis of the liver	Coccidioidomycosis	Diabetes mellitus
	Coccidioidomycosis	Diabetes mellitus	Lactose intolerance	Thalassemia
Stomach cancer	Lactose intolerance			
Coccidioidomycosis	Thalassemia			
Lactose intolerance				

Source: Adapted from Spector, R. E. (2000). Cultural Care Guides to Heritage Assessment and Health Traditions. Reprinted by permission of Pearson Education, Inc. Upper Saddle River, NJ 07458.

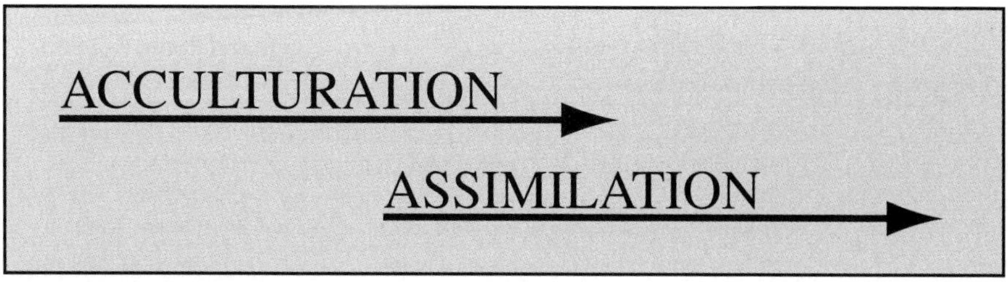

Figure 20–1. Acculturation–assimilation continuum.

trendy American clothes, you probably see this as evidence that the patient has adopted the ways of his or her new culture and is fully assimilated. However, when this patient shows no interest in learning about health needs and self-care, you may become very frustrated. You have failed to realize that in some cultures, health care is centered around one family member. Therefore, the individual has no reason to learn self-care. You have misplaced the client's position on the acculturation–assimilation continuum. Table 20–2 presents examples of health beliefs and practices held by several different cultures.

So, how long does it take for an individual to become "Americanized"? Generally, the process covers two generations and follows this sequence:

- **First generation:** Adult immigrants arrive with a "basket" that is full to the brim with values, beliefs, and attitudes of their home country. Over the years, selected traditional items from the basket are discarded and replaced with the American counterparts as adjustment to the new environment is made.
- **Second generation:** Eventually, these immigrants have a child and the child inherits the basket with its mixed contents. As this child grows, more traditional, cultural items are replaced.
- **Third generation:** Eventually, the second child has a child whose basket contains mostly American values, beliefs, and attitudes. By the time this child (grandchild of the original immigrants) reaches adulthood, the few remaining traditional cultural patterns have been discarded from the basket and the individual is functioning fully as an American.

It takes time to adjust to a new and different culture. Many nurses are very surprised to learn that not all individuals believe that illness is due to physical or biological problems that can be altered by humans. For example, most Americans view a fever, sore throat, and cough as due to some "bug." They go to a physician who gives them a medication that alters the bug in some way and they are better. Andrews and Boyle (1995) point out that in addition to this **biomedical–scientific** view of health and illness, there are two other major views.

Table 20–2. Comparison of Health Beliefs and Practices of Specific Cultural Groups

Subculture	Concepts of Health	Origins of Illness	Type of Healer, Prevention, and Healing Practices
African American	Health is measured by one's ability to work. React to poor health only when there is a crisis, such as high fever or bleeding.	Illness may be punishment from God for wrongdoing, or is due to voodoo, spirits, or demons.	Prevention through good diet, rest, cleanliness, and laxatives to clean the system. Wear copper and silver bracelets to prevent illness. Also use some herbs. Some believe in voodoo and religious healing.
Hispanic American	Health is a gift from God, and is also due to good luck. Healthy person has robust appearance and feels well.	Illness may be punishment from God for wrongdoing; or caused by an imbalance between "hot" and "cold" properties of the body.	*Curandero* cures hot illness with cold medicine and vice versa. Illness is prevented by eating well, praying, being good, working, and wearing religious medals.
Asian/ Pacific Island American	Health involves the balance of *yin* and *yang* (negative and positive energy forces). Healthy body is gift from parents and ancestors.	Illness is caused by imbalance of *yin* and *yang*.	Healers include herbalist, spiritual healer, and physician. Food is essential for harmony with nature and is important in cause and treatment of disease. Acupuncture and moxibustion restore balance of yin and yang. Herbal remedies, such as ginseng, are also used.
Native American	Health is harmony between the individual, Earth, and the supernatural, as well as the ability to survive difficult circumstances.	Illness is disharmony and can be caused by violation of taboos, witchcraft, displeasing holy people, annoying the elements, disturbing plant and animal life, neglecting the celestial bodies, or misusing sacred Native American ceremony.	Healer is the medicine man. Illness is prevented through elaborate religious rituals and charms consisting of fetishes and pollen carried in a bag. Medicine and religion are closely related. Do not believe in the germ theory.

Source: Berger, K. J., & Williams, M. B. (1999). Fundamentals of nursing: Collaborating for optimal health *(2nd ed.). Stamford, CT: Appleton & Lange.*

Personal Care and Family Life	Use of Health Care Delivery System	Health Problems	Death and Dying
African-based family with large extended families, flexible family roles and responsibilities. Strong religious orientation.	May receive inadequate health care. May experience segregation and racism when seeking care. Often use home remedies because of effectiveness and also because they are less expensive.	Hypertension, sickle-cell anemia, some cancers (e.g., lung, oral). High infant—maternal mortality, drug and alcohol abuse, obesity, and AIDS.	Believe in life after death.
Extended family is important. Value helping each other. Patriarchal family, with men making all decisions. Family honor is important. Children are a great source of pride.	Experience barriers to health care because of language (inability to speak English). May seek care from a physician, a folk practitioner, or both. May be late or miss appointments for care because of present time orientation.	Poverty-related diseases, such as tuberculosis, malnutrition, lead poisoning, and drug addiction.	View death and dying as "God's will." Believe in rewards from God in afterlife for good behavior.
Patriarchal family. Women are subservient to men. Ancestor worship and respect and obedience to parents are observed. Divorce is considered a disgrace.	Language barriers may exist: family spokesman may accompany client to Western physician. Prefer physicians from own cultural group if available in the community. May resist painful diagnostic tests. Having to have blood drawn is upsetting.	Respiratory diseases, immunization deficiencies, dental caries, tuberculosis, lactose intolerance.	Believe in reincarnation.
Extended family and tribal ties are strong. Cooperation is emphasized within the family and tribe.	Speak tribal language and may not understand English. Often seek care from medicine man first. General beliefs incompatible with those of health care system. Native Americans living in the eastern United States and most urban areas are not covered by the Indian Health Service.	Cirrhosis of the liver, alcoholism, high infant mortality, shortened life span, suicide, homicide, domestic violence. Leading causes of death are heart disease, accidents, malignant neoplasms, and cirrhosis.	Fear spirits of the dead. Children and family should be with dying person. Many rules and customs surround the dying. Do not believe in life after death.

Two Major Views of Health and Illness

1. **Magicoreligious:** Health and illness are in the control of a force beyond nature such as a god or gods; that health is restored as the result of a supernatural agent.
2. **Holistic:** Health results from a balance and harmony with nature. If this balance is disrupted, the result is illness.

Thus, if nurses were to interact with all patients assuming that they subscribed to the biomedical perspective of illness, this would probably result in inadequate nursing interventions for patients who hold another view.

One nursing intervention that frequently offers a great challenge is adjusting an individual's culturally determined dietary practices to conform to a health need. Because food has such significance beyond providing sustinance for the body for all cultures, altering dietary habits to meet health care needs can at times seem like an impossible task. Keithley, Keller, and Vazquez (1996) have provided a unique way to use the Food Guide Pyramid as a foundation for patients with different cultural and ethnic food preferences (Figures 20–2 and 20–3).

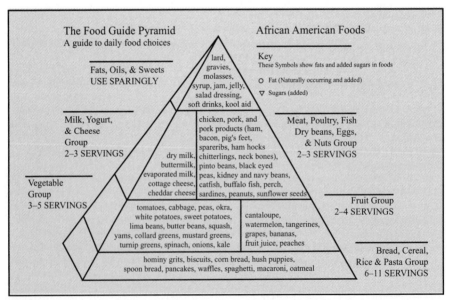

Figure 20–2. The Food Guide Pyramid: African American foods. (*From Keithley, J. K., Keller, A., & Vazquez, M. G. (1996). Promoting good nutrition: Using the food pyramid in clinical practice.* MEDSURG Nursing, 5(6): 401. Reprinted with permission of the publisher, Jannetti Publications, Inc.)

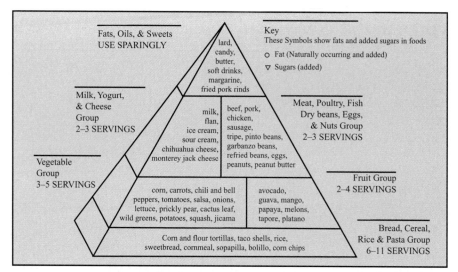

Figure 20–3. The Food Guide Pyramid: Mexican American foods. *(From Keithley, J. K., Keller, A., & Vazquez, M. G. (1996). Promoting good nutrition: Using the food pyramid in clinical practice.* MED-SURG Nursing, 5(6): 401. *Reprinted with permission of the publisher, Jannetti Publications, Inc.)*

Therefore, to give culturally sensitive and competent nursing care, knowledge of many aspects of a particular ethnic group is essential. However, beware of the trap of assuming that because your patient belongs to a specific cultural or ethnic group, they believe and act like the group. The word for this assumption is *stereotyping*, also known as *generalizing*. If you fall into this trap, you will make some grave errors and the quality of care to your patients will be substandard.

So, how do you avoid the trap and give culturally competent care? Here are the basic steps required to answer that question.

1. **Learn about your own heritage and culture.** Because you have grown up and have been socialized into a cultural environment, it may seem to you that you do not have a heritage basket. But you do have a basket, and analysis of its current and past contents will expand your horizons.
2. **Recognize that you are also a part of the health care provider culture with its own beliefs and practices.** Table 20–3 provides a brief outline of this culture. Note how the headings can be compared to belief and practice headings used to describe cultures in most literature.
3. **Come to terms with ethnocentrism, the belief that some, if not all, of the values and ways of behaving of your culture or ethnic group are better that of another group.** This can be a destructive force and can interfere with competent care. Yet, it is often an unconscious and pervasive force in delivery of health care.

> **Table 20–3.** Characteristics of the Health Care Provider's Culture

1. Beliefs
   a. Standardized definitions of health and illness
   b. The omnipotence of technology
2. Practices
   a. The maintenance of health and the protection of health or prevention of disease through such mechanisms as the avoidance of stress and the use of immunizations
   b. Annual physical examinations and diagnostic procedures, such as Pap smears
3. Habits
   a. Charting
   b. Constant use of jargon
   c. Use of a systematic approach and problem-solving methodology
4. Likes
   a. Promptness
   b. Neatness and organization
   c. Compliance
5. Dislikes
   a. Tardiness
   b. Disorderliness and disorganization
6. Customs
   a. Professional deference and adherence to the pecking order found in autocratic and bureaucratic systems
   b. Handwashing
   c. Employment of certain procedures attending birth and death
7. Rituals
   a. Physical examination
   b. Surgical procedure
   c. Limiting visitors and visiting hours

Source: Spector, R. E. (2000). Cultural diversity in health illness (5th ed.). Reprinted by permission of Pearson Education, Inc. Upper Saddle River, NJ 07458.

4. **Research information about your patient's cultural background.** This will probably mean that you should add at least one book on transcultural nursing to your personal library (see additional reading list at end of chapter).
5. **Assess where your individual patient fits on the acculturation–assimilation continuum.** Several formal assessment tools are available to help

you do this (Table 20–4 and Figure 20–4). Also, if you are in the patient's home, use the information that your senses of sight, hearing, and smell provide. These senses may give clues to cultural practices of the members of the household.

6. **Carefully analyze your patient's health behaviors.** Are they truly detrimental to the patient's health or just different from your own or the health care provider culture? This may be a very difficult question to honestly answer because our individual ethnocentric traits often cloud our analysis!

In addition, you face many challenges when you and your patient speak different languages, both with and without an interpreter. When you converse in English with the patient or interpreter, be very conscious of the words you use. You already know the pitfalls of speaking "Nurse-ese" to patients. But, are you aware of your use of idioms and colloquialisms? To English-speaking people, they are natural and immediately placed in context and understood. However, we would like to add a personal experience regarding this type of miscommunication.

One of us participated as an instructor in a literacy project helping adults to speak and read English as a second language. Before class formally began one evening, the instructor said, "Boy, it sure rained cats and dogs yesterday."

Table 20–4. Cultural Assessment of Health Care Practices

- What has made you ill?
- What do you ordinarily do to keep well or take care of yourself?

  Special diet
  Herbs
  Rituals
  Amulets
  Other

- What drugs, tablets, or foods did you use or are you using? What did you use them for?
- What ceremonies or rituals do you perform to get well?
- Who took care of you when you were sick?
- What did he or she do for you when you were sick?
- When did you last see this person?
- Will you take medication from me today?

Information compiled from Berger, K. J., & Williams, M. B. (1999). Fundamentals of nursing: Collaborating for optimal health. *Reprinted by permission of Pearson Education, Inc. Upper Saddle River, NJ 07458.*

Heritage Assessment Tool

This set of questions can be used to investigate a given client's or your own ethnic, cultural, and religious heritage.

It can help you to perform a heritage assessment to determine how deeply a given person identifies with a particular *tradition*. It is most useful in setting the stage for understanding a person's HEALTH traditions. The greater the number of positive responses, the greater the person's identification with a traditional heritage. The one exception to positive answers is the question about family name change. This question may be answered negatively.

1. Where was your mother born? _____

2. Where was your father born?_____

3. Where were your grandparents born? _____
    a. Your mother's mother?_____
    b. Your mother's father? _____
    c. Your father's mother? _____
    d. Your father's father? _____

4. How many brothers_____ and sisters _____ do you have?

5. What setting did you grow up in? Urban _____ Rural _____
    Suburban _____

6. What country did your parents grow up in?
    Father_____
    Mother _____

7. How old were you when you came to the United States? _____

8. How old were your parents when they came to the United States?
    Mother _____
    Father_____

9. When you were growing up, who lived with you?_____
    _____

10. Have you maintained contact with
    a. Aunts, uncles, cousins?   (1) Yes _____   (2) No _____
    b. Brothers and sisters?   (1) Yes _____   (2) No _____
    c. Parents?   (1) Yes _____   (2) No _____
    d. Your own children?   (1) Yes _____   (2) No _____

11. Did most of your aunts, uncles, cousins live near your home?
    (1) Yes_____   (2) No _____

12. Approximately how often did you visit your family members who lived outside your home?
    (1) Daily_____   (2) Weekly _____   (3) Monthly _____
    (4) Once a year or less _____   (5) Never _____

13. Was your original family name changed?
    (1) Yes_____   (2) No _____

Figure 20–4. Heritage assessment tool. (*From Spector, R. E. [2000]. Cultural Care Guides to Heritage Assessment and Health Traditions. Reprinted by permission of Pearson Education, Inc. Upper Saddle River, NJ 07458.*)

14. What is your religious preference?
    (1) Catholic _____   (2) Jewish_____
    (3) Protestant _____   Denomination _____
    (4) Other _____   (5) None _____

15. Is your spouse the same religion as you?
    (1) Yes_____   (2) No _____

16. Is your spouse the same ethnic background as you?
    (1) Yes_____   (2) No _____

17. What kind of school did you go to?
    (1) Public _____   (2) Private_____   (3) Parochial_____

18. As an adult, do you live in a neighborhood where the neighbors are the same religion and ethnic background as yourself?
    (1) Yes_____   (2) No _____

19. Do you belong to a religious institution?
    (1) Yes_____   (2) No _____

20. Would you decribe yourself as an active member?
    (1) Yes_____   (2) No _____

21. How often do you attend your religious institution?
    (1) More than once a week _____   (2) Weekly_____
    (3) Monthly_____   (4) Special holidays only _____
    (5) Never_____

22. Do you practice your religion in your home?
    (1) Yes_____   (2) No_____   (if yes, please specify)
    (3) Praying _____   (4) Bible reading _____
    (5) Diet _____   (6) Celebrating religious holidays _____

23. Do you prepare foods of your ethnic background?
    (1) Yes_____   (2) No _____

24. Do you participate in ethnic activities?
    (1) Yes_____   (2) No_____   (if yes, please specify)
    (3) Singing _____   (4) Holiday celebrations_____
    (5) Dancing _____   (6) Festivals _____
    (7) Costumes _____   (8) Other _____

25. Are your friends from the same religious background as you?
    (1) Yes_____   (2) No _____

26. Are your friends from the same ethnic background as you?
    (1) Yes_____   (2) No _____

27. What is your native language?

28. Do you speak this language?
    (1) Prefer _____   (2) Occasionally_____   (3) Rarely _____

29. Do you read your native language?
    (1) Yes_____   (2) No _____

Figure 20–4. (Continued)

This made sense to the instructor but not the students! They understood the individual words but not the meaning.

We have hundreds of such phrases in the English language. Based on where your patient is on the acculturation–assimilation continuum, the use of idioms can be very confusing and frustrating to the patient. Thus, providing culturally competent care to your patients will not come naturally. It will require work on your part. The rewards, however, are great.

Books to Consider Adding to Your Personal Library

Andrews, M. M., & Boyle, J. S. (1995). *Transcultural Concepts in Nursing Care* (2nd ed.). Philadelphia: J.B. Lippincott.

Geissler, E. M. (1994). *Pocket Guide to Cultural Assessment*. St. Louis, MO: Mosby.

Spector, R. E. (2000). *Cultural Diversity in Health and Illness* (5th ed.) and companion, *Culture Care Guides to Heritage Assessment and Health Traditions*. Upper Saddle River, NJ: Prentice Hall Health.

Fadiman, A. (1997). *The Spirit Catches You and You Fall Down*. New York: Farra, Straus and Giroux.

RESOURCE WEB SITES

American Holistic Nurses' Association, *www.ahna.org*
DiversityRX, *www.diversityrx.org/HTML/DIVRX.htm*

21

Alternative Therapies

Use of Alternative Therapies

Many health care consumers today rely on some form of alternative therapy. Consumers often use a combination of traditional medicine and alternative or complementary medicine. A recent study in a Brooklyn, New York, hospital found that 56% of patients had, at one time, used some form of alternative therapy. Eighty-seven percent believed that the therapy they used had helped. The most common alternative treatments used were: massage (31%), chiropractic (30%), herbs (24%), meditation (18%), acupuncture (15%), and hypnosis (10%). The essential thing that nurses need to be aware of is that 70% of these patients did not inform their physician that they had used alternative therapy. This is important because herbs and supplements in particular are the most likely to cause problems by interacting with medications and causing serious side effects (Drug Watch, 2000).

What is alternative therapy? You may have heard the terms alternative or complementary therapy (medicine) used to describe many forms of treatment, but the most common are:

- Herbs and nutritional supplements
- Chiropractic manipulation
- Homeopathy
- Acupuncture
- Mind–body techniques
  - Yoga
  - Meditation
  - Hypnotherapy
  - Biofeedback
  - Movement-oriented therapy

185

Most patients use alternative treatments in addition to conventional medical treatment rather than as a substitute for it. Alternative treatments are a way for patients to take some control and make some decisions about their own health care. Unfortunately, some mainstream physicians still ascribe to the "I'm the doctor, therefore, I know the answers, you will do what I tell you to do," rather than including the patient in the decision-making process.

Let's consider how the American public has embraced alternative therapies:

- In 1992, the National Institutes of Health (NIH) established the Office of Alternative Medicine. In 1998, the NIH made the office a National Center for Complementary and Alternative Medicine (NCCAM). This gave NCCAM a much larger budget as well as the power to direct its own research. In 1999, the National Cancer Institute established its own Office of Complementary and Alternative Medicine.
- In an attempt to regulate herbs and supplements, the Food and Drug Administration (FDA) wanted to place them in the same category as pharmaceuticals. This would have given the FDA the ability to limit consumer access to herbs and supplements. In 1994, Congress passed the Dietary Supplement Health and Education Act (DSHEA), which allows manufacturers of supplements to sell products and make some claims on the packaging with little intervention by the FDA.
- In 1999, 67% of health maintenance organizations (HMOs) offered at least one type of alternative treatment.

Although alternative treatments have been widely accepted by the American public, they are not without their problems. Herbs and supplements tend to cause the most problems with regard to conventional medicine for the following reasons:

A CASE IN POINT

Mrs. Dean, a 75-year-old grandmother, is seen by a parish nurse during a blood pressure screening at St. Ann's Catholic Church. The nurse finds that Mrs. Dean has a blood pressure reading of 90/58. The nurse asks Mrs. Dean if she is taking any antihypertensive medications or any other medications. Mrs. Dean responds that she does take blood pressure medication and she also takes several herbs to control her blood pressure as well. After listing all of the medication and herbs that Mrs. Dean is taking, the nurse asks if her doctor is aware of the herbs that she takes in addition to her other medications. Mrs. Dean answers that she tried to tell her doctor about them but that he "cut me off" and said, "I don't care about any of that trees and bark stuff, all I want to know is about your prescription medication." The nurse informs Mrs. Dean that she will contact the physician in order to clarify her medication order and explain that there is some concern because of Mrs. Dean's low blood pressure reading.

- **Lack of regulation.** In 1995, *Consumer Reports* studied ginseng and in 1999 they looked at ginkgo biloba and echinacea. In both studies, they found that there was a wide variation in the amount of herbs present in different brands and also in different bottles of the same brand.
- **Lack of research.** Although there is more research being done on certain herbs and supplements, the studies are not always as rigorous as they need to be.
- **Side effects.** Herbs and supplements can cause side effects just like any pharmaceutical drug.
- **Need for better communication.** Patients do not always inform their health care provider that they are taking herbs/supplements.

Some common herbal products can prolong the sedative effects of anesthesia and cause increased bleeding and fluctuations in blood pressure. Doctors and especially anesthesiologists need to be made aware of all medicines, over-the-counter drugs, and herbs and supplements that the patient is taking. Table 21–1 lists herbs that have been known to cause problems in surgery.

Be sure that you inform patients who are scheduled to undergo surgery to inform their health care providers of any herb or supplement use. Also, patients need to be told to stop taking herbal products and supplements at least 2 weeks prior to surgery.

A CASE IN POINT

Mr. Purdy was scheduled to undergo a bunionectomy as an outpatient procedure. He was seen the morning of surgery by the anesthesiologist who asked whether Mr. Purdy was taking any prescription or any other medication. Mr. Purdy said that he was not currently taking any medication of any kind. After the anesthesiologist left, Mrs. Purdy asked her husband about whether he should have told the doctor about the herbs he takes on a regular basis (ginkgo biloba, ginseng, and garlic, as well as vitamins C and E and a multivitamin). Mr. Purdy told his wife that the doctor was only asking about prescription medications. During surgery, the orthopedic surgeon noticed prolonged and excessive bleeding from the operative site. He became concerned and ordered a prothrombin time (PT) and partial thromboplastin time (PTT) (to check clotting factors). The surgeon discovered that Mr. Purdy had delayed clotting and was able to make adjustments in treatment. Following surgery, the surgeon discussed his findings with Mrs. Purdy and told her that in the future she and her husband need to make all doctors aware of not only prescription medication, but all medication, herbs, and supplements. The surgeon also warned them that a more extensive procedure could have led to disastrous results.

Table 21–1. Common Herbal Products Associated with Surgical Problems

Garlic	May increase bleeding and prevent clots from forming
Ginkgo biloba	May increase bleeding and prevent clots from forming
Ginger	May increase bleeding and prevent clots from forming
Ginseng	May increase bleeding and prevent clots from forming
Kava kava	Has a prolonged sedative effect
St. John's Wort	Has a prolonged sedative effect
Valerian	Has a prolonged sedative effect

Some of these same herbs and supplements, as well as others, can also have side effects. Patients need to be made aware of potential problems when relying on herbs and supplements. Table 21–2 lists some common herbs and supplements and the potential side effects or problems associated with their use.

Herbs and supplements also have many positive effects. With further controlled research studies and some regulation of the amount of herb present in each dose, herbs and supplements will be more widely accepted. According to Fontaine (2000), the following herbs and supplements have been found through research to have specific effects on certain conditions:

- Ginkgo has been found to improve memory, concentration, and confusion, as well as treating sexual dysfunction including erectile dysfunction, delayed ejaculation, anorgasmia, and decreased sex drive.
- St. John's Wort is effective in treating mild to moderate depression.
- Garlic lowers cholesterol levels and may lower diastolic blood pressure.
- Feverfew may be effective in preventing migraines.
- Topical capsaicin can be helpful in treating the pain of diabetic neuropathy and fibromyalgia.
- Saw palmetto improves urinary flow rates of men with mild to moderate benign prostatic hyperplasia.
- Echinacea enhances the immune system, helps reduce the side effects of cancer therapies, and also helps prevent and/or cure upper respiratory infections.
- Milk thistle may speed the production of new liver cells and slow entry of liver-damaging toxins.
- Ginger is helpful in treating nausea and vomiting associated with anesthesia, morning sickness, and motion sickness.
- Valerian has a positive effect on subjective quality of sleep.
- Cranberry has a positive effect on urinary tract infections.

Some of the more common herbs and their dosages and what they are used for are listed in Table 21–3.

Table 21–2. Common Herbs and Supplements and Their Side Effects

Astralagus	Should not be used with immune suppressing drugs or autoimmune disorders such as arthritis, lupus, and multiple sclerosis.
Beta carotene	Can increase the risk of lung cancer in smokers.
Echinacea	Should not be used by people with autoimmune disorders or those taking immune-suppressing drugs. Should only be taken for 7 to 10 days at first signs of illness, not for long periods of time.
Ephedra	Can increase blood pressure—can cause death (heart attacks, stroke, seizures) in healthy young people and is currently being considered for removal from the market in all forms including Ma Huang.
Feverfew	Can enhance the action of blood thinners and may cause severe bleeding.
Garlic	Can enhance the action of blood thinners and may cause severe bleeding.
Ginger	Can enhance the action of blood thinners and may cause severe bleeding.
Ginkgo biloba	Can enhance the action of blood thinners and may cause severe bleeding.
Ginseng	Can enhance the action of blood thinners and may cause severe bleeding. Can also increase blood pressure and decrease blood sugar.
Goldenseal	Should not be used by people with autoimmune disorders or those taking immune suppressing drugs. Should only be taken for 7 to 10 days at first signs of illness, not for long periods of time.
Kava kava	Should not be combined with alcohol or sedatives. Can worsen Parkinson's disease. With long-term use, can cause skin problems such as rash and dryness.
Licorice	Should not be taken with immune-suppressing drugs such as corticosteroids. May increase blood pressure.
Saw palmetto	Can partially block iron absorption from foods.
St. John's Wort	Can decrease the effectiveness of birth control pills. May interfere with asthma and heart medication as well as cyclosporin and blood thinners. Can also partially block iron absorption. Recent studies suggest that the use of St. John's Wort in combination with light therapy (frequently used to treat seasonal affective disorder [SAD]) may cause cataracts to form.
Valerian	Should not be combined with alcohol, antihistamines, sedatives, or barbiturates because of increased sleepiness and drowsiness.
Vitamin A	Has been linked to cleft palates, cleft lips, and birth defects of the brain and heart if taken during pregnancy.

Source: WHO monographs on selected medicinal plants v.1, World Health Organization. Geneva World Health Organization, 1999. CCASS Mark QV 766 99 WH.

Table 21-3. Common Herbs

Name	Properties/Use
Capsaicin	For tenderness and pain of osteoarthritis, fibromyalgia, diabetic neuropathy, shingles
Chamomile	For anxiety, stomach distress, stomach ulcers, infant colic, drug withdrawal
Chondroitin	Helps slow cartilage degradation in osteoarthritis
Echinacea	Antiviral, antibiotic for colds, flu, and other infections
Evening Primrose oil	For PMS, mastalgia, hypertension, multiple sclerosis, alcoholism
Feverfew	For prevention of migraines
Garlic	Antibiotic, antiviral, antifungal, anticoagulant; for any infection, hypertension, high blood lipid levels
Ginger	For nausea and vomiting of various causes, hypertension, high cholesterol; enhances insulin
Ginkgo	For attention and memory problems, headaches, tinnitus, intermittent claudication, erectile problems
Ginseng	For mood swings, improved physical performance, reduction of fasting blood glucose, stimulation of immune system, ease cocaine withdrawal
Glucosamine	Improves pain and movement in osteoarthritis
Goldenseal	Antibiotic, antiseptic, antiinflammatory for wound healing, colds and flu, hypertension, uterine bleeding, enhances insulin
Green tea	Antioxidant, protects against cancer, lowers cholesterol, helps regulate blood sugar and insulin levels
Kava	For anxiety, insomnia, low energy, muscle tension
Milk thistle	Antioxidant for all liver disorders; psoriasis

Form/Dose	Contraindications/Side Effects
Cream topically applied	May be a brief burning or stinging sensation with first use Wash hands after applying; avoid touching eyes
Infusion; Tincture: 1 teaspoon TID	NOT for those allergic to ragweed
400 mg TID	

400 mg for 5–14 days,
  peaks at 5 days
	NOT for people with autoimmune disease, NOT for
	  pregnant and lactating women
	Bitter taste

250–500 mg/day	
0.2% parthenolide 100–300 mg/day	NOT for use with prescription headache drugs NOT for use by pregnant and lactating women Chewing leaves can cause mouth sores and loss of taste; capsule preferred
Varying recommendations	NOT for people with clotting disorders May cause stomach upset

500–1,000 mg q 4 hrs
Motion sickness:
  1,500 mg 30 prior
	People taking anticoagulant should check with MD
	  prior to use

24% flavonoids and 6% terpenes. 60–80 mg TID or QID	May cause mild GI upset
200 mg BID. Minimum 4–6 weeks	NOT for use when acutely ill with cold or flu NOT to be used with hypoglycemia Nervousness, insomnia, euphoria, hypertension
500 mg TID	People taking diuretics may need higher doses of herb

2 capsules TID for
  maximum 3 weeks
	NOT for use during pregnancy—may cause premature
	  uterine contractions
	Only for short-term use; long-term use may irritate or
	  inflame mucosa

3–4 cups/day	NOT to be used in large quantities during pregnancy People with anxiety disorder or irregular heartbeat should limit use to no more than 2 cups daily
100 mg TID	In large amounts—intoxicating and potential for abuse
Varying recommendations	No known side effects

(Continued)

Table 21–3. Common Herbs (Concluded)

Name	Properties/Use
St. John's Wort	For mild to moderate depression, viral infections including HIV and herpes
Saw palmetto	Urinary antiseptic, for benign prostatic hyperplasia
Selenium	Antioxidant especially when combined with vitamin E, may prevent some types of tumors, aids in production of antibodies, protects liver
Tea tree oil	Antifungal, antiseptic, for acne, minor burns and cuts, athlete's foot, nail infections, herpes, douche for yeast infections
Valerian	For insomnia, muscle pain, menstrual and intestinal cramps, benzodiazepine withdrawal
Yohimbe	For decreased sex drive, erectile problems

As you can see, herbs and supplements have many positive benefits. Unfortunately, they can also cause problems. It is vital that you keep an open mind when talking with patients about their use of herbs and supplements. Be sure that you ask your patients if they are taking any, how much, and for what reason. In this way, you will be better able to keep the health care team informed and also be aware of any possible combined effect with conventional pharmaceuticals.

Other Alternative/ Complementary Therapies

You may already be familiar with some of the common alternative/complementary therapies (Table 21–4). Since none of these have the potential to cause the

Form/Dose	Contraindications/Side Effects
900 mg/day Minimum 4–8 weeks	NOT for pregnant and lactating women, not for children NOT for use with other antidepressants May cause photosensitivity; avoid foods with tyramine and OTC cold and flu remedies, amino acid supplements
160 mg BID	Use only after proper diagnosis from primary practitioner May cause dizziness, dry mouth, tachycardia, angina, testicular pain
200 µg	Metallic taste in mouth, garlicky breath odor Excessively high levels may lead to liver and kidney impairment
Full strength or dilute in water or oil	Do NOT ingest
400 mg before bed 0.5% essential oil	NOT to be used with alcohol Nonaddictive; bitter taste
Varying recommendations	NOT for people with hypertension, kidney disease NOT to be used with tyramines, OTC cold remedies, caffeine, amphetamines May cause hypertension, anxiety, panic attacks, hallucinations

Source: Fontaine, K. L. (1999). Healing practices: Alternative therapies for nursing. *Reprinted by permission of Pearson Education, Inc. Upper Saddle River, NJ 07458.*

problems that herbs and supplements may, we will give just a brief decription of each therapy. For further information about alternative or complementary therapies, see the resources listed at the end of this chapter.

Whether you take or use alternative/complementary therapies, be aware that many of your patients will. Be certain that when you care for patients in any setting, you ask about their use of alternative therapies. Be open-minded in your asking and be careful about making judgments, as patients will perceive your feelings and may not tell you everything you need to know about what therapies they are using. Alternative therapies are here to stay and their use will continue to grow. You need to learn more about them so that you can be informed and keep your patients safe.

Table 21–4. Other Forms of Alternative Therapies

Chiropractic	Chiropractors are licensed in 44 states and the District of Columbia although they are not allowed to prescribe medication. Chiropractic is a system of treating disease by physically manipulating the spinal column. The chiropractor believes that diseases are caused from pressure on the nerves due to faulty alignment of the vertebrae. As a result of this misalignment, many parts of the body, including internal organs, may not receive transmission from various nerves.
Homeopathy	Homeopathy is a system that was developed in the mid-1700s. Homeopaths give patients highly diluted natural remedies that, in larger doses, would cause the symptoms that the patient is having. This is thought to increase the body's ability to heal itself. Homeopaths study at homeopathic colleges and are not licensed.
Acupuncture	Acupuncture is widely accepted in Chinese medicine and is the practice of inserting tiny sharp needles into specific points along "meridians" that flow throughout the body. Acupuncture can be used to treat numerous painful conditions, induce anesthesia, and prevent or treat disease. Acupuncture is used to unblock or rectify an imbalance in the flow of chi that circulates throughout the body along the meridians. Many physicians are incorporating acupuncture into their practice as it becomes more widely accepted. Acupuncturists are licensed to practice, and a number of colleges exist within the United States.
Yoga	There are many different forms of yoga. They all use breath training and movement (a series of stretches and poses). Yoga can increase flexibility, improve balance, help improve breathing, and lower one's stress level. Yoga is a great form of exercise as well as therapeutic.
Meditation	There are many forms of meditation. Most use some focus on the here and now as well as breath control. Through meditation one learns to let go of worry and preoccupation and gain perspective. Most people use meditation to decrease stress although it has also been shown to slow breathing, heart rate, and oxygen consumption and ease muscle tension.
Biofeedback	Biofeedback is a learned process used to control autonomic bodily functions. This control is taught through the use of skin temperature, muscle tone, cardiovascular signs, or electroencephalogram. The patient practices the desired response under the supervision of a trained professional. Biofeedback has been used to successfully retrain muscles and treat insomnia, phobias, and some types of seizures.
Movement therapy	There are a number of therapies that focus on movement. Most focus on movement, body awareness, and breathing. The idea is to maintain health and also to correct specific problems. Most help to retrain the body to improve coordination and balance, release or change postural problems, and relieve structural or functional stress. Some types of movement therapy are Tai Chi, Feldenkrais Method, Trager Approach, and the Alexander Technique.

RESOURCE WEB SITES

Herbs/Supplements

American Botanical Council, *www.herbalgram.org*
American Herbalists Guild, *www.healthy.net/herbalists*
Herb Research Foundation, *www.herbs.org*
FDA site on dietary supplements,
http://vm.cfsan.fda.gov/~dms/supplement.html

Chiropractic

American Chiropractic Association, *www.amerchiro.org*
Federation of Chiropractic Licensing Boards, *www.fclb.org/fclb*

Acupuncture

www.acupuncture.com
www.medicalacupuncture.org
www.acupuncture.edu

Homeopathy

Homeopathic Educational Services, *www.homeopathic.com*
National Center for Homeopathy, *www.homeopathic.org*

Yoga

www.yogaclass.com/central.html
www.yogasite.com

Meditation

American Meditation Institute, *www.americanmeditation.org*
www.mindtools.com

Biofeedback

Biofeedback Certification Institute, *www.aapb.org*
Biofeedback Certification Institute of America, *www.bciaorg/*

RESOURCE WEB SITES (CONT.)

Massage/Movement Therapies

American Massage Therapy Association, *www.amtamassage.org*
Massage Network, *http://masagenetwork.com*
Feldenkrais Guild, *www.feldngld@peak.org*
Alexander Technique, *www.Alexandertech.com*
Trager Institute, *www.trageradmin@trager.com*

OTHER RESOURCES

Fontaine, K. L. (2000). *Healing practices: Alternative therapies for nursing.* Upper Saddle River, NJ: Prentice Hall.

22

Spirituality

Spirituality

All human beings are spiritual beings. We all have an inherent sense of meaning and understanding about the significance of our being human. Some of us attribute this sense of significance to a higher being and express a belief in God. Others derive this sense of significance from relationships with others and with the environment.

Some of us choose to express our spirituality in a formalized manner through affiliation with a specific religion; others believe that formalized religion gets in the way of their spiritual expression. Either way, spiritual well-being is an essential component of well-being in general. Spiritual beliefs can help people cope with life stressors and crises as well as provide a sense of purpose. Spiritual beliefs can also help us to develop a sense of inner tranquility that allows us to love and trust others and have an abiding sense of peace, hope, and faith. Physical illness forces all of us to face loss, fears, grief, our own mortality, and questions of meaning.

Our knowledge of research in health care has expanded to include the mind's role in the development of illness. Many health problems can be traced to an individual's lifestyle. Therefore, is it so unrealistic to think that a strong spiritual base can lead individuals toward health, and in some instances even a miraculous recovery?

Nurses often have difficulty recognizing and intervening when patients experience spiritual distress. We believe that this difficulty stems from feelings of discomfort and lack of information about how to intervene. Some nurses would rather refer all matters of a spiritual nature to a minister, priest, or rabbi. Unfortunately, many patients are unable to time their spiritual distress to coincide with a visit from a spiritual advisor. Some nurses also believe that in order to assist a patient in spiritual distress they must be of the same religion. A similar problem is that health care providers sometimes believe that science and religion "do not mix."

Another difficulty in dealing with spiritual distress is that it tends to remind us of our own human frailty. For us to feel comfortable, we must first confront our own limitations. We must accept that illness, suffering, and death are all natural occurrences of the human condition. We must also come to terms with our own spirituality. What are your beliefs? What gives you a sense of hope, peace, and spiritual well-being? Only after answering these questions for ourselves can we begin to help patients.

Behaviors Suggestive of Spiritual Distress

Individuals will express spiritual distress differently. If the nurse does not specifically ask about spiritual concerns, the patient may be unwilling to bring them up. There are certain behaviors that may be suggestive of spiritual distress and may require referral to a spiritual leader. According to Murray and Zentner (2001, p. 148), consider referring a patient who exhibits any of the following behavior patterns:

- Withdrawn, sullen, silent, depressed
- Restless, irritable, complaining
- Restless, excitable, garrulous, wants to talk a lot
- Shows by word or other signs undue curiosity and anxiety about self
- Takes a "turn for the worse," critical, terminal
- Shows conversational interest, curiosity in religious questions, issues; reads religious materials
- Specifically inquires about a chaplain, chapel worship, religious materials
- Has few or no visitors; has no cards or flowers
- Has had, or faces, particularly traumatic or threatening surgical procedure

Most larger hospitals have chaplains that are on duty 24 hours a day. You should familiarize yourself with what spiritual avenues of referral are available at your facility. Facilities also have chapels available and other spiritual leaders are available through telephone contact. Consider contacting someone if the patient is going through any major trauma. Even if the patient doesn't need someone to talk with, the family or friends might.

Questions for Spiritual Assessment

To help patients deal with spiritual distress, it is important to first assess what their beliefs are. It is important to determine what spiritual and religious beliefs patients have and how these beliefs relate to their current health situation. There are many spiritual assessment forms available. Murray and Zentner (2001, p. 141) recommend that the following questions be used for spiritual assessment.

It is important for you to intervene when patients experience spiritual distress because it allows you to gain deeper insights into your patients' experiences. It can also allow you to share in the awesome life experiences of birth, death, illness, and recovery. Sharing in these life experiences and emotions

1. What is your concept of God? What is your God like? (Or, what is your religion? Tell me about it.)
2. Do you believe that God or someone is concerned for you?
3. Who is the most important person to you? Is that person available?
4. Has being sick (what has been happening to you) made any difference in your feelings about God? In the practice of your faith? If it has, could you explain how it has changed?
5. Do you believe that your faith is helpful to you? If it is, how? If it is not, why not?
6. Are there any religious beliefs, practices, or rituals that are important to you now? If there are, could you tell me about them? May I help you carry them out by showing you where the chapel is? By telling the dietary department about your vegetarian preference? By allowing you specific times for prayer or meditation?
7. Is there anything that would make your situation easier? (Such as a visit from the minister, priest, rabbi, or chaplain? Someone who would read to you? Time for reading your religious book or praying? Someone to pray with you?)
8. Is prayer important to you? (If so, has being sick made a difference in your practice of praying?) What happens when you pray?
9. Do you have available religious books or articles such as the Bible, prayer books, phylacteries, or a crucifix that mean something to you?
10. What are your ideas about illness? About life after death?
11. Is there anything especially frightening or meaningful to you right now?
12. If these questions have not uncovered your source of spiritual support, can you tell me where you do find support?

Source: Murray, R., & Zentner J. (2001). Health promotion strategies through the life span (7th ed.). Reprinted by permission of Pearson Education, Inc. Upper Saddle River, NJ 07458.

with your patients will help you further develop your role as patient advocate. You will develop a more accurate perception of exactly what the patient needs and desires. Another reason to intervene in spiritual distress is that you will allow the patient to express spiritual pain that can help in healing that individual's spirit. This healing of the spirit can occur long after the need for technology and physical care has subsided.

Prayer is one of the most significant spiritual experiences for the majority of people. According to a 1997 Gallup survey, over 90% of Americans pray daily and believe that prayer has an effect on their lives (Bacon, 1995; Byrd & Sherrill, 1995; Dossey, 1994; Hughes, 1997). A number of research studies have suggested that prayer can speed healing. Praying for and with patients are two of the most direct ways for nurses to be involved in patients' spiritual experiences. Other ways of being involved include reading spiritual books with or to your patient, providing quiet time for meditation and prayer, and being certain that religious articles are close at hand. Remember, your patient may belong to one of the religions listed in Table 22–1, but do not assume that the patient adheres to all of the practices common to that religion.

Occasionally, you may care for patients who follow more nontraditional religions. We have met patients who follow Voodoo practices in the Southeast

Table 22–1. Summary of Major Health Care Implications of Selected Religious Cultures and Subcultures

Religion	Food Preference	Responsibility Related to Patient Belief/Need
Hinduism	Vegetarian; no alcoholic beverages; other restrictions conform to sect doctrine; fasting important part of religious practice, with consequences for person on special diet or with diabetes or other diseases regulated by food	Medical care is last resort; patient considers help will come from own inner resources. Nurse should treat patient with respect and convey sense of dignity. Reinforce need for medical care and explain care measures. Patient may reject help and be stoic. Assess carefully for pain. Provide privacy. Assist to maintain religious practices. Cleanliness and dietary preferences are important. Certain prescribed rites are followed after death. The priest may tie a thread around the neck or wrist to signify blessing; the thread should not be removed. Immediately after death, the priest will pour water into the mouth of the corpse; the family will wash the body. They are particular about who touches

Table 22–1. Summary of Major Health Care Implications of Selected Religious Cultures and Subcultures (Continued)

Religion	Food Preference	Responsibility Related to Patient Belief/Need
Hinduism (cont.)		their dead. Bodies are cremated. Loss of limb is considered sign of wrongdoing in previous life.
Buddhism Zen, sect of Buddhism Shintoism, Japan's state religion	Vegetarian; no intoxicants; moderation in eating and drinking	Family help care for ill member and give emotional support. Religion discourages use of drugs; assess carefully for pain. Cleanliness important. Question about feelings regarding medical or surgical treatment on holy days. Prepare for death; help patient remain alert, resist confusion or distraction, and remain calm. Last Rite chanting is often practiced at bedside soon after death. Contact the deceased's Buddhist priest or have the family make contact.
Islam	No pork or pork-containing products; no intoxicants	Members are excused from religious practices when ill but may still want to pray to Allah and face Mecca. There is no spiritual advisor to call. Family visits are important. Cleanliness is important. After 130 days, fetus is treated as fully developed human. Members maintain a fatalistic view about illness; they are resigned to death, but encourage prolonging life. Patient must confess sins and beg forgiveness before death, and family should be present. The family washes and prepares the body, folds hands, and turns the body to face Mecca. Only relatives or friends may touch the body. Unless required by law, no postmortem or no body part should be removed.
Black Muslim (Nation of Islam)		There is no baptism. Procedure for washing and shrouding dead and performing funeral rites is carefully prescribed. Cleanliness is important.

(Continued)

Table 22–1. Summary of Major Health Care Implications of Selected Religious Cultures and Subcultures (Continued)

Religion	Food Preference	Responsibility Related to Patient Belief/Need
Judaism	Orthodox eat only kosher (ritually prepared) foods; milk consumed before meat, or meat eaten 6 hours before milk consumed; does not eat pig, horse, shrimp, lobster, crab, oyster, birds of prey if Orthodox. Others may restrict diet. Special utensils and dishes for Orthodox. Fasts on Yom Kippur and Tishah-b'Ab; may fast other times but excluded if ill	There is no infant baptism. Baby boys are circumcised on eighth day if Orthodox. Preventative measures, avoiding illness, are important. Members are concerned about future consequences of illness and medication. They are preoccupied with health; will convey that pain is present and want relief. Nursing measures for pain are important. On Sabbath, Orthodox Jews may refuse freshly cooked foods, medicine, treatment, surgery, and use of radio or television. Orthodox male may not shave. Nurse should avoid loss of yamulka, prayer books, or phylacteries. Nurse must arrange for kosher or preferred food; food may be served on paper plates. Check consequences of fasting on person's condition. Visits from family members are important. If patient is without family, notify synagogue so other people may visit. Family or friends should be with dying person. Artificial means should not be used to prolong life if patient is vegetative. Confession by dying person is like a rite of passage. Human remains are ritually washed following death by members of the Ritual Burial Society. Burial should take place as soon as possible. Cremation is not permitted. All Orthodox Jews and some Conservative Jews are opposed to autopsy. Organs or other tissues should be made available to the family for burial. Parts of the body are not donated to medical science or removed, even during autopsy. Donation or transplantation of organs requires rabbinical consultation. A fetus is to be buried, not discarded.

Table 22–1. Summary of Major Health Care Implications of Selected Religious Cultures and Subcultures (Continued)

Religion	Food Preference	Responsibility Related to Patient Belief/Need
Christianity		All will wish to see spiritual advisor when ill and to read Bible or other religious literature and follow usual practices.
Roman Catholic	Nothing special, except fasting or abstaining from meat on Ash Wednesday and Good Friday; some Catholics may fast every Friday and other holy days	Rosary, Bible, prayer book, crucifix, and medals are important. Infant baptism is mandatory, and especially urgent if prognosis is poor. Baptism is demanded if aborted fetus may not be clinically dead. For baptismal purposes, death is a certainty only if there is obvious evidence of tissue necrosis. Tell priest if you baptize baby; it is done only once. Inquire about dietary preferences and fasting. Members may want information on natural family planning. The Rite for Anointing of the Sick is mandatory. If the prognosis is poor, the patient or his or her family may request it. In sudden death, priest is called to anoint and administer Viaticum, if possible, or special prayers are said. Amputated limb may be buried in consecrated ground; there is no blanket mandate but it may be required within a given diocese. Donation or transplantation of organs is approved providing the recipient's potential benefit is proportionate to the donor's potential harm.
Orthodox		
Eastern Orthodox (Turkey, Egypt, Syria, Cyprus, Bulgaria, Rumania, Albania, Poland, Czechoslovakia)	Fasting each Wednesday, each Friday, and 40 days before Christmas and Easter; avoid meat, dairy products, and olive oil	Prayer book and icons are important. Infant is baptized if death is imminent. Check consequences of fast days on health; fasting is not necessary when ill. Blessing for the sick (unction) is not Last Rite but a form of healing by prayer. Last Rites are obligatory if death is impending; cremation is discouraged.

(Continued)

Table 22–1. Summary of Major Health Care Implications of Selected Religious Cultures and Subcultures (Continued)

Religion	Food Preference	Responsibility Related to Patient Belief/Need
Greek	Fasting periods on Wednesday, Friday, and during Lent; avoid meat and dairy products.	Prayer book and icons are important. Infant is baptized if death is imminent. Patient prepares by fasting for Holy Communion and Sacrament of Holy Unction. Fasting is not mandatory during illness. Members oppose euthanasia. Every reasonable effort should be made to preserve life until terminated by God. Cremation or autopsies that may cause dismemberment are discouraged. Last Rites are administered for the dying.
Russian Orthodox	Fasting on Wednesday, Friday, and during Lent; no meat or dairy products	Prayer book and icons are important. There is no baptism of infant. Check consequences of fasting on health. Cross necklace is important; it should be replaced immediately when patient returns from surgery. Do not shave male patients except in preparation for surgery. Patients do not believe in autopsies, embalming, or cremation. Traditionally, after death, arms are crossed, and fingers are set in a cross. Clothing at death must be of natural fiber so that the body will change to ashes sooner.
Protestantism (Many denominations and sects)		
Baptist	Some groups condemn coffee and tea; most condemn alcoholic beverages; some groups may fast on Sundays or other special days, especially in Black Baptist churches	There is no infant baptism. Client may be fatalistic; may believe illness is punishment from God; and may be passive about care. Inquire about effect of fasting if client is on special diet, is a diabetic, or has disease dependent on dietary regulation.

Table 22–1. Summary of Major Health Care Implications of Selected Religious Cultures and Subcultures (Continued)

Religion	Food Preference	Responsibility Related to Patient Belief/Need
Brethren (Grace) (Plymouth)	Most abstain from alcohol, tobacco, and illicit drugs	There is no infant baptism. Anointing with oil is done for physical healing and spiritual uplift. There are no Last Rites.
Church of Christ, Scientist (Christian Scientist)	Avoid coffee and alcoholic beverages	There is no infant baptism. If hospitalized or receiving medical treatment, guilt feelings may be intense. Be supportive. Allow practitioner or reader to visit freely as desired. Use nursing measures to alleviate pain. Patient may refuse blood transfusions as well as intravenous fluids and medication. There are no Last Rites or autopsy, unless sudden death.
Church of Christ	Avoid alcoholic beverages	There is no infant baptism. Anointing with oil and laying on of hands are done for healing. There are no Last Rites.
Church of God	Most avoid alcoholic beverages	There is no infant baptism.
Church of Jesus Christ of Latter Day Saints (Mormon)	Eat in moderation; limit meat; avoid coffee and tea; no alcoholic beverages; avoid use of tobacco	There is no infant baptism, but baptism of dead is essential; living person serves as proxy. Laying on of hands is done for healing. White undergarment with special marks at navel and right knee is to remain on; it is considered a safeguard against danger.
Episcopalian	May fast from meat on Friday	Infant baptism is mandatory, but not for aborted fetus or stillbirth. Patient fasts in preparation for Holy Communion, which may be daily; thus, check effects on disease. Rite for Anointing Sick (Last Rites) is not mandatory.
Friends (Quakers)	Moderation in eating; most avoid alcoholic beverages and drugs	There is no infant baptism. Health teaching is important. Give explanations about medical technology used in care. Share information about condition as indicated.

(Continued)

Table 22–1. Summary of Major Health Care Implications of Selected Religious Cultures and Subcultures (Concluded)

Religion	Food Preference	Responsibility Related to Patient Belief/Need
Jehovah's Witnesses	Avoid food to which blood is added, e.g., certain sausages and lunch meats	There is no infant baptism. Members are opposed to blood transfusion. (Hospital administrator or doctor may seek court order to be appointed guardian of child in times of emergency need for blood.) There are no Last Rites.
Mennonite	Most avoid alcoholic beverages	There is no infant baptism. Shock therapy, psychotherapy, and hypnotism conflict with individual will and personality.
Nazarene	Avoid alcoholic beverages	There is no need to baptize infant. Stillborn is buried. Laying on of hands is done for healing. There are no Last Rites.
Pentecostal	Avoid alcoholic beverages	There is no infant baptism. Prayer, anointing with oil, laying on of hands, speaking in tongues, shouting, and singing are important for healing of patient.
Unitarian/ Universalist		Infant baptism is not necessary. Cremation is preferred to burial. Check before calling clergy to visit.
Seventh-day Adventists	Vegetarian (no meat) or lacto-ovo-vegetarian (may eat milk and eggs but not meat); pork and fish without fins and scales prohibited; avoid coffee and tea; avoid alcoholic beverages	There is no infant baptism. Health measures, prevention, and health education are important. Some believe in divine healing and anointing with oil. Avoid administering narcotics and stimulants. Use nursing measures for pain; medication is last resort. Check on food preferences. Sabbath is from Friday sundown until Saturday sundown for most groups. Client may refuse medical treatment and use of secular items, such as television, on Sabbath.

Source: Murray, R., & Zentner J. (2001). Health promotion strategies through the life span *(7th ed.). Reprinted by permission of Pearson Education, Inc. Upper Saddle River, NJ 07458.*

and Southwest, as well as patients who practice Wiccan and other religions. These religions are not uncommon and their practitioners have beliefs that could interfere with traditional medical practices. Most of the practitioners believe in spells that can be either good or bad. Illness can be caused by bad spells. For the patient to improve, a healer may be needed to remove the spell. Healers tend to rely on objects, powders, herbs, incantations, and prayer to remove spells. We would encourage you to work with the healer to bring the patient every type of healing possible. Rarely do healers refuse to work with the health care team for the improvement of their patient. Unfortunately, the reverse is not always true. Many health care workers balk at nontraditional forms of healing. For the patient to benefit, you may need to open your heart and mind to new ways of healing. Remember, if your patient believes that the spell can make them ill, then chances are the patient will remain ill regardless of medical intervention. If the patient believes that a healer removes a spell, chances are improvement for whatever reason (healer or medical) will surely follow. There are many things that cannot be explained in our world. Open yourself to new experiences for your own benefit and for your patient's benefit.

People who do not deny but doubt the existence of God because it cannot be proved are agnostics. Atheists deny the existence of a god and reject all religious beliefs. Remember, just because a person says that he or she is an agnostic or an atheist does not mean that he or she has no spiritual beliefs. It is still important for you to consider the patient's spiritual beliefs when providing health care.

It is important for nurses to address a patient's spirituality whether the patient follows a specific religion or not. As nurses, we can provide spiritual comfort and we can see that spiritual resources are available to the patient. Remember that spirituality is much more important than checking a box on a required form!

RESOURCE WEB SITES

Web Sites
The following Web sites may assist you in finding answers to spiritual questions or direct you to further information about a religion that you are not familiar with.

1. A–Z of Jewish and Israel Related Resources: *www.ort.org:80/anjy/a-z*
2. CyberMuslim Information Collective: *www.uoknor.edu/cybermuslim*
3. CyberZen: *www.indy.net/~bdmoore/cyberzen.html*
4. Distinctive Churches: *www.best.com/~nodakid/church.html*

RESOURCE WEB SITES (CONT.)

5. Global Hindu Electronic Network:
   www.rbhatnagar.csm.uc.edu:8080/hindu_universe.html
6. Library of God: *www.convex.uky.edu:80/~rtcrit00/atemple.html*
7. Yahoo Religion Subdirectory: *www.yahoo.com/society_and_culture/religion*
8. Latter-day Saints: *www.LDS.org*

23

Death and Dying

Death As Part of Life

Death and dying may or may not be part of your nursing curriculum. If you do learn about death, it will most likely be incorporated into various nursing courses. Some schools offer electives in death and dying. Whether or not you learn about death and dying in school, we can guarantee that you will be exposed to it during your nursing career.

American society in general would have us believe that death is something to be avoided at all costs. We should not discuss it, we should avoid people who are dying, and most of all, we should not admit that we ourselves will die. Our society is so focused on youth, vitality, and immortality that we often lose sight of the meaningfulness of the dying experience. Other cultures embrace dying people and use the death experience for renewal and growth. As nurses, if we choose to fear death and avoid it, we will treat dying patients in the same manner. If, however, we choose to embrace death and learn from dying patients, we can provide the support, love, and understanding that they need.

Death Across the Life Span

As stated, all of us will die, and death occurs at all ages and throughout the life span. Although we all have our own individual reaction to death, most of us find it particularly hard to face the death of a child. It is also difficult to face the death of someone close to our own age and the deaths of close relatives and loved ones. Although none of us wants anyone to die, most of us can rationalize the death of someone who is ill and elderly. Table 23–1 shows how various age groups conceptualize death and how society reacts to the death of someone in that age group.

Table 23–1. Death of a Child, Adult, or Elderly Person

Perception of Death	Society's Response
Child	
• The very young child (under age 3) has no perception of the permanence of death. By age 3–6, a child understands loss by separation (not permanence). By age 6–9, the child understands that death is permanent. At age 10–12, the child understands death and realizes that it can happen to anyone at anytime (Burgess, 1997).	• The death of a child causes much grief and anger.
	• Why have they died young?
	• How could God take such a young child?
• Most children are very perceptive and know when they are dying.	• Ongoing pain for parents and loved ones.
• Children may try to protect their parents by not discussing death with them. They need to be encouraged to talk with family members.	• Loss of continuance of the human race.
	• More of a tragedy than the death of someone who has "lived a full life."
• Often children will openly discuss death with other children or with health care givers.	
Adult	
• Young adults are aware of the possibility of death, but rarely think it will happen to them.	• Depends on the age of the individual. Once again, most are more affected by and wonder about the loss of the young adult.
• As people age, they become more familiar with death and think about the financial and legal ramifications of an early death.	• As people age, they accept that death can occur at any time. Many people believe in the hope of an eternal resting place.
• A majority of adults face the loss of their parents and, sometimes, siblings and spouses.	
Elderly	
• The elderly realize that death is a common event but continue to live their lives to the fullest.	• Our society correlates aging with death.
	• People tend to accept the death of an aged person more easily than the death of a child.

Death and Nursing

All living things will die. It is a fact of nature. Where, when, and how we will die, none of us know. The same holds true for our friends, family, and loved ones. Most of us learn about death at an early age through the loss of a pet, or perhaps a grandparent. Some of us are shielded from death and do not experience a death until we are adults. As a nurse, you will definitely experience a patient's death, so you will need to learn to prepare for it and grow from it.

Occasionally, nursing students experience their first death during a clinical rotation. As difficult as it is to lose a patient, it happens to be a good time to experience a death. During your clinical rotation you will have the support of your instructor and fellow students.

1. **What feelings do you think Terri is experiencing?**
   - **Sadness** that the patient died
   - **Anger** that the patient had to die, or that the medical team could not save her
   - **Guilt** that she might not have done everything she could to save the patient
   - **Fear** that she might not be able to save other patients or that her loved ones will die also

A CASE IN POINT

Terri is a 22-year-old sophomore nursing student in her second week of her emergency room (ER) rotation. The ambulance pulls up with a 48-year-old woman who was in an automobile accident. The woman's husband was driving the car. He is dead on arrival (DOA). The patient has a fractured pelvis, a compound fracture of the right femur, a left pneumothorax, and multiple lacerations and contusions. Terri observes the doctors and nurses working on the patient and helps monitor vital signs. The patient seems to be stabilizing so the doctor orders a magnetic resonance image (MRI) to determine if there is any internal bleeding. Terri offers to accompany the woman to the MRI so that she will not be alone and so that Terri can see an MRI in process. During the MRI, the patient complains of severe chest pain and suddenly experiences a respiratory arrest. Terri calls for help and begins cardiopulmonary resuscitation (CPR). Unfortunately, the patient dies from a suspected pulmonary embolus.

Terri is very upset by the patient's death and returns to the ER. One of the ER nurses recognizes Terri's distress and calls her instructor. The instructor finds Terri sitting on a chair in the patient's room with the woman's body on the gurney.

2. **What factors might affect Terri's reaction to the patient's death?**
   - The age of the patient who died (close in age to Terri's parents)
   - The suddenness of the patient's death
   - Whether Terri had experienced other deaths in the past
   - Terri's general psychological makeup
   - Terri's experience with other losses
3. **What would help Terri at this point?**
   - To experience her feelings and talk about them
   - To feel supported
   - To know that she did not cause the patient's death and that she did everything she could to save her
   - To understand that sometimes people die even though we do our best
4. **What can Terri learn from this experience?**
   - That life is very fragile
   - That not all patients will live
   - How to experience loss and the death of a patient
   - That others will support her when she has bad experiences in the future (Sometimes we have to ask for that support!)

Working with the dying can be challenging for nurses. Dying people can teach us many things about ourselves. As nurses, we are not immune to death and we will have to learn how to relate to dying patients.

- Some nurses are very good with dying people, while others are not.
- We must learn to show compassion to all patients.
- If you are afraid of dying patients, then take the opportunity to find out why.
- If the dying patient makes you angry, then you need to learn to control your anger.
- If you cannot handle the thought of your own death, then try to come to some understanding of why that is.
- Some nurses need to seek the help of a counselor to come to terms with their feelings about death and dying.

Preparation for Death

There are a number of things that must be considered prior to our deaths. Some people are lucky enough and wise enough to attend to all the details of dying. Others die unprepared and leave family or friends to cope with the details of their death.

Funeral

The majority of individuals in our society will have a funeral or memorial service. The service will depend on the religious affiliation of the deceased as well as personal and family desires. Most nurses are not involved with planning a funeral for patients, but you may need to encourage some patients to consider planning a funeral. Many nurses who work with dying patients have participated in the funeral process. Some things to consider when planning a funeral are:

- Burial or cremation
- Setting of service
- Religious readings or favorite passages
- Who will read or speak
- Music

Will

A will is an important legal document that helps us to distribute our property upon our deaths.

- A will must comply with the legal statutes in the state in which the person resides.
- Two witnesses who have no beneficiary interest in the estate must sign it.
- If a person dies without a will (intestate), the estate will usually pass to a surviving spouse or children, although this may vary depending on the state in which the person resides.
- Any person who has specific ideas about the distribution of their property should be encouraged to make a will.
- If a patient has no will, a lawyer can be found who will make a hospital visit and complete the document for approval and signatures.

Advanced Health Care Directives

In 1992, Congress enacted the Patient Self-Determination Act (PSDA) (Burke & Walsh, 1992). All federally funded health care institutions are required to provide patients with written information about the right to execute advanced health care directives at the time of admission. These advanced directives, if enacted, are to be placed in the patient's chart on admission. If the patient chooses not to enact them, a signed form stating such should also be included in the chart. All of the advanced directives are used to indicate what type of medical care or how much life-sustaining treatment is desired if physical or mental incapacitation occurs. In most states, these forms must be in writing and are witnessed by two individuals (sometimes notarization is required).

It is important to note that each state requires different forms and may even refer to the forms by different names. For example, the state of Florida has a Living Will form; however, in Texas the form is called Directive to Physicians and Family or Surrogates. It is essential that you familiarize yourself with the state-specific forms from the state in which you are employed or going to school. Also be aware that you may use different terminology when describing the forms. Please note that the forms used in this text are only examples. If you would like further information, or desire a copy of the forms for your state, please contact Partnership For Caring (formerly Choice in Dying) at 800-989-9455 or access the forms on the Web site at *www.partnershipforcaring.org*.

LIVING WILL

1. The living will allows competent individuals to state how much life-saving medical intervention they desire if they become unable to make their wishes known (Figure 23–1).
2. Most living wills state that the individual wishes to be kept pain-free, but that extraordinary means of keeping one alive are not desired.
3. The language is often vague. The patient may wish to add in specific information such as:
   - No CPR
   - No respirator
   - No tube feedings
   - No dialysis
4. Living wills require the signatures of two witnesses.
5. There is no legal requirement forcing physicians to follow a living will.
6. There is also no protection from criminal or civil liability for physicians, so many physicians choose to ignore the patient's wishes (Guido, 2001).

NATURAL DEATH ACT

1. The natural death act is a living will that is legally recognized and has statutory enforcement (Figure 23–2).
2. In most states, individuals over the age of 18 are able to sign a natural death act if they are of sound mind and capable of understanding the document.
3. In most states, the document requires the patient's signature and the signature of two witnesses who will not benefit from the patient's death. The witnesses cannot be related to the patient.
4. Some states have a mandatory form that must be filled out; others do not. Be sure that you are familiar with the laws in your state (Guido, 2001).

Florida Living Will

Declaration made this _____ day of _____, _____,
(day)   *(month)*   *(year)*

I, _____, willfully
and voluntarily make known my desire that my dying not be artificially
prolonged under the circumstances set forth below, and I do hereby
declare that:

If at any time I am incapacitated and
_____ I have a terminal condition, or
_____ I have an end-stage condition, or
_____ I am in a persistent vegetative state

and if my attending or treating physician and another consulting
physician have determined that there is no reasonable medical
probability of my recovery from such condition, I direct that life-
prolonging procedures be withheld or withdrawn when the application of
such procedures would serve only to prolong artificially the process of
dying, and that I be permitted to die naturally with only the
administration of medication or the performance of any medical
procedure deemed necessary to provide me with comfort care or to
alleviate pain.

It is my intention that this declaration be honored by my family and
physician as the final expression of my legal right to refuse medical or
surgical treatment and to accept the consequences for such refusal.

In the event that I have been determined to be unable to provide express
and informed consent regarding the withholding, withdrawal, or
continuation of life-prolonging procedures, I wish to designate, as my
surrogate to carry out the provisions of this declaration:

Name: _____

Address: _____

_____ Zip Code: _____

Phone: _____

Figure 23–1. Florida Living Will. *Reprinted by permission of Partnership for Caring, 1620 Eye Street, NW, Suite 202, Washington, DC 2006 (800) 989-9455.*

I wish to designate the following person as my alternate surrogate, to carry out the provisions of this declaration should my surrogate be unwilling or unable to act on my behalf:

PRINT NAME, HOME ADDRESS AND TELEPHONE NUMBER OF YOUR ALTERNATE SURROGATE

Name: _____

Address: _____

_____ Zip Code: _____

Phone: _____

ADD PERSONAL INSTRUCTIONS (IF ANY)

Additional instructions (optional):

I understand the full import of this declaration, and I am emotionally and mentally competent to make this declaration.

SIGN THE DOCUMENT

Signed: _____

WITNESSING PROCEDURE

Witness 1:

TWO WITNESSES MUST SIGN AND PRINT THEIR ADDRESSES

Signed: _____

Address: _____

Witness 2:

Signed: _____

Address: _____

Courtesy of **Partnership for Caring, Inc.**   6/00
1035 30th Street, NW Washington, DC 20007 800-989-9455

Figure 23–1. (Continued)

DECLARATION OF A DESIRE FOR A NATURAL DEATH

I, _____ being of sound mind, desire that, as specified below, my life not be prolonged by extraordinary means or by artificial nutrition or hydration if my condition is determined to be terminal and incurable or if I am diagnosed as being in a persistent vegetative state. I am aware and understand that this writing authorizes a physician to withhold or discontinue extraordinary means or artificial nutrition or hydration, in accordance with my specifications as set forth below:

(Initial any of the following as desired):

If my condition is determined to be terminal and incurable, I authorize the following:

_____ My physician may withhold or discontinue extraordinary means only.

In addition to withholding or discontinuing extraordinary means if such means are necessary, my physician may withhold or discontinue either artificial nutrition or hydration, or both.

If my physician determines that I am in a persistent vegetative state, I authorize the following:

_____ My physician may withhold or discontinue extraordinary means only.

In addition to withholding or discontinuing extraordinary means if such means are necessary, my physician may withhold or discontinue either artificial nutrition or hydration, or both.

This the _____ day of _____ , 1999.

I hereby state that the Declarant, _____ , being of sound mind, signed the above Declaration in my presence and that I am not related to the Declarant by blood or marriage and that I do not know or have a reasonable expectation that I would be entitled to any portion of the estate of the Declarant under any existing Will or Codicil of the Declarant or as an heir under the Interstate Succession Act if the Declarant died on this date without a Will. I also state that I am not the Declarant's physician, or an employee of any health facility in which the Declarant is a patient, or an employee of a nursing home or any group-care home where the Declarant resides. I further still state that I do not now have any claim against the Declarant.

WITNESS our hands and seals this the _____ day of _____ , 1991.

_____ (SEAL)
Witness

_____ (SEAL)
Witness

CERTIFICATE

I, _____ , Notary Public for _____ , hereby certify that _____ , the Declarant, appeared before me and swore to me and to the witnesses in my presence that this instrument is his/her Declaration of a Desire for a Natural Death, and that he/she had willingly and voluntarily made and executed it as his/her free act and deed for the purposes therein expressed.

I further certify that _____ and _____ , witnesses, appeared before me and swore that they witnessed _____ , the Declarant, sign the attached Declaration, believing him/her to be of sound mind; and also swore that at the time they witnessed the Declaration (i) they were not related within the third degree to the Declarant or to the Declarant's spouse, and (ii) they did not know or have reasonable expectation that they would be entitled to any portion of the estate of the Declarant upon the Declarant's death under any Will of the Declarant or Codicil thereto then existing or under the Interstate Succession Act as it provides at that time, and (iii) they were not a physician attending the Declarant or an employee of an attending physician or an employee of a nursing home or any group-care home where the Declarant resided, and (iv) they did not have a claim against the Declarant. I further certify that I am satisfied as to the genuineness and due execution of the Declarant.

This the _____ day of _____ , 1999.

_____
Notary Public for Mecklenburg
County, North Carolina

(Notary Seal)

My Commission expires: _____

Figure 23–2. Declaration of desire for a natural death. (*From Murray, R. B., & Zentner, J. P. [1997]. Health assessment & promotion strategies through the life span [6th ed.]. Reprinted by permission of Pearson Education, Inc. Upper Saddle River, NJ 07458.*)

DURABLE POWER OF ATTORNEY FOR HEALTH CARE (DPAHC) OR MEDICAL DURABLE POWER OF ATTORNEY (MDPA)

1. The DPAHC and MDPA allow a competent person to give decision-making authority about medical interventions to another individual (Figure 23–3).
2. The durable DPAHC and MDPA are only enacted when patients are mentally incapable of making decisions for themselves.
3. This document allows the person who holds the durable power of attorney to:
   - Ask questions.
   - Select and remove physicians from the patient's care.
   - Assess risks and complications.
   - Select treatments and procedures.
   - Refuse care and/or life-sustaining procedures.
   - Act in full authority as the patient would act if he or she were able to.
4. Whoever is given the durable power of attorney is responsible for making medical determinations and does not need to consult with other interested parties.
5. Health care providers are protected from liability if they act in good faith on the agent's decisions (Guido, 2001).

A CASE IN POINT

Tony was 32 years old when he was diagnosed with testicular cancer that had metastasized to his liver. His closest relative was his partner, Karl. They had lived together for 9 years. Tony was not close to his family because they did not approve of his lifestyle. Tony discussed all of the details of his wishes with Karl and he decided to make Karl his durable power of attorney for health care. They also knew that this would ensure that Karl would be able to visit him in the hospital at any time.

As Tony became more and more debilitated, he was admitted to the hospice unit of the hospital. Tony's family arrived and requested that Karl not be allowed to visit their son. The hospice staff explained that Karl would be allowed to visit and make medical decisions regarding Tony's care. Although the family was not pleased, they were forced to recognize the legal implications of the situation. Tony and his family were able to reconcile their differences before his death, and Karl was allowed to make funeral arrangements for Tony.

Do Not Resuscitate (DNR) Directives

Some facilities have institutional guidelines regarding do not resuscitate (DNR) or no code orders. Physicians are allowed to place a DNR or no code order in the patient's chart after consultation with the patient or the patient's health care proxy (Guido, 2001).

Directive to Physicians

Some states recognize a document called a *directive to physicians*. This document complements the living will and DPAHC (Figure 23–4). The document is directed specifically to physicians and spells out the patient's desires with regard to medical treatment should the individual become incapacitated. This document is similar in legality to the living will in that the physician can choose to follow it or not.

Hospice

Hospice offers terminally ill patients an alternative to dying in a hospital environment with a host of life-sustaining equipment. Hospice also allows the patient to forego signing a living will or other medical directive, as the philosophy behind the hospice movement is that death is a natural part of life. Hospice organizations believe that it is important to offer nursing and medical care to maintain comfort without life-sustaining measures. For example, the patient will not be resuscitated and other life support systems will not be used when death is imminent. Hospice personnel provide comfort and support to the family as well as to the individual who is dying. One of the many benefits of hospice care is that it allows the family some respite from caring for the terminally ill individual. After the patient dies, the hospice personnel continue to provide the family with support during their period of bereavement. The objective of hospice care is to keep the patient at home for as long as possible and make the patient's last days as comfortable and meaningful as possible.

Most hospices require the patient to be competent to make a decision to choose hospice care. Many also require that the patient be in a terminal condition with a maximum number of months left to live (e.g., one hospice treats patients with less than 6 months to live). In 1982, Congress recognized the need for alternative terminal care and authorized Medicare reimbursement for hospice care (Public Law 97-248, 1982). Many hospices are affiliated with hospitals, but there are also a number of hospice home health agencies that are affiliated with hospitals or other health care facilities.

FLORIDA DESIGNATION OF HEALTH CARE SURROGATE

Name:_____

(Last)   *(First)*   *(Middle Initial)*

In the event that I have been determined to be incapacitated to provide informed consent for medical treatment and surgical and diagnostic procedures, I wish to designate as my surrogate for health care decisions:

Name:_____

Address: _____

_____ Zip Code: _____

Phone: _____

If my surrogate is unwilling or unable to perform his or her duties, I wish to designate as my alternate surrogate:

Name: _____

Address: _____

_____ Zip Code: _____

Phone: _____

I fully understand that this designation will permit my designee to make health care decisions and to provide, withhold, or withdraw consent on my behalf; to apply for public benefits to defray the cost of health care; and to authorize my admission to or transfer from a health care facility.

Additional instructions (optional):

Figure 23–3. Florida Designation of Health Care Surrogate. *Reprinted by permission of Partnership for Caring, 1620 Eye Street, NW, Suite 202, Washington, DC 2006 (800) 989-9455.*

FLORIDA DESIGNATION OF HEALTH CARE SURROGATE — PAGE 2 OF 2

I further affirm that this designation is not being made as a condition of treatment or admission to a health care facility. I will notify and send a copy of this document to the following persons other than my surrogate, so they may know who my surrogate is:

PRINT THE NAMES AND ADDRESSES OF THOSE WHO YOU WANT TO KEEP COPIES OF THIS DOCUMENT

Name: ______________________________

Address: ______________________________

Name: ______________________________

Address: ______________________________

SIGN AND DATE THE DOCUMENT

Signed: ______________________________

Date: ______________________________

WITNESSING PROCEDURE

TWO WITNESSES MUST SIGN AND PRINT THEIR ADDRESSES

Witness 1:

Signed: ______________________________

Address: ______________________________

Witness 2:

Signed: ______________________________

Address: ______________________________

Courtesy of **Partnership for Caring, Inc.** 10/99
1035 30th Street, NW Washington, DC 20007 800-989-9455

Figure 23–3. (Continued)

MEDICAL DIRECTIVE

I, _____ being of sound mind, make this statement as a directive to be followed if I am ever unable to participate in decisions regarding my medical care. Should I become mentally incompetent because of a medical condition like a coma or persistent vegetative state or severe dementia and my doctors do not expect me to recover, I direct the following treatment decisions be made in my behalf. These directions express my legal right to refuse treatment.

	YES	NO	UNSURE
1. CPR: Use drugs, electric shock, and artificial breathing to bring me back to life when my heart stops.	___	___	___
2. Mechanical breathing: Use a machine to do my breathing for me when I cannot breathe unaided.	___	___	___
3. Artificial nutrition: Give me food through a tube in my vein or stomach	___	___	___
4. Artificial hydration: Give me liquid through a tube in my vein.	___	___	___
5. Hospitalization: Move me from my home or hospice or nursing home to a hospital.	___	___	___
6. Major surgery: Operate on something like a blockage in my stomach or remove my gallbladder.	___	___	___
7. Kidney dialysis: Have a machine do the work of my kidneys —cleansing my blood—when they stop working on their own.	___	___	___
8. Chemotherapy: Give me drugs to fight cancer.	___	___	___
9. Minor surgery: Operate on something minor like an infected toe.	___	___	___
10. Major tests: Do tests like heart catheterization or colonoscopy to see what is wrong inside me.	___	___	___
11. Blood: Transfuse blood or blood products into me if I am in need of them.	___	___	___
12. Antibiotics: Give me drugs to fight diseases like pneumonia or a kidney infection.	___	___	___
13. Minor tests: Do an x-ray or a blood test to see what is wrong with me.	___	___	___
14. Pain medication: Give me enough medication so that I am not in pain.	___	___	___
15. Home: Move me from the hospital so that I can die at home.	___	___	___

16. Other: _____
_____
_____
_____
_____   ___ ___ ___

I provide this directive in addition to my living will.

Signed_____ Date _____

Witness _____

Witness _____

Figure 23–4. Medical directive. (*From Murray, R. B., & Zentner, J. P. [1997]. Health assessment & promotion strategies through the life span [6th ed.]. Reprinted by permission of Pearson Education, Inc. Upper Saddle River, NJ 07458.*)

A CASE IN POINT

Connie, age 52, was diagnosed with pancreatic cancer in February 1998. A wife and mother of three children, she decided that it would be best for the whole family to meet with the oncologist to discuss treatment options. Her oncologist offered three options: radical experimental treatment that was yet unproven, a course of chemotherapy that might prolong her life for 2 months, or allow the cancer to continue to spread and treat her symptoms. Connie is an avid vegetarian who was unwilling to "poison her body with chemicals." Her family is supportive of her decision to choose the third option. Her oncologist put her in touch with a hospice center. The hospice nurse makes an initial home visit and does a complete assessment. She tells Connie that she and a volunteer will be seeing Connie throughout her illness. She also explains that Connie or any member of the family can call her 24 hours a day. She tells Connie and her family some of the concepts of hospice care.

- Pain control
- Nutrition support
- Physical relaxation methods
- Emotional support
- Spiritual support
- Grief and bereavement support

The hospice nurse meets with other hospice personnel to develop a plan of care for Connie and her family. The hospice nurse will check on Connie once a week, and a hospice volunteer will visit with Connie daily. The nurse contacts Connie's oncologist to get orders for pain management and nutrition supplements. Connie and her family are given daily support during the next 7 weeks until Connie's death. Connie was able to die at home with her family around her. She continued receiving pain management up until the time of her death, and died peacefully in the arms of her husband. The hospice personnel attended Connie's funeral and visited the family once a week for the first month following her death. Connie's family developed an ongoing friendship with the hospice volunteer, whom they continue to see.

Terminally Ill People

Once a person receives a terminal diagnosis, intense emotional reactions are normal. The individual often experiences the following turbulent emotions:

- Emptiness
- Disbelief
- Rage
- Loss of control
- Fear of pain and suffering
- Isolation
- Alienation
- Fear of abandonment
- Fear of financial ruin

These feelings are quite normal and to be expected (Varcarolis, 1994). The individual usually vacillates between feelings and may seem calm one minute and very angry the next. In 1969, Kübler-Ross published a classic text, *On Death and Dying*. Kübler-Ross studied dying patients and learned about the dying process. As a result of this work, Kübler-Ross determined that there are five stages to the dying process.

1. **Denial:** The patient cannot accept the terminal diagnosis. Denial is healthy and gives the patient time to adjust to the diagnosis.
2. **Anger:** The patient wants to know "why me." Anger may be kept in or it may be displaced onto family, friends, and health care givers.
3. **Bargaining:** The patient usually bargains with God, offering to be a better person or to live a better life.
4. **Depression:** Once the anger and denial have worn off, the patient begins to feel a great sense of loss. Depression occurs when the patient realizes that no amount of medicine, surgery, or alternative therapy can cure his or her illness.
5. **Acceptance:** The patient has finished mourning his or her losses and becomes physically weaker. Often, the patient withdraws and stops communicating with loved ones in preparation for death, although he or she may be comforted by having someone in the room or by someone holding his or her hand.

The nurse needs to intervene with the dying patient depending on which stage the patient is in. In other words, we would not treat a patient in the anger stage in the same way we would treat a patient in the bargaining stage (Table 23–2).

The dying patient has many tasks that need to be accomplished. Some of these tasks are affected by Kübler-Ross's stages of dying, although they are not related. Humphrey (1986) identified the following adaptation tasks:

- Getting affairs in order
- Coping with the loss of both loved ones and self
- Considering future health care needs

Table 23–2. Nursing Interventions and Rationales: Working with a Person Who Is Dying

Intervention	Rationale
Stage One: Denial and Isolation	
1. Examine own feelings about death.	1. Personal defenses and fears can be projected onto dying person if not identified and worked out.
2. Encourage the patient's expression of feelings, concerns, and fears: • Sit at bedside. • Actively listen and reflect patient's feelings. • Hold hand or touch shoulder when appropriate.	2. Provides presence and decreases feelings of abandonment. • Lessens feelings of isolation and keeps channels of communication open. • For some, physical touch provides comfort and demonstrates concern.
3. Provide small amount of information at a time. Encourage questions when patient is ready.	3. Having correct information can decrease anxiety and clarify information.
4. Encourage decisions regarding self-care.	4. Increases feelings of control and encourages functioning at optimum level.
Stage Two: Anger	
1. Acknowledge person's right to be angry.	1. Increases feelings of support and being understood.
2. Understand that anger directed at staff and family is not personal.	2. Feelings of helplessness and loss stimulate anger, which is often projected onto staff and loved ones.
3. Work with patient to rechannel anger into positive channels, e.g., making decisions, setting goals, and fighting disease.	3. Can help rechannel energy in ways that help increase self-esteem, feelings of control, and sense of being supported by staff and others.
Stage Three: Bargaining	
1. Offer to contact clergy or rabbi.	1. May assist in dispelling irrational religious beliefs.
2. Encourage discussion of feelings, especially guilt and loss.	2. Decreases feelings of guilt and possible thoughts of being punished for past actions.
3. Encourage patient's positive coping strategies used in the past.	3. Positive reinforcement can strengthen positive behaviors.
4. Encourage periods of time to focus on more satisfying areas of life.	4. Periods of time away from discussion of disease and death helps person put life in broader terms.
Stage Four: Depression	
1. Focus on daily short-term *obtainable* goals.	1. Emphasizes positive functioning and areas of independence.
2. Continue to spend time with patient on regular basis.	2. Staff awareness of tendency to withdraw can help staff modify own behaviors.
3. Encourage patient to participate in usual activities.	

(Continued)

Table 23–2. Nursing Interventions and Rationales: Working with a Person Who Is Dying (Continued)

Intervention	Rationale
4. Encourage patient to participate in support groups.	3. Can decrease time spent in brooding and offer broader focus of experience.
5. Maintain adequate pain control.	4. Discussion with others in similar circumstances can decrease feelings of isolation and increase feelings of being understood.
	5. Physical comfort can increase ability to interact with others and may diminish tendency to withdraw.
Stage Five: Acceptance	
1. Sit with person—even when person does not want to talk.	1. Provides presence and support and decreases feelings of abandonment.
2. Allow appropriate privacy, e.g., during toileting and bathing.	2. Allow appropriate privacy, e.g., during toileting and bathing.
3. Continue pain control.	3. Provides comfort during final stages of dying

Source: Varcarolis, E. M. (1994). Foundations of psychiatric–mental health nursing. Philadelphia: Saunders.

- Planning for the time remaining
- Anticipating future pain and physical losses, contributing to a loss of identity
- Considering being a nonperson
- Deciding to speed up or slow down the dying process

Most human beings want to feel that their time on earth has not been wasted, and that they leave something of themselves behind. The dying patient may want to participate in developing an activity to help keep their memories alive for family and friends. For example, they might choose one of the following:

- Writing a journal
- Recording shared times on videotape
- Recording personal messages on audiotape
- Distributing photographs
- Distributing personal possessions to loved ones (Burgess, 1997, p. 248)

Grief and Grieving

Grief begins as soon as a threat of loss occurs. Individuals experience anticipatory grief at the time of a terminal diagnosis or of a terminal diagnosis of a loved one. Whenever an individual anticipates a loss, or experiences a loss, it is a reminder of all the other losses he or she has ever experienced. Grief is a very private experience. Each individual grieves in his or her own way, depending on background experiences as well as psychological, sociocultural, and spiritual factors. It is important to realize that since we all grieve differently, there is no specific formula for assisting an individual through the grieving process.

The Grieving Family

One factor that affects the family is the type of death that has occurred. Some family members have the opportunity to grieve over a longer period of time than others do. For example, a person dying of cancer may live 2 to 3 years; someone else might die unexpectedly in an automobile accident. Either death is traumatic for the family, but if a death is protracted, the family has the ability to begin working through the grief process while the patient is still living.

Rando (1993) identified six stages of the mourning process. These six stages occur in three phases: avoidance, confrontation, and accommodation (Table 23–3). Rando's phases are similar to Kübler-Ross's stages of dying in that the individual moves back and forth between stages.

The nurse can help the family deal with their grief by developing an awareness of the family's response to dying and death. To help guide a family through the grieving process, you will need to be aware of what the family is experiencing (Table 23–4).

The Grieving Child

Children are extremely sensitive to family dynamics and will know when something is wrong. Young children will experience distress when separated from a parent or loved one who is very ill or hospitalized. According to Siegel and colleagues (1992), children experience distress related to:

- Increasing limitations of parents' physical or emotional availability
- Loss or separation from parent
- Changes in parents' role functioning
- Changes in family routines
- Changes in family emotional climate
- Decreases in financial resources due to caring for an ill family member

Table 23–3. Rando's Six "R" Processes of Mourning

Avoidance phase

Recognize the loss
- Acknowledge the death
- Understand the death

Confrontation phase

React to the separation
- Experience the pain
- Feel, identify, accept, and give some form of expression to all of the psychological reactions to the loss
- Identify and mourn secondary losses

Recollect and reexperience the deceased and the relationship
- Review and remember the relationship realistically
- Revive and reexperience the feelings in the relationship

Relinquish the old attachments to the deceased and the old assumptive world

Accommodation phase

Readjust to move adaptively into the new world without forgetting the old
- Revise the assumptive world
- Develop a new relationship with the deceased
- Adapt new ways of being in the world
- Form a new identity

Reinvest personal energies

Reprinted with permission from Rando, T. A. (1993, p. 45). Treatment of complicated grief. *Champaign, IL: Research Press.*

Children need to be made aware of the situation and should be allowed to ask questions. Since children are often very intuitive and sometimes blunt, parents need to be aware that it is not possible to hide their feelings or emotions. Table 23–5 offers some dos and don'ts for discussing death with children.

One thing that we have learned through many years of working with suicidal patients is that children have difficulty understanding suicide. The death of a parent is traumatic, but when that death is by suicide, the family is often reluctant to discuss it with a child. Many times, families glorify death by saying things like "Daddy is in heaven," or "Daddy has gone to a wonderful place to be with God," or "Daddy is in a better place and he is happy." Whatever is said, be certain that the child does not think that heaven is a better place to be than earth. We have had very young children decide to join Daddy because heaven sounded much nicer than living. It is difficult to get this concept across

Table 23–4. Family's Response to Dying and Death

Four Main Stages	Family Experiences	Nurse Can Foster
Living with Terminal Illness		
Person learns diagnosis, tries to carry on as usual, undergoes treatment	*Impact:* Emotional shock, despair, disorganized behavior	Hope as different treatment methods are used, communication, seeking helpful resources, family cohesiveness
	Functional disruption: Much time spent at hospital (if traditional surgery or treatment chosen), ignoring of home tasks and emotional needs, weakening of family structure, emotional isolation	
	Search for meaning: Questioning why this happened; casting blame on various persons, deity, institutions, habits; realization that "Someday I will die too"	Security
	Informing others (family and friends): ascent from isolation, with moral and practical support—or feeling of rejection: others do not understand, do not care, or are afraid; possible need to retreat again into emotional isolation	Courage, reliable help, understanding of why some people cannot help
Living–Dying Interval	*Engaging emotions:* Beginning grieving, fearing loss of emotional control, assumption of roles once carried by dying person	Problem solving; idea that life will change but will be ongoing
Person ceases to perform family roles, is cared for either at home or in hospital; person needs to come to terms with accomplishments and failures and to find renewed meaning in life	*Reorganization:* Firmer division of family tasks	Cooperation instead of competition; analysis to see if new role distribution is workable
	Framing memories: Reviewing life of dying person—what he or she has meant and accomplished, new sense of family history, relinquishment of dependency on dying member	Focus on life review rather than only on what person is now

(Continued)

Table 23–4. Family's Response to Dying and Death (Continued)

Four Main Stages	Family Experiences	Nurse Can Foster
Bereavement Death occurs	*Separation:* Absorption in loneliness of separation as person becomes unconscious *Mourning:* Guilt, "Could I have done more?"	Intimacy among family members; release of grief as normal
Reestablishment	Expansion of the social network: overcoming feelings of alienation and guilt	Looking back with acceptance and forward to new growth and socialization with a reunited, normally functioning family

Source: Murray, R. B., & Zentner, J. P. (2001). Health promotion strategies through the life span (7th ed.). Reprinted by permission of Pearson Education, Inc. Upper Saddle River, NJ 07458.

A CASE IN POINT

Jessie was a neonatal nurse who worked within a neonatal intensive care unit (NICU). Jessie was also pregnant and due to deliver her first child in 3 months. At 25 weeks' gestation, Jessie went into premature labor. Despite intervention, she delivered a baby girl with spina bifida by cesarean section. The spinal malformation was severe and the baby died of sepsis shortly after birth.

All of the nurses in the unit who knew Jessie were devastated that the baby had died. No one knew what to do for Jessie. Several nurses felt that Jessie should see and hold the baby, while others felt that she should be spared the sight of her malformed child.

- What would you do in this situation?
- Would you encourage Jessie to see and hold her baby or not?
- If she wants to see her baby, should it be wrapped in a blanket? Or lay in a bassinet?
- How soon should she be allowed to see the baby?
- What if her husband does not want Jessie to see the baby?
- How would you handle this conflict?

Table 23–5. Do's and Don'ts for Discussing Death with Children

Do
- Ask the child what he or she is feeling. Bring up the subject of death naturally in the context of a dead pet, a book character, television show, movie, or news item.
- Help the child have a funeral for a dead pet.
- Help the child realize he or she is not responsible for the death.
- Tell the child what has happened on his or her level (but not in morbid detail).
- Explain the funeral service briefly beforehand; attendance depends on the child's age and wishes.
- Answer questions honestly, with responses geared to the child's age.
- Remember that expressions of pain, anger, loneliness, or aloneness do not constitute symptoms of an illness but are part of a natural process of grieving.
- Help the child realize that the adults are also grieving and feel upset, anger, despair, and guilt.

Do Not
- Admonish the child not to cry; it is a universal way to show grief and anxiety.
- Tell a mystical story about the loss of the person; it could cause confusion and anxiety.
- Give long, exclusively detailed explanations beyond the level of understanding.
- Associate death with sleep, which could result in chronic sleep disturbances.
- Force the child to attend funerals or ignore signs of grieving in the child.

Source: Murray, R. B., & Zentner, J. P. (2001). Health promotion strategies through the life span (7th ed.). Reprinted by permission of Pearson Education, Inc. Upper Saddle River, NJ 07458.

to children, but it is important that they know that "Daddy" is dead and that it will be difficult to live without him.

The Nurse and Grief

Everyone grieves, and nurses are no exception. Most nurses believe that they should be able to maintain their "professional demeanor" and not give in to their feelings. When the death of a patient occurs, we have a right to grieve our loss and express our feelings. We also need to comfort other nurses who are grieving. Remember that there is no "right" or "wrong" when it comes to grieving.

Be prepared to experience grief as a nurse. Some nurses react to grief by avoidance and refuse to acknowledge their feelings. Other nurses are vulnerable and expose themselves to the grief experience. You will need to learn to experience grief. The most important thing is to put yourself in your patient's shoes. Be empathetic and feel what your patient is feeling.

We have cried with parents at the loss of a child and hugged and held the mother of a young man dying of AIDS. For each loss we experience, we know pain, and for the pain we experience, we learn to know joy. Loss is not easy but just be yourself and offer your heart to the grieving, be they patient or nurse.

Impulsive Suicide

At some point, you may work with a suicidal patient or even be faced with a suicidal family member, friend, or coworker. The thought of suicide tends to bring out strong feelings in most people. Some of us believe that suicide is immoral, while others understand that suicide is the result of severe psychological distress. Regardless of your beliefs, suicide happens and suicide rates in our country continue to rise. Suicide among teenagers and the elderly continue to rise exponentially (Table 23–6).

Clues to Suicidal Behavior

Did you ever wonder why it is that the general public often know the warning signs for cancer, or how to recognize a heart attack, but they have no idea about clues to suicidal behavior.

Table 23–6. Summary of Suicide Statistics

- Suicide is the ninth leading cause of death in the United States.
- Suicide is the third cause of death among young people 15–24 years of age.
- The highest suicide rate is for persons over 65 years of age.
- It is estimated that there are about 10 attempted suicides to 1 completion.
- Of *all* suicides, 72% are committed by white males.
- The gender ratio is 4 males to 1 female (4:1).
- Suicide by firearms is the most common method (60% of all suicides).
- Nearly 80% of all firearm suicides are committed by white men.
- Professional persons, including lawyers, dentists, military men, and physicians, have higher-than-average suicide rates.
- Suicide is less frequent among practicing members of most religious groups.

Source: Varcarolis, E. M. (1998, p. 727). Foundations of psychiatric–mental health nursing. (3rd ed.). Philadelphia, PA: Saunders.

1. **Actual** (verbal) **clues**
   - I'm going to kill myself.
   - I wish I were dead.
   - My family would be better off without me.
   - You're going to regret how you've treated me.
   - I'm tired of living.
   - Here, take this (valued object). I won't be needing it anymore.
   - I don't need to study for the final exam, I won't be around to take it.
2. **Behavior clues**
   - Previous suicide attempt
   - Giving away valued possessions
   - Drug or alcohol abuse
   - Loss of a loved one
   - Loss of job/money/prestige
   - Prolonged physical illness
   - Buying a gun
   - Writing a suicide note
   - Sudden recovery from a severe depression
   - Withdrawal from social activities
   - Crying for no apparent reason
   - Changes in typical behavior
3. **Catastrophic clues** (something that is catastrophic for the individual)
   - A student on a football scholarship survives an automobile accident, but is paralyzed from the neck down and unable to play football
   - A young aspiring model breaks her nose and receives several facial scars in a house fire
4. **Depressive clues** (think of how you feel or act when depressed)
   - Insomnia
   - Anorexia/overeating
   - Sloppiness
   - Inability to concentrate (drop in grades)
   - Feeling worthless
   - Feeling hopeless
   - Loss of self-esteem
   - Rage/anger/hostility
   - Preoccupation with death
   - Chronic minor illness or accidents

It is important for everyone to be familiar with suicidal clues. An individual who is suicidal will most likely give more than one clue. For example, someone might decide to make a will or plan a funeral after the death of a friend, but that individual is being prudent, not suicidal. However, if the person makes out a will, plans a funeral, says "I wish I were dead," appears depressed, and buys a gun, that person is probably suicidal.

Once it is apparent that the individual may be suicidal, you need to ask them, "Are you thinking about harming yourself?" or "Are you considering suicide?" or a similar question. Asking the question does not give the individual the idea to commit suicide. They already have the idea. Once you ask the question, the individual will either admit that they are feeling suicidal, or deny it. Most people will be honest with you.

Sometimes all it takes is for someone to care enough to ask one tough question. Have you ever had a major problem that you felt you could not share with anyone else? The distress of carrying that burden alone is often very difficult to handle. During that time, did anyone ask you what was wrong? When we are carrying a heavy burden alone and someone cares enough to ask us about it, we are usually able to share the problem. Once you share the problem with someone else, the burden becomes lighter. The same is true of suicidal thoughts. Sometimes, when they are shared with someone else the suicidal individual feels better and may be willing to seek help in sorting out the problem.

Suicide Intervention Dos and Don'ts

If the person tells you that they are considering suicide, here are some intervention dos and don'ts.

Do's	Don'ts
Be direct	Dare the person to go through with it
Talk openly	Leave the person alone
Be matter of fact about suicide	Tell the person they are a coward or selfish
Listen attentively	Promise unrealistic things
Allow the person to express feelings	Engage in philosophical discussion (you'll lose)
Be nonjudgmental	Debate or lecture
Accept the person's feelings	Promise not to tell anyone (you may need to in order to save a life)
Offer alternatives (not false reassurance)	
Take action to remove harmful objects	
Get help from a suicide specialist	

Suicide Plan

Once it is known that a person is considering suicide, you need to determine the seriousness or lethality of the plan. The following things need to be considered:

- Does the person have a plan?
- Is the method of suicide (hanging, guns, or pills, etc.) available?
- How lethal is the proposed plan (higher risk of death with guns, automobile accidents, drowning, and electrocution; lower risk with pills, wrist cutting, and carbon monoxide)? Remember that combining two lower risk methods of suicide—for example, taking barbiturates and using carbon monoxide—may place the person at higher risk.

The higher the lethality, the higher the risk of suicide. For example, consider the following individuals.

Stephanie is a 32-year-old nurse who is depressed over the breakup of her marriage. Stephanie lives alone and has a variety of pills at her disposal including Seconal and Xanax. She also has access to her mother's Lasix, Digoxin, and potassium. Stephanie plans to eat supper, make a pill cocktail of all of the above pills, and drink alcohol with them. She then plans to lay down, disconnect the phone, and place a plastic bag over her head before she falls asleep.

Marie is a 15-year-old high school student who has decided to commit suicide by overdosing on birth control pills. She is not aware that birth control pills are not lethal.

A Case in Point

Marty was a 54-year-old female who called the suicide hotline every Thursday night. Tom, a volunteer, was usually on duty when Marty called. Over time, Marty and Tom developed a trusting relationship and one night Tom asked Marty why she called every Thursday. Marty explained that she enjoyed talking with Tom. She asked Tom, "If I ever intended to kill myself, do you really think I would call first?" She then said, "I'm not stupid, when I'm going to do it I'm going to do it, I won't be calling you first!" Marty continued calling for months until one Thursday night when Tom did not hear from her. Wondering whether Marty was ill, Tom asked other volunteers if they had spoken with Marty. No one had. Tom read Marty's obituary in the paper 2 days later. True to her promise, Marty did not call the hotline before she killed herself.

Jane is a 40-year-old flight attendant who also skydives. She recently lost her job due to airline cutbacks. She lives alone and decides to commit suicide. Janet plans to take a bath with a radio plugged in beside the tub. She intends to drink two or three glasses of wine while listening to her favorite radio station. Prior to getting out of the tub, she plans to "accidentally" drop the radio in the tub with her.

Which of these three women has the least lethal plan? The answer is Marie. Remember that electrocution is more lethal than overdosing. However, if Stephanie is able to swallow and keep down her pill cocktail, she will certainly die as well. It would be necessary to intervene with all three women, although more intense intervention is needed for both Jane and Stephanie. Remember that even though Marie has a plan that is not lethal, she will still require intervention. Any threat of self-injury needs to be taken seriously!

After determining whether a patient has a plan and how lethal that plan is, it is necessary to develop a plan for dealing with suicidal behavior. Most suicidal individuals need intervention from a crisis center, emergency room, suicide hotline, or mental health provider. Direct the suicidal individual to the closest available site in your area. Accompany them to the hospital or crisis center. Encourage them to seek help from a suicide or crisis hotline. When suicide is imminent, it is up to you to get help. If in doubt, it is better to err on the side of caution than to wait too long and have someone die.

Even though you intervene in suicidal behavior, it is important to realize that the choice to live or die is left to the suicidal individual. By that we mean that you can intervene, but the person may still commit suicide. Although in health care we talk about a "safe environment," there is no such thing. Patients have committed suicide on locked psychiatric units in padded seclusion

A CASE IN POINT

George was a nursing student who had a good friend in high school, Lee, who threatened suicide frequently. Every time Lee was feeling suicidal he would call George for help. George tried many times to intervene and get Lee some help, but Lee would never follow through. The more Lee called, the more frustrated George became. Finally, George told Lee that if he really wanted to die, he should cut his wrists lengthwise to sever the arteries and lie in a bathtub of warm water to encourage the blood flow. Within 2 weeks, Lee was dead. He left a note thanking George for the information on how to die. To this day, George has not fully recovered from the guilt of having helped his friend to commit suicide. Although George attempted to help Lee, he allowed his anger and frustration to take over.

rooms. If someone wants to commit suicide badly enough, they will eventually succeed.

If you happen to work in an area where suicidal individuals are brought for treatment, be compassionate. We have worked in the ER and have seen suicidal patients being treated disrespectfully. If you observe other staff members treating suicidal (or for that matter any patient) disrespectfully, report it! We have witnessed doctors requesting oversized nasogastric tubes for lavage of patients who have overdosed so that the patient will not attempt suicide again. All patients deserve to be treated with respect.

If you become angry and frustrated when caring for suicidal patients, you need to determine why. Nurses are not allowed to abuse patients, and verbal abuse is just as harmful as physical abuse. When someone is desperate enough to consider suicide, the health care giver should not add to that distress.

Suicide Survivors

If you have ever experienced a suicide, you know how difficult it is to accept. Survivors of suicide (SOS) are confronted with the social stigma that surrounds suicide as well as the loss of a loved one. Most of us find it difficult to comfort someone who is grieving, but we are more uncomfortable when that person has lost someone to suicide. Often, SOS face their loss alone because they are unsure of how to seek support. Because of the nature of suicide, many survivors end up feeling abandoned and left alone to mourn their loss.

Suicide Survivors and Grief

Points to consider when dealing with SOS include:

- An SOS experiences a great deal of anger and guilt that is not always associated with the grief process.
- Nurses need to be available and to actively listen to the SOS.
- Do not think about what you should say, but rather listen to what the survivor is telling you.
- Let the survivor come to conclusions about why the individual committed suicide.
- There is no reason for you to try to offer explanations because chances are you do not know why it happened either.
- The death needs to be talked about openly with all family members.
- Sometimes families avoid discussing the suicide because they are afraid to break the silence that follows.
- Often the family is dysfunctional and silence is the way that they have dealt with other problems.

- To reach all family members, you may need to relate to each one on an individual basis to allow the individual to express their grief.

An SOS may take longer to heal because of the nature of their loss. Be patient! There are a number of organizations that provide support to the SOS. If the SOS has access to the Internet, these two sites might be of help.

RESOURCE WEB SITES

1. American Foundation for Suicide Prevention: *www.afsp.org*
2. Survivors of Suicide: *www.members.xoom.com/sos5/*

Rational Suicide

We stated earlier that no matter how you intervene in a suicidal crisis, the decision to live or die remains with the suicidal individual. Some individuals believe in the right to die and believe that they have the right to choose when and how they die. Quality of life, personal dignity, and self-control all lead a person to rational suicide.

When an individual is in a terminal condition and plans for death by their own hand, it is called *rational suicide*. Many suicides occur in this fashion. Most health care givers are not informed prior to a rational suicide because the individual and their family do not want any intervention. Another reason is that when a person commits suicide, insurance companies may refuse to pay benefits.

Assisted Suicide

Assisted suicide is similar to rational suicide in that the individual is experiencing a prolonged and terminal illness. With both rational and assisted suicide, the individual consciously chooses to die at a time and place that they choose. In rational suicide the individual has the means for suicide at their disposal; in assisted suicide the dying individual requests assistance from a physician who prescribes a lethal dose of a medication. The primary difference between assisted and rational suicide is that, with assisted suicide, the physician is made aware of the patient's desires.

Assisted suicide is illegal in most states, although Oregon passed the Death with Dignity Act in 1994 and then reviewed judicially, and on November 4,

A CASE IN POINT

Leona is a 95-year-old widow in failing health who lives alone in her own home. Her husband died 6 months ago of lung cancer. Leona and her husband had been married 65 years and they had no children. When Leona's husband died, her niece decided that Leona could no longer live on her own and that she should be placed in a nursing home. Leona knows that she is dying and refuses to leave her home of 65 years. Leona chooses to die in her own bed, in her own home. One evening, Leona takes an overdose of barbiturates and dies in her sleep. Since Leona is 95 years old, the coroner determines that she died of old age and natural causes. No autopsy is ordered.

1997, it was reasserted by a 60 to 40% margin when the voters opposed repeal of the act (Guido, 2001). Dr. Jack Kevorkian and his "death machine" have forced the state of Michigan to consider the issue as well. Initiatives for assisted suicide have been sponsored by the Hemlock Society, Choice in Dying, and Americans against Human Suffering in California and Washington. According to the Oregon Death with Dignity Act, certain provisions must be met prior to writing a prescription for assisted suicide. The provisions are:

- Both the attending physician and a consulting physician must certify that the patient has no more than 6 months to live.
- The patient must make both an oral and a written request for the prescription, followed by a second oral request 15 or more days after the original request.
- The attending physician must refer the patient for counseling if a psychological illness or depression is suspected.
- The doctor must wait at least 48 hours after the third request before prescribing the medication (Guido, 2001).

To date, most nursing organizations have agreed that nurses should not encourage assisted or rational suicide. Nurses are in a difficult position because they have been taught to be an advocate for patient rights, yet to prevent suicide. Many nurses believe that they should be allowed to respect the patient's right to die rather than face a life of disease with pain and unrelieved suffering. Ironically, the patient is more likely to ask a nurse for information about suicide than a physician. Whether or not you sympathize with the patient's request, it is up to you to provide a sounding board for patients who wish to discuss rational suicide. Burgess (1997) offers the information in Table 23–7 for assessing whether or not a patient is considering rational suicide.

Table 23–7. Assessment of Rational Suicide

1. The purpose and motives of the person considering suicide
   Is the person making a request for help?
   Why is the person consulting a health professional?
   Is the request for help in suicide a request for someone else to decide?
   Is the suicide plan financially motivated?
   What has kept the person from committing suicide so far?
   Does the person fear becoming a burden?
2. Stability of request
   How stable is the request?
   Has suicide been planned for a long time or is it a response to a recent event?
3. Is the request consistent with the person's basic values?
4. Are the medical and nonmedical facts cited in the request accurate?
5. Has the person considered the effects of suicide on others?
6. Suicide plan and options
   How far in the future would this take place?
   Has the person picked a method of suicide?
   Would the person be willing to tell others about his or her suicide plan?
   Does the person see suicide as the only way out?
7. What cultural influences are shaping a person's choices?
8. Are the person's affairs in order? Have arrangements been made for a funeral or durable power of attorney? In most states a health professional's relationship with a patient implies a legal and professional duty to refrain from assisting suicide. Terminally ill patients with suicide plans, however, deserve thoughtful evaluation of their rational and irrational requests and appropriate treatment options for their depression, pain, or symptom distress. Clinicians need to understand the ethical issues and criteria for evaluating rational suicide.

Source: Burgess, A. W. (1997, p. 579). Psychiatric nursing promoting mental health. *Reprinted by permission of Pearson Education, Inc. Upper Saddle River, NJ 07458.*

Although patients frequently ask for assistance from nurses, there are legal and ethical concerns. Nurses are expected to try to determine the cause of the patient's request.

- Is the patient depressed?
- Is the patient's pain uncontrolled?
- Is the patient afraid of dying?
- Is the patient afraid of suffering?

- Does the patient need information about advance medical directives?
- Is the patient concerned about dying alone?

The nurse can deal with each of these situations by offering to contact resources, request more pain medication, or just spend time with the patient listening to concerns.

Although nurses are legally and ethically unable to assist the patient with suicide, many nurses are not adverse to the idea. In other countries, nurses are part of the assisted suicide team who help patients end their lives with dignity. As the issue becomes more commonplace and legal parameters are put into place, it is likely that the nurse will have to come to terms with the process.

Assisted suicide occurs when a patient seeks help to die. With active euthanasia, the patient is not always a part of the decision-making process. Many disabled people and others with chronic illness fear that the more society approves of assisted suicide, the more likely euthanasia is to follow. No matter how compassionate and ethical our society claims to be, deciding whether or not a person should die and taking that person's life is still murder at this time. There are other countries, however, where active euthanasia is practiced.

Nurses are involved with life and death decisions on a daily basis. You will hear the term *slow code,* meaning that a patient is allowed to die before a code is called, or little is done to resuscitate the patient when a code is called. This occurs when some family members wish their loved one to be allowed to die and others cannot agree. It is also done when the doctor believes that no further intervention will prolong life and the patient is suffering.

When one of us was a member of the code team, she was told by another team member that a slow code meant we should walk backwards rather than run as we usually did. You may also be given doctor's orders to give a patient a high dose of pain medication that the pharmacist may tell you is "not compatible with life." In both of these instances, you will need to make a decision as to what you plan to do.

Death is a subject that we are all familiar with but that few people want to discuss. Whether or not we discuss death, it will continue to occur. All of us need support when someone dies, although we all grieve privately and in our own way. It is important for nurses to support dying patients, grieving families, and other nurses when a death occurs.

The Hemlock Society has chapters in every state (P.O. Box 11830, Eugene, OR 97440. Telephone: 503-342-5748). The goal of the Hemlock Society is to disseminate information about rational and assisted suicide. Through books and literature, including the book *Final Exit,* the Hemlock Society provides clear and precise information on how to die.

A CASE IN POINT

A young military nurse worked on an oncology unit. One patient forced her to come to terms with what she believed about living and dying. Joe was a 22-year-old Air Force corporal when he was diagnosed with bladder cancer. By the time he was 23 years old, it had metastasized to all parts of his body. During the night shift, Joe and the nurse would talk because they were both the same age. They had a great time talking about music, school, and dating. Joe knew that he was dying and talked with the nurse about his wishes. He did not want to suffer and requested that he be allowed to die without intervention. (This occurred before living wills were common.) His request was charted and the nurse spoke with his attending physician. One night, she arrived at the hospital and was told that Joe had coded five times during the prior shift. Each time, his doctor resuscitated him. The nurse was appalled that Joe's wishes were being ignored and that such heroic methods were being used to keep him alive. About 20 minutes into the shift, Joe coded again. His physician yelled to begin resuscitation immediately. He was reminded of Joe's wishes. The nurse told him that she would have nothing to do with further resuscitation attempts. A nurse from another unit was called in to assist him, but Joe died despite all of their intervention. The nurse was extremely angry with the physician for continuing to revive a patient who was so debilitated and who had expressed a desire to die with dignity. She felt guilty that she had let Joe down in allowing this to continue and prayed that he was beyond knowing. This was the first situation in which the nurse had to come to terms with what she believed about dying.

RESOURCE WEB SITES

Partnership For Caring: *www.partnershipforcaring.org*
Hemlock Society: *www.hemlock.org*

24

ABGs—The Basics Contained in 10 Questions

Arterial blood gases (ABGs) are usually ordered on patients in emergency departments and critical care units. ABG values provide an objective assessment of arterial blood oxygenation, aveolar ventilation, and acid–base balance. In addition to identifying problems, the information is used to monitor the effectiveness of medical and nursing interventions. The following 10 questions will walk you through the essentials for understanding ABG results.

Questions

1. **Is there one pH for the body?** No. Various body tissues and fluids have their own pH value. For example, saliva has a pH range of 6.6 to 7.5, while urine's pH range is 4.6 to 8.0. However, the value that is crucial to health is pH of arterial blood. Normal arterial blood has a pH range of 7.35 to 7.45. This is a very narrow range and values outside this range quickly lead to acute illness and if uncorrected, can be fatal. When someone speaks of a patient's **pH value,** the reference is being made to arterial blood.

2. **How does the body achieve this pH value?** As long as there is a **1:20 ratio** of carbonic acid to bicarbonate arterial, pH will remain within normal limits (WNL). You should remember some essential facts from chemistry.
   - H_2CO_3 = carbonic acid
   - Carbonic acid can change into carbon dioxide and water and back to carbonic acid. $H_2CO_3 \leftrightarrow CO_2 + H_2O$
   - HCO_3 = bicarbonate

243

Following are the basic combinations for carbon dioxide and bicarbonate.

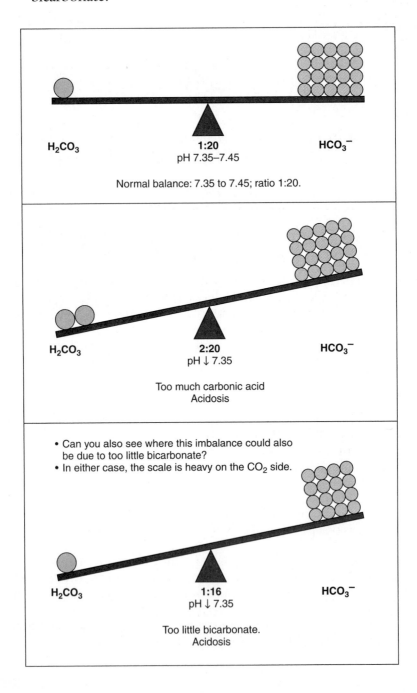

H_2CO_3 **1:20** HCO_3^-
pH 7.35–7.45

Normal balance: 7.35 to 7.45; ratio 1:20.

H_2CO_3 **2:20** HCO_3^-
pH ↓ 7.35

Too much carbonic acid
Acidosis

- Can you also see where this imbalance could also be due to too little bicarbonate?
- In either case, the scale is heavy on the CO_2 side.

H_2CO_3 **1:16** HCO_3^-
pH ↓ 7.35

Too little bicarbonate.
Acidosis

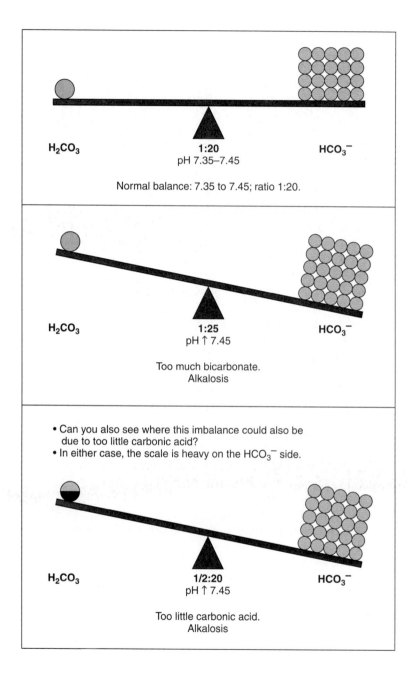

Normal balance: 7.35 to 7.45; ratio 1:20.

Too much bicarbonate.
Alkalosis

• Can you also see where this imbalance could also be
  due to too little carbonic acid?
• In either case, the scale is heavy on the HCO_3^- side.

Too little carbonic acid.
Alkalosis

Note: In all cases once the pH goes **over** 7.45 it is called
alkalosis and once the pH goes **below** 7.35 it is called **acidosis.**

3. **How does the body maintain this delicate balance?** Two body organs accomplish the balance between carbonic acid and bicarbonate.
   - The **lungs** control the **carbonic acid** side of the ratio by controlling the body's level of carbon dioxide. (Recall the carbonic acid to carbon dioxide equation in question 2.)
   - The kidneys control the **bicarbonate** and **H⁺** ion concentrations by various chemical reactions in the kidney tubules. The balance between these controls is reflected in the **arterial blood gas** values.
4. **What information is indicated in an ABG report?** An ABG report will have at least the following information.
   - **pH:** How acid or alkaline the arterial blood is.
   - **CO_2:** The pressure exerted by the carbon dioxide dissolved in the arterial blood (carbon dioxide tension). Note that carbonic acid is not directly measured. Instead, CO_2, its gaseous state, is measured.
   - **HCO_3^-:** The amount of bicarbonate dissolved in the arterial blood.
   - **O_2:** The pressure exerted by the oxygen that is dissolved in arterial blood (oxygen tension).
   - **SaO_2:** Oxygen saturation, which represents the percentage of hemoglobin that is carrying oxygen.
        The oxygen values (O_2 and SaO_2) are essential in evaluating how well the patient's body is being oxygenated. However, these values *do not* influence the pH value. The pH value is determined by the ratio of carbonic acid to bicarbonate.
5. **What are the normal values for ABGs?**
   - pH: 7.35 to 7.45
   - CO_2: 35 to 45 mm Hg
   - HCO_3^-: 24 to 28 mEq/L
        Remember that the CO_2 and HCO_3^- determine arterial pH. However, ABG reports also include two additional values that evaluate the patient's oxygen status.
   - O_2: 80 to 100 mm Hg
   - SaO_2: 95 to 100%
6. **How do I know if an abnormal pH is due to the lungs (respiratory) or to the kidneys (metabolic)?**
   - Check the pH value. Where is it in comparison to normal—alkaline or acid?
   - Check the CO_2 value. High CO_2 means more of the gas is available for conversion to carbonic acid. Low CO_2 indicates less carbon dioxide is available for conversion to carbonic acid. The CO_2 represents the lungs' side of the balance, **respiratory control.**
   - Check the HCO_3^- value. A high value means a large amount of bicarbonate build-up, while a low value indicates bicarbonate loss. The HCO_3^- represents the kidneys' side of the balance, **metabolic control.**
   - Determine which value (CO_2 or HCO_3^-) can create the patient's pH.
   - Here are four examples of laboratory values to illustrate each of the main pH imbalances.

Example 1: pH = 7.31 CO_2 = 50 mm Hg HCO_3^- = 24 mEq/L

—*Analysis:* pH is less than 7.35, so the condition is **acidosis.**
CO_2 is above 45 mm Hg.
HCO_3^- is normal.

Conclusion: This is an example of **respiratory acidosis.** (*Note:* A pH of 7.31 could not be caused by a bicarbonate value that is WNL.)

Example 2: pH = 7.31 CO_2 = 44 mm Hg HCO_3^- = 20 mEq/L

—*Analysis:* pH is less than 7.35 so the condition is **acidosis.**
CO_2 is normal.
HCO_3^- is less than 24 mEq/L.

Conclusion: This is an example of **metabolic acidosis.** (*Note:* This is the same pH as the first example, but it is due to too little bicarbonate. Refer to page 244 if you need help visualizing this.)

Example 3: pH = 7.48 CO_2 = 33 mm Hg HCO_3^- = 24 mEq/L

—*Analysis:* pH is more than 7.45 so the condition is **alkalosis.**
CO_2 is below 35 mm Hg.
HCO_3^- is normal.

Conclusion: This is an example of **respiratory alkalosis.** (*Note:* A pH of 7.45 could not be caused by a bicarbonate value that is WNL.)

Example 4: pH = 7.48 CO_2 = 43 mm Hg HCO_3^- = 33 mEq/L

—*Analysis:* pH is more than 7.45 so the condition is **alkalosis.**
CO_2 is normal.
HCO_3^- is above 28 mEq/L.

Conclusion: This is an example of **metabolic alkalosis.** (*Note:* This is the same pH as the third example, but it is due to too much bicarbonate. Refer to page 245 if you have difficulty visualizing this.)

---

7. **Can I tell by looking at an ABG report if the body is attempting to get the pH back into balance?** Yes. But sometimes it is tricky. What you are asking about is called **compensation.** As one system goes out of balance, the other system kicks in to restore and maintain the all important ratio of 1 part carbonic acid to 20 parts bicarbonate.

When you look back at the four examples, you see imbalances without evidence that the body is attempting to regain the ratio. These are examples of **uncompensated** situations. The following is an example of a compensated situation.

$$pH = 7.4 \qquad CO_2 = 60 \text{ mm Hg} \qquad HCO_3^- = 37 \text{ mEq/L}$$

Note that the carbon dioxide and bicarbonate values are both abnormal, but the pH is WNL. In this case, the kidneys are retaining bicarbonate to counter the lungs' retention of carbon dioxide, thus keeping the 1 to 20 ratio and a pH that is WNL.

Compensation can be full or partial. In **full compensation,** the pH is WNL but both carbon dioxide and bicarbonate are abnormal. In **partial compensation,** the pH is still abnormal as well as the carbon dioxide and/or the bicarbonate values. Remember, compensation takes time. Acid–base imbalances with a respiratory etiology are generally corrected quicker than imbalances with a metabolic etiology.

8. **What is base excess that I see on ABG reports? Base excess** (BE) is a value that indicates the sum of the body's buffer **anions**—that is, negative ions. Bicarbonate accounts for only about half of the body's anions. (Total buffer anions are in the range of 45 to 50 mEq/L, while total bicarbonate range is 24 to 28 mEq/L.) Therefore, base excess gives a better view of the **metabolic** side of the acid–base balance.

Normal values for base excess are −3 to +3 mEq/L. Positive values, those above +3 mEq/L, indicate base excess. Negative values, those below −3 mEq/L, indicate base deficit. The following are two ABG examples that include BE values.

Example: #1

$$pH = 7.16 \qquad CO_2 = 57 \text{ mm Hg} \qquad HCO_3^- = 25 \text{ mEq/L} \qquad BE = +1$$

Both the bicarbonate and BE values are WNL. This is a case of **respiratory acidosis** with no evidence that compensation has begun.

Example: #2

$$pH = 7.18 \qquad CO_2 = 41 \text{ mm Hg} \qquad HCO_3^- = 14 \text{ mEq/L} \qquad BE = -4$$

The respiratory value (carbon dioxide) is WNL, while the bicarbonate is below normal. Note that the base excess is actually a deficit (−4). This value indicates that there is a true deficit of bicarbonate. This example is typical of one that might be seen in an individual with diabetic ketoacidosis. So this represents **metabolic acidosis** where, as yet, there is no compensation by the lungs.

9. **Can you determine the 1:20 ratio from the ABG values?** Yes. But you do not need to. The pH tells you about the CO_2 and HCO_3^- balance. Once the pH is beyond the norm in either direction, the 1:20 ratio has been lost. Although carbonic acid is seldom measured, its normal blood value is 3% of the carbon dioxide value, or 1.05 to 1.35 mEq/L. Remember that normal bicarbonate is 22 to 26 mEq/L. Using these normal ranges, the ratio of carbonic acid to bicarbonate can be calculated.

   Note that in this calculation we are using carbonic acid, *not* carbon dioxide. You *cannot take* the carbon dioxide value and divide it into the bicarbonate value to determine the ratio. So, although calculating the ratio is possible, it is not practical to do so.

10. **When should I be alert for possible acid–base imbalance?** Table 24–1 provides an overview of each of the four basic acid–base imbalances with common etiologies and assessment findings.

   When the pH has a metabolic etiology, the pH values and the bicarbonate value go together; that is, high pH plus high HCO_3^- in metabolic alkalosis and low pH plus low HCO_3^- in metabolic acidosis. When the imbalance has a respiratory etiology, the pH value and the carbon dioxide values are opposite; that is, low pH and high CO_2 in respiratory acidosis and high pH and low CO_2 in respiratory alkalosis.

Table 24–1. Four Basic Acid–Base Imbalances

Imbalance	Common Etiologies	Assessment Findings
Metabolic acidosis: pH less than 7.35, HCO_3^- will be ↓	Diabetic acidosis, shock, renal failure, intestinal fistulas, lactic build-up as in cardiac arrest	Apathy, disorientation, weakness, stupor, coma, Kussmaul's respiration
Metabolic alkalosis: pH more than 7.45, HCO_3^- will be ↑	Nasogastric drainage, prolonged vomiting	Shallow and slow respirations, lethargy, irritability, tetany, convulsions
Respiratory acidosis: pH less than 7.35, CO_2 will be ↑	Respiratory depression (drugs, CNS trauma, any condition leading to hypoventilation), COPD, pneumonia	Dyspnea, disorientation, tachycardia, arrhythmias
Respiratory alkalosis: pH more than 7.35, CO_2 will be ↓	Any situation leading to hyperventilation (emotions, pain, respirator overventilation)	Lightheadedness, inability to concentrate, numbness and tingling, loss of consciousness

CNS, central nervous system; COPD, chronic obstructive pulmonary disease.

SPEED BUMP

A memory tip to help to make this connection is MeTRO.

Metabolic (e)
Together
Respiratory
Opposite

You should now have a solid foundation for understanding ABGs. The next time you look at ABG values, please refer to these guidelines to help you understand what mechanisms are taking place. With practice, the need to refer to this information will become less and less.

25

Endocrine Highlights

▌ Production and Secretion of Hormones

The endocrine system (also referred to as the hormone system) consists of organs with secretions that go directly into the circulatory system. The main actions of the system center on regulating three body functions: metabolic activity, growth, and reproduction. There are nine endocrine glands in women and seven in men (Figure 25–1). (Remember, men will not have ovarian and placental hormones.) Although the number of endocrine glands is small, the number of hormones that they secrete is large. Table 25–1 presents an overview of the *most commonly* seen dysfunctions that occur in the endocrine system.

The production and secretion of hormones from the endocrine glands is controlled by negative feedback loop actions (see Figure 32–2). The hypothalamus and pituitary gland regulate almost all of the glands. Because of this regulatory pathway, disorders of an endocrine gland may be due to a problem at one of several points: the hypothalamus, pituitary, or the gland itself.

Two major exceptions to the hypothalamus–pituitary gland and hormone–serum levels loop are the parathyroids and the pancreas. Hormone levels from these two glands respond to serum levels and do not involve the hypothalamus–pituitary loop.

Students often have difficulty with hypo- and hyperfunction of endocrine glands. This is one of those times when mastering knowledge of the normal actions of the hormones will be worth the study time.

251

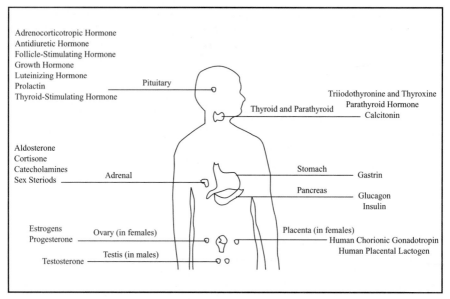

Figure 25–1. Endocrine glands.

Diabetes

Of all the endocrine dysfunctions, the two most frequently encountered are hypothyroidism and diabetes mellitus, which is usually referred to simply as diabetes. (When referring to diabetes insipidus, the disorder of the posterior pituitary, the entire name is used.)

Because diabetes is such a prevalent health problem, you will be learning about it in almost all of your nursing courses. As you look at the texts for the various nursing courses, notice the vast amount of space devoted to diabetes. Be prepared, therefore, for many classes and test questions on the topic. In addition, you will no doubt have many clinical assignments in which diabetes is one of the patient's health care needs. As some topics are covered in school, students tend to put the knowledge gained on a back burner as they move into other courses. This cannot be done with diabetes!!

We will look at the most recent information on diabetes classification. Over the years diabetes has had several classification systems. The terms *juvenile-onset* and *adult-onset* were used up until the late 1970s. In 1979, these terms were replaced. Juvenile-onset diabetes became *insulin-dependent diabetes mellitus* (IDDM), also called *Type I diabetes;* while adult-onset became *non–insulin-dependent diabetes mellitus* (NIDDM), also called *Type II diabetes.*

Table 25–1. Commonly Seen Endocrine Dysfunctions

Major Endocrine Gland/Hormone	Hypofunction Disorder	Hyperfunction Disorder
Pancreas Insulin	Hyperglycemia = diabetes mellitus Based on severity, can be life threatening	Rare natural occurrence Excess external insulin = hypoglycemia/insulin reaction
Thyroid Thyroxine (T_4); thyronine (T_3)	Undetected at birth can lead to cretinism Adult onset leads to myxedema	Graves' disease Severe hyperthyroidism (can be life threatening): thyrotoxicosis, thyroid storm
Adrenal cortex Glucocorticoids (chief one: cortisol, also called hydrocortisone); mineralocorticoids (chief one: aldosterone)	Addison's disease If etiology is at the adrenal cortex, both glucocorticoids and mineralocorticoids are deficient; if etiology is at the pituitary level, glucocorticoids are major deficiency (*note:* if exogenous glucocorticoids are administered for periods of 10–14 days or longer and suddenly stopped [versus dosage being tapered off], adrenal insufficiency[a] may result)	Cushing's disease, a syndrome usually due to excess amounts of glucocorticoids
Growth hormone	Dwarfism (several forms)	In children: gigantism In adults: acromegaly

[a] Adrenal insufficiency from any etiology can be life threatening.

The Four Diabetes Groups

In 1997, the American Diabetes Association developed a new classification system based on the cause, not insulin use. The new system now has four diabetes groups.

1. **Type 1 diabetes:** This type has two categories.
   - **Type 1 immune-mediated.** Individuals in this group have beta-cell destruction (and thus no insulin production) due to an autoimmune process.
   - **Type 1 idiopathic.** Individuals in this group have no evidence of an autoimmune process.
2. **Type 2 diabetes:** In this group are individuals with some insulin production by the pancreas but the amount is not sufficient to maintain normal blood glucose levels. In addition, insulin receptors on cell surfaces are resistant to letting what insulin is available into the cells for use.

Note the change from Roman numerals to Arabic numerals (old Type I and Type II, and new Type 1 and Type 2)

3. **Other specific types:** This category includes individuals whose diabetes is due to such etiologies as drugs or chemicals, genetic defects, and pathologies of other endocrine glands that stress the pancreas.

4. **Gestational diabetes:** Diabetes that develops during pregnancy.

As you look at this new classification system it may seem to be the same as the current system. To help you understand how it is different from the IDDM and NIDDM classification system, we will look at a clinical situation. You are talking to your clinical instructor about your patient who is a Type II diabetic. You proudly tell your instructor that the patient has received her morning dose of long-acting insulin. Your instructor looks at you with a puzzled look and asks, "If she is a Type II diabetic, why is she receiving insulin?" Up to now, this was confusing. Although we know that over time many individuals who have Type II diabetes need exogenous insulin to maintain blood sugar levels, these patients were never reclassified as Type I diabetics.

Because the foundation of the new nomenclature is etiology of the underlying pathology, it should make understanding this patient easier. This patient would initially be in the new classification system as a Type 2 diabetic. (In the old system she would fit the profile of Type II.) However, as her metabolic needs change, insulin may be added to her health care regime without confusion as to what type she is. The etiology of her condition has not changed, therefore, her classification has not changed. The patient remains a Type 2 diabetic who requires insulin.

It will take time for this new classification system to become known and used. In the meantime, realize that if you are reading about diabetes and the reference is to adult-onset or juvenile-onset diabetes, you are reading old material. Reference to Types I and II should be expected for several years because it takes time to bring textbooks up to date. Conversion to the updated classification will take several years.

Diabetes is one of our most prevalent health problems. Keeping up with advances in diabetic care will be essential to your professional practice.

26

Drug Calculations and Medication Issues

◼ The Basics

Regardless of the area of practice, all nurses administer medications. One of the major responsibilities associated with this nursing action is preparing and administering the correct medication dose. Almost from your first nursing course to your last, faculty will expect you to demonstrate competency in calculating drug doses. This chapter will provide you with highlights that you will need to better understand how to calculate drug dosages.

Before going to these basic guidelines, let us first go to the grocery store and get some milk. In the milk section we find milk with different amounts of fat: 3%, 2%, 1½%, 1%, and 0% fat (Figure 26–1). In addition, the milk is available in several sizes: half-pints, pints, quarts, half-gallons, or gallons. So, although you can buy 3% milk in five different size containers, the strength (fat content) of the milk remains the same (Figure 26–2).

Now that you realize that the "strength" of milk (its percent of fat) is not related to the size of the container, let's take a trip and buy some milk. You are now in France buying milk. At the checkout counter all you have is U.S. currency. The clerk makes you go to the bank and exchange your money for French currency and now you can buy the milk. You now are in England and try to buy milk with your French currency. Again, the clerk makes you exchange the French currency for British currency before you can buy the milk. Finally, back home in the United States you go to the store to get milk, and guess what? All you have is British currency. So you must make another trip to the bank to exchange the British money into its equivalent in U.S. currency (Figure 26–3).

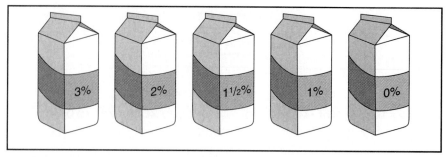

Figure 26–1. Milk—same size container—with different percentages of fat content.

Keeping this milk analogy in mind, let's look at a typical drug calculation problem:

- A patient is to have 100 mg of a medication. The bottle indicates that there is 0.1 g of the medication in one tablet. What do you give the patient?

Faced with this question, students often experience a mild panic attack and research indicates that many practicing nurses might also have problems solving it correctly. If you follow the basics of medication calculation, you will not be among this group.

The following is the most widely used calculation formula for basic calculations so you might as well let it become part of you.

$$\frac{D \times V}{H} = X$$

D is the desired strength of the medication, what the patient is to receive, or what percent milkfat you want.

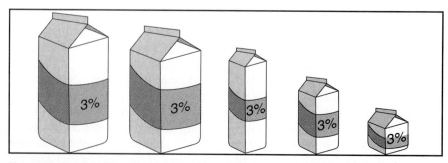

Figure 26–2. Milk—different size containers—with same percentages of fat content.

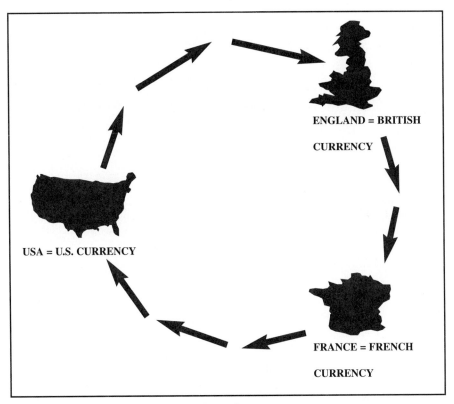

Figure 26–3. Money exchange required to buy milk.

V is the vehicle, or how the medication is packaged, such as pill, liquid, suppository, or skin patches, or the size of the milk container.

H is the on-hand strength, the strength that is on the shelf or in the drawer, or the percent of milkfat currently in the refrigerator.

X is the amount (volume) of the medication that the nurse will actually give to the patient.

Important: **X** will *always* be how much of the vehicle or volume is given to the patient.

Remember: The strength of any medication is one of the following: grains, grams, milligrams, units, or milliequivalents (Table 26–1). *All other* values are for the way the medication is packaged.

You will notice that many exchange tables are more complex than Table 26–1; however, if you master these nine basic values, you can always do ratio and proportion to figure out an equivalent value. For example, you need 5 grains and have on hand a bottle with a label that reads, "325 milligrams in 5

Table 26–1. Strength of a Medication

Apothecary System	Metric System			
Grains	Grams (g)	Milligrams (mg)	Units (U)	Milliequivalents (mEq)
15	1.0	1,000		
7½	0.5	500		
1	0.06	60		

Note: The units and mEq areas are blank. That is because units and mEq are never exchanged into another system of measure. You may, however, have to calculate the amount to give. For example, you are to give 15 mEq and have on hand 30 mEq per 6 cc. Once you place the numbers into the basic drug calculation formula, you will be able to determine that you will need to administer 3 cc.

mL of medication." The basic ratio formula to convert between grains and milligrams is:

$$\frac{1,000 \text{ mg}}{15 \text{ grains}} = \frac{X \text{ mg}}{5 \text{ grains}}$$

$$X = 333 \text{ mg}$$

$$5 \text{ grains} = 325 \text{ mg}$$

Therefore, administer 5 mL of the medication.

Note: Most exchange tables list 5 grains as equal to 300 mg.

What bothers you now is that 333 does not equal 325, let alone 300. So in actuality, the exchange tables are approximate equivalents. Nurses and doctors understand that they are not exact exchanges. Now that you know this, the exact values that pharmaceutical companies place on their labels will not confuse you. Just to be sure, let's do another problem. You need ½ grain and have on hand 30 milligrams in 1 tablet. Since grains and milligrams are not the same measure, we must first make them the same by changing grains to milligrams.

$$\frac{1,000 \text{ mg}}{15 \text{ grains}} = \frac{X \text{ mg}}{½ \text{ grain}}$$

$$X = 33 \text{ milligrams } (33 \text{ mg} = ½ \text{ grain})$$

Again, 33 does not equal 30 but, because we are working with approximates, the ½ grain order is equivalent to the 30 milligram tablet on hand. So, by knowing the nine basic values, you can calculate exchange values.

Important Points to Remember

- The units used to indicate a medication's strength in the metric (grams and milligrams) and apothecary systems (grains) in Table 26–1 do not have an even rate of exchange. That is why you have to convert, or exchange, between the metric system and the apothecary system. (Remember, you could not buy milk in France until you had exchanged the U.S. money for French currency.)
- The two systems listed in Table 26–1 (units and mEq) are two systems unto themselves. They do not and cannot be exchanged into any other system or between each other.
- A medication—*in whatever form*—has a specific strength in a specific vehicle (package or container).
- The strength of any medication is *always* in grams, milligrams, micrograms, grains, units, or milliequivalents!
- Everything else—pills, ounces, suppositories, ampoules, milliliters, minim, teaspoons, or tablespoons—is the vehicle package or container for the medication.

Now we return to the basic formula and the original problem. The patient is to have 100 mg of a medication. The bottle indicates 0.1 g per tablet. What do you give to the patient? The basic formula:

$$\frac{D \times V}{H} = X$$

Put the numbers into the formula:
  D = 100 mg—dose (strength) the patient is to receive
  V = 1 tablet—the way the medication is packaged
  H = 0.1 g/tablet—dose (strength) of the medication you have available
  D and **H** in this sample are not the same system. One needs to be exchanged for the other. Now exchange grams for milligrams by using the basic ratio and proportion-type formula used earlier and you find that 0.1 g is the same as 100 mg.

$$D = 100 \text{ mg}$$
$$V = 1 \text{ tablet}$$
$$H = 100 \text{ mg}$$

With the exchange complete, we can now put the numbers in the formula.

$$\frac{[\text{D}]\ 100 \times [\text{V}]\ 1}{[\text{H}]\ 100} = \text{X}\ [\text{tablet}]$$

$$\text{X} = 1$$

The patient should be given 1 tablet.

One more example is given to be sure you have the basics down. The patient is to receive 7½ grains of a medication. The bottle indicates there are 250 mg in each 15 mL. (*Note:* In medication administration, 1 cc and 1 mL have an equal volume. However, mL is becoming the abbreviation used most in print.)

Putting the numbers in their proper places we have:

$$\text{D} = 7\tfrac{1}{2}\ \text{grains}$$
$$\text{V} = \text{mL}$$
$$\text{H} = 250\ \text{mg}/15\ \text{mL}$$

Again, **D** and **H** are **not** in the **same system,** so exchange one for the other. In this case, change grains to milligrams. The exchange chart shows that 7½ grains exchanges for 500 mg. So, we can put the numbers in their proper places:

$$\text{D} = 500\ \text{mg}$$
$$\text{V} = \text{mL}$$
$$\text{H} = 250\ \text{mg}/15\ \text{mL}$$

The calculation formula now looks like this:

$$\frac{500 \times 15}{250} = \text{X}\ [\text{mL}]$$

$$\text{X} = 30\ \text{mL}$$

When you take 30 mL from the container you will be giving the patient 7½ grains of the medication.

Here is another common problem.

The patient is to have 15 mg of medication per kg (kilogram) of body weight. You weigh the patient and find he weighs 143 lbs (pounds). The first thing you notice is kg and lb are not the same. In this case, pounds need to be exchanged for kilograms. The rate of exchange is 2.2 lbs equals 1 kg.

$$\frac{2.2}{1} = \frac{143}{\text{X}}$$

$$\text{X} = 65$$

This patient weighs 65 kg.

Next:

$$\frac{15 \text{ mg}}{1 \text{ kg}} = \frac{X \text{ mg}}{65 \text{ kg}}$$

$$X = 975 \text{ mg}$$

This patient should receive 975 mg of the medication. You have now discovered **D**—*desired*—only, since the problem does not give you information on **V** and **H**.

Using the example of **V** is ampoules (small containers) with 2 mL of medication and **H** is 750 mg per 2-mL ampoule, the numbers fit in as follows:

$$D = 975 \text{ mg}$$

$$V = \text{mL}$$

$$H = 750 \text{ mg}/2 \text{ mL}$$

D and **H** are in the same system, so there is no need to exchange. The numbers are ready to put into the formula:

$$\frac{975 \times 2}{750} = 2.6 \text{ mL}$$

To get the ordered strength of 975 mg, you will need one full ampoule (2 mL) and 0.6 mL from the second ampoule. Again, **be careful** to note that **V** is mL. You want 2.6 mL, **not** 2.6 ampoules, which would overdose the patient by 450 mg. You avoid this type of error by **always** using the vehicle or volume of the on-hand dose and remembering that **X** will **always** be in that vehicle.

Steps for Basic Drug Calculations

Follow these steps for basic drug calculations.

- Find the parts.

  D = the strength of the medication ordered by the physician
  V = the package or form of the strength on hand (pill, liquid, etc.)
  H = the strength of the medication available

- Make sure that **D** and **H** are in the same system.
- Place the numbers in the formula and solve.

Here is a little test. You have an order that reads: "give 4 mL of medication." What part of the calculation formula (**D**, **V**, or **H**) do you have? If you said, "none of the above," you are correct. This order means the physician knows the strength and vehicle of the medication (the **H** and **V** in the basic formula), has done the math, and has provided you with **X**. *Caution:* Good nursing requires that you work backward to determine the strength of the medication in those 4 mL. Why? To be sure that the strength of the medication the patient will receive in those 4 mL is within therapeutic range. **Do not assume** that because the physician wrote the order the dose is correct. This could be a very costly assumption.

SPEED BUMP

- Master the difference between the three parts—**D**, **V**, **H**—and you will always place the right information in its proper formula space!
- Make sure the strength of the desired (**D**) is the same as the strength on hand (**H**). Remember how you tried to buy milk in the various countries but had to exchange one currency for another? Strength desired and strength on hand in the formula **must be in the same system.**

Common Errors of Students Making Drug Calculations

There are two common errors made by students when making drug calculations.

1. Errors in basic arithmetic—decimals, fractions, percentages.
2. Overlooking the parts; placing nonrelated material in the formula.

For example, you need 100 mg and the medication label instructions are, "add 5 mL of sterile water to yield 25 mg per 1 mL." This gives us:

$$\mathbf{D} = 100 \text{ mg}$$
$$\mathbf{V} = \text{mL}$$
$$\mathbf{H} = 25 \text{ mg/mL}$$

Students tend to mistake the 5 mL for V. But, read the label until you find the strength per a specific vehicle or volume! Remember, somewhere on the medication label, the strength **per unit** will be written.

■ Calculating Intravenous Drip Rates

In today's nursing, most IV infusions are delivered using an electrical IV infusion pump (Figure 26–4). With a pump, the nurse enters required pieces of information to control the speed at which a volume of IV will flow over a specified period of time (usually per hour or half-hour). These devices are wonderful, but they cannot work without human input. They require that the nurse:

- **Know and follow proper operating instructions.** With electronic equipment changing frequently, this will require learning the "ins and outs" of new or upgraded equipment frequently, so learn and follow equipment instructions.
- Follow specific steps when the IV tubing is unthreaded from the pump to do things such as change the patient's gown. If the nurse does not follow specific steps, the patient will receive the IV fluid at the wide-open rate. This can be very detrimental to the patient's health.

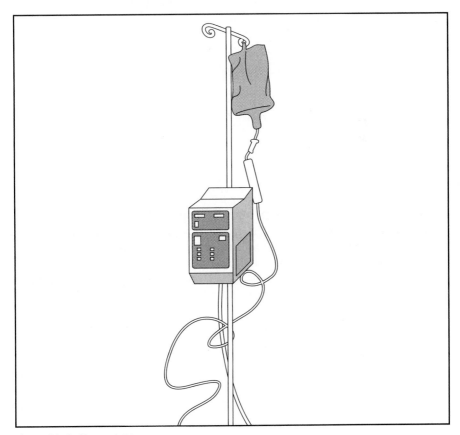

Figure 26–4. Electronic IV pump.

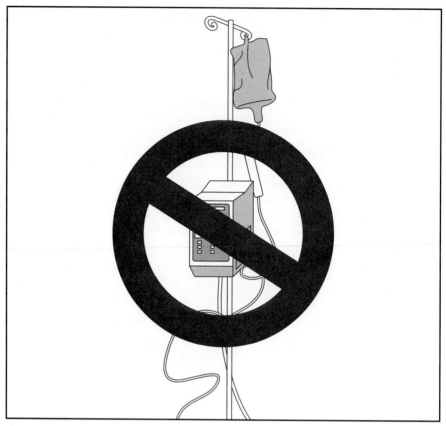

Figure 26–5. No pump available.

There will be times, however, when your patient is receiving an infusion without a pump (Figure 26–5). This means that you will need to calculate the rate. One of the main factors influencing the flow rate of an IV is the "drip/drop factor" of the infusion tubing. Look at the following common drop factors: 10 drops = 1 mL; 15 drops = 1 mL; 60 drops = 1 mL. So, as it turns out, "a drop is not a drop." Some drops are larger than others (Figure 26–6).

What you need to know for manual control of an IV flow rate:

- The drop factor—how many drops equal 1 mL? This information is always on the tubing box (you just have to look for it).
- How many mL of fluid the patient is to receive over what period of time (i.e., the number of mL of IV fluid the patient is to receive per hour or per half-hour).
- Place the information in the basic IV flow rate formula and solve.

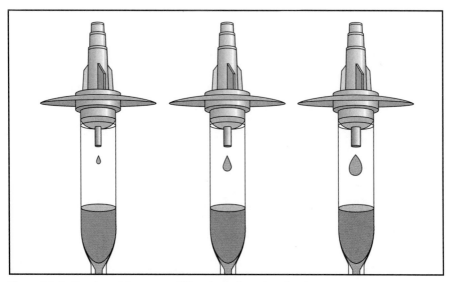

Figure 26–6. Number of drops per milliliter depends on drip chamber.

The basic IV flow rate calculation formula is:

$$\frac{\# \text{ mL} \times \text{drop factor}}{\text{total time the solution}} = \text{number of drops per time of solution}$$

Example:

The patient is to receive 1,000 mL of IV fluid over 8 hours. The drop factor is 15. Putting the information in its proper place:

$$\frac{1,000 \times 15}{8 \text{ hours}} = \text{X drops per hour}$$

Note: At this point you can work with large or small numbers. Let's work with small numbers. One thousand mL in 8 hours breaks down to 125 mL in 1 hour; 1 hour equals 60 minutes.

The numbers in the formula now become:

$$\frac{125 \times 15}{60} = \text{X (drops per minute)}$$

$$X = 31.25$$

If this IV drips between 31 and 32 drops per minute, the patient will receive 125 mL per hour.

Example:

The patient is to receive 250 mL over a half-hour. The drop factor is 10. Putting the numbers in their places:

$$\frac{250 \times 10}{30} = \text{X drops per minute}$$

$$\text{X} = 83 \text{ drops per minute}$$

Example:

The patient is to receive 500 mL over 4 hours and the drop factor is 60.

$$\frac{500}{4} = 125 \text{ mL per hour}$$

$$\frac{125 \times 60}{60} = \text{X drops per minute}$$

$$\text{X} = 125 \text{ drops per minute}$$

Remember 60 drops per cc—means they are very small drops.

Medication Administration—
Adverse Consequences

True, when analyzed, a failure by the nurse to follow all of the basic medication administration "rights" (right patient, medication, dose, route, time, and documentation) can be identified. However, it is also true that errors seldom occur in a vacuum. In the fall of 1999, the Institute of Medicine (IOM) released a report about errors in health care settings and looking beyond the actions of the individual who made the error. In addition, the Joint Commission on Accreditation of Healthcare Organizations (JCAHO) periodically sends out a publication that advises member health care organizations about system strategies that can be implemented to avoid serious medication errors. So you will now find that many institutions are now looking at ways to decrease errors by analyzing all events surrounding the error. In addition to correcting the error in the human action, could the system be redesigned so that the error is preventable in the future? Where can the chain of unintended consequences be broken?

In October 1996, the consequences of a medication error took a major turn: A newborn died as a result of a medication error. The difference here was the fact that three nurses were indicted on criminal charges of negligent homicide. Up to this time, nurses who have made errors have been involved in malpractice lawsuits and disciplinary action by the board of nursing only. This was the first time criminal charges had ever been made by a government agency. In January 1988, two of the nurses accepted a plea bargain agreement. The third nurse did not accept the agreement and was later acquitted. On analysis of this incident, *multiple system and human errors* were detected! But, do remember that you, the nurse, are at the end of the chain when you administer the medication. **Your vigilance must be constant and stringent!**

27

Highlights of Fluids, Electrolytes, and IV Medications

Among the many factors contributing to normal homeostasis of the body are fluid and electrolytes (F/E). This chapter has been divided into three parts. The first part presents some common questions regarding fluid and electrolytes. The second part explores essential material if you are giving IV medications. Finally, highlights regarding IV complications are presented.

The Basics of Fluid and Electrolytes

Some of the more frequently asked questions concerning fluids and electrolytes are as follows.

1. **What are electrolytes?** **Electrolytes** are a specific group of chemical compounds that separate into **ions** (atoms with an electrical charge) when placed in solution. Ions that carry a positive charge are **cations,** while those that carry a negative charge are called **anions.**

2. **What are the body's main electrolytes?** In the body, electrolytes are most often hooked-up with a companion (i.e., sodium chloride [NaCl] and magnesium sulfate [$MgSO_4$]) (Figure 27–1). Electrolytes are measured in milliequivalents per liter (mEq/L) and in the healthy individual, the number of cations equals the number of anions. Fluid and electrolyte balance is primarily maintained by actions of the kidneys. However, other

CATIONS	ANIONS
+ CHARGE	– CHARGE
SODIUM -------- Na$^+$	CHLORIDE ------- Cl$^-$
POTASSIUM ----- K$^+$	PHOSPHORUS---- PO$_4$
CALCIUM ------- Ca^{2+}	BICARBONATE --- HCO$_3$
MAGNESIUM ---- Mg^{2+}	SULFATE -------- SO$_4$

Figure 27–1. The body's main electrolytes.

regulating mechanisms include antidiuretic hormones, rennin, angiotensin, aldosterone, and the parathyroids. When one or more of these regulating mechanisms cannot keep up or malfunctions, indications of fluid and electrolyte imbalance will occur.

3. **Where are the main electrolytes located?** The main electrolytes are located in the body's three main fluid compartments.
   • **Intracellular:** within cells
   • **Interstitial:** between cells
   • **Intravascular:** within blood vessels
   Fluid and electrolyte balance within and between these fluid compartments is controlled by many mechanisms (Figures 27–2 and 27–3). One of the primary control systems is **osmosis.**

4. **What is the difference between isotonic, hypertonic, and hypotonic fluids?** The concentration of electrolytes and other body substances such as glucose, plasma proteins, and urea are what create in plasma the phenomenon of **osmolality.** The osmolality of plasma is a measure of its pulling or drawing power on water. Normal plasma osmolality is in the range of 280 to 300 mOsm/kg (milliosmoles per kilogram). The greater the amount of glucose, proteins, and urea in plasma, the higher the serum osmolality value and the greater the pulling power on water. In the body, we are concerned with the solute concentrations (pulling power) between plasma and intracellular fluid. The main mechanism that keeps solute concentrations between the body's fluid compartments in balance is osmosis.
   When the concept of pulling power is applied to a solution outside the body (such as intravenous solutions), it is referred to as **osmolarity.** As with plasma, solutions with high solute to particle concentration have a high osomolarity value (pulling power) on water. When these solutions

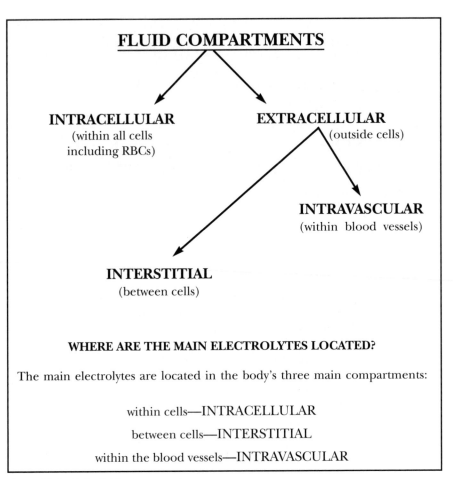

Figure 27–2. Major fluid compartments.

are administered intravenously, they pull water into the intravascular space through the cell's semipermeable membrane in an attempt to equalize the concentration of the particles on both sides of the cell membrane.

Three facts associated with osmosis are:

- Osmosis requires a membrane with holes that are big enough to let some particles (solutes) through but not others, thus the term **semipermeable membrane**—cell walls are semipermeable membranes.
- In osmosis, it is the water, or solvent (what the particles are dissolved in), that moves.
- The water moves through the semipermeable membrane (cell walls) to the compartment with the most particles and solutes.

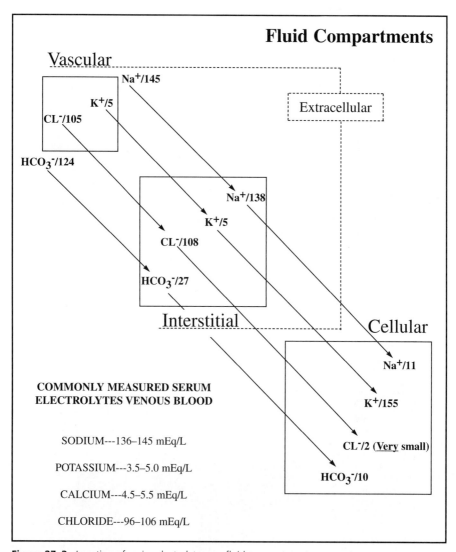

Figure 27–3. Location of major electrolytes per fluid compartment.

5. **Where do I find a patient's osmolality value?** You will not find it. Although the laboratory can determine serum osmolality, it is seldom an ordered test. Instead, it is estimated using one of several techniques. One of the more common means is by the following formula (Kee, 1999):

$$\text{Serum osmolality} = (2 \text{ serum sodium}) + (\text{blood urea nitrogen} \div 3) \\ + (\text{serum glucose} \div 18)$$

The following is an example (adult):

Serum Na = 142   BUN = 13   Glucose = 108

$(2 \times 142) + (13 \div 3) + (108 \div 18)$

284   +   4.33   +   6   = 294 osomolarity value

SPEED BUMP

Moses sounds like osmosis.
Moses moved the water.
Osmosis is movement of water (Figure 27–4).

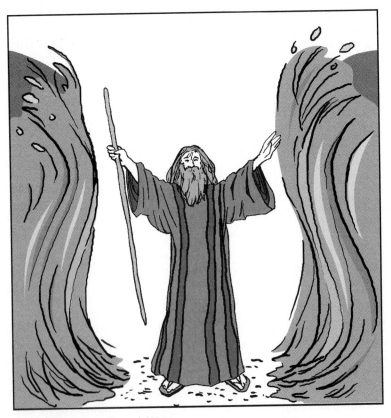

Figure 27–4. Moses/Osmosis/Water.

Another way to estimate serum osmolality is to double the serum sodium value. This *will be less accurate* than the formula but still provides basically accurate and useful information. In the previous example, 2 times the Na value of 142 would be 284 which is close to the calculated 294.

When serum osmolality is decreased (< 280 mOsm/kg), assess for signs associated with overhydration. With increased levels (> 300 mOsm/kg), assess for signs associated with dehydration. Critical levels are generally considered less than 240 and more than 320 mOsm/kg. That is, these serum osmolality levels indicate potentially life-threatening situations and should be reported to the physician without delay.

6. **What are the effects of the three major categories of tonic solutions on the body?** As you care for patients who have IVs, it becomes apparent that there are many kinds of solutions that are available and that can be ordered. These solutions can be placed into one of the following three basic groups; each group has a specific osmotic action.

- **Isotonic solution:** This solution has the same concentration of solutes to particles as in another solution. In the body, the comparison is between plasma and normal body cells. Thus, just enough fluid passes in and out of the cells to maintain equilibrium with plasma values; like two children who weigh the same on a teeter-totter. They move just enough to keep the board level. Plasma is 0.9% sodium chloride, or **normal saline (NS)**. Cells surrounded by normal saline remain unchanged, like the balanced teeter-totter. Table 27–1 contains common hypertonic intravenous solutions with therapeutic uses.

- **Hypotonic solution:** This solution has fewer particles than the cells. So when a hypotonic solution surrounds cells, fluid will move into the cells (they have the most particles) in an attempt to make the ratio of fluid to particles the same on both sides of the cell wall. The result is that the cells fill with additional water and swell. Table 27–2 contains common hypertonic intravenous solutions with therapeutic uses.

- **Hypertonic solution:** When this solution surrounds cells it has more particles than the cells. Again, the key facts with osmosis indicate that fluid will now move out of the cells in an attempt to create concentration equilibrium. The effect on the cells? They shrink. Table 27–3 contains common hypotonic intravenous solutions with therapeutic uses.

7. **Besides osmosis, are there other factors that cause fluid and electrolyte shifts?** Yes. Three of the most common factors are (1) diffusion, (2) active transport, and (3) hydrostatic pressure. Although these are covered in anatomy and pathophysiology texts, here are their basic definitions.

- **Diffusion:** The movement of ions and molecules from areas of high concentration toward areas of low concentration. This is a passive action.

- **Active transport:** The movement of ions and molecules from areas of low concentration to areas of higher concentration. This is not a passive movement; it requires energy.

Table 27–1. Common Isotonic Solutions[a]

Solution[b]	Common Therapeutic Uses
Sodium chloride	• Fluid loss and rehydration
	• Hypernatremia
	• Metabolic alkalosis
	• Only fluid used with blood transfusions
5% Dextrose in water	• Hydration
	• Minimal calories
Lactated Ringer's[c]	• Hydration
	• Burns
	• Acute blood loss

[a] 280–300 mOsm/L, expand the intravascular compartment only.
[b] These fluids, by remaining in the vascular space, can lead to fluid overload. Do careful assessments on patients with increased blood pressure and congestive heart failure.
[c] Has high potassium content. Question if ordered for a patient with renal failure.

- **Hydrostatic pressure:** The pressure that results when a fluid is in a confining space. It is a "pushing-type" pressure.
8. **How are intravenous fluids classified and used?** Intravenous fluids can be grouped into one of the three tonic groups. These groups are based on normal plasma osmolality of 280 to 300 mOsm/kg. Remember, however, the term for IV solutions is osmolarity. Intravenous solutions are grouped into three groups based in their osmolarity range as follows (osmolarity values can be found on the intravenous solution container).

Table 27–2. Common Hypotonic Solutions[a]

Solution[b]	Common Therapeutic Uses
0.45% NS (normal saline)	• Cellular hydration
	• Electrolyte replacement
2.5% D/W (dextrose in water)	• Hydration
5% D (dextrose) in 0.45% NS (normal saline)	• Hydration
Normosol M	• Hydration
	• Electrolyte replacement

[a] < 280 mOsm/L moves fluid out of intravascular space into intracellular and interstitial compartments.
[b] These fluids, by shifting fluid into cells, can lead to increased intracranial pressure. Use with caution in patients with cerebrovascular accident, head trauma, neurosurgery, as well as those at risk for third-space shifting.

Table 27–3. Common Hypertonic Solutions[a]

Solution[b]	Common Therapeutic Uses
5% Dextrose in normal saline	• Hydration
	• Shock until plasma expanders are available
5% Dextrose in 0.45 normal saline	• Progressive treatment of diabetic ketoacidosis
5% Dextrose in lactated Ringer's	• Hydration
5% Dextrose in 0.33 normal saline	• Hydration
10% Dextrose in water	• To provide a small amount of nutritional glucose[c]

[a] > 300 mOsm/L, pull fluid from intracellular and interstitual spaces into the intravascular space.
[b] Because these solutions pull fluids into the vascular space they can lead to expanded intravascular volume. Do careful assessments on patients at risk for circulatory overload.
[c] Remember, it takes 50 g of glucose to create a 5% dextrose solution. Therefore, at 4 calories per gram, 1 liter (1,000 cc) of 5% dextrose provides only 200 calories and a 10% solution will yield only 400 calories. So the belief that an IV is providing the patient with nutrition is incorrect. IVs mainly provide fluid and, based on the solution, various electrolytes.

- **Isotonic:** 280–300
- **Hypotonic:** below 180
- **Hypertonic:** above 300

9. **What are some examples of fluid and electrolyte imbalances?** Let us look at some examples of fluid and electrolyte imbalances. Although the pathophysiology of each imbalance is similar, there are many etiologies that create each type of imbalance.

   - **Isotonic imbalances:** Occur when intravascular sodium and water increase or decrease in tandem, thus, maintaining the (approximate) normal sodium-to-water ratio. When they decrease, **hypovolemia** occurs; while increase leads to **hypervolemia.**
   - **Hypotonic imbalances:** Occur when intravascular sodium falls below normal. This can happen when there is (1) water excess or (2) a sodium deficit. In either case, the patient will have **hyponatremia.**
   - **Hypertonic imbalances:** Occur when intravascular sodium increases beyond normal. This can happen when there is (1) a water deficit or (2) a sodium excess. In either case, the patient will have **hypernatremia.**
   - **Drowning:** The effects of aspirating water will depend on the type and amount of fluid aspirated. Saltwater is hypertonic compared to the body. When aspirated into the lungs, it will draw fluid into the alveoli, creating pulmonary edema, hypoxemia, hypovolemia, and hemoconcentration. Freshwater is hypotonic compared to the body. When aspirated into the lungs, it is absorbed into the bloodstream, creating hemodilution, hypervolemia, and hemolysis.

- **Edema:** Abnormal shift of fluid into interstitial space. Four common etiologies for edema are osmotic pressure, as overload with hypotonic intravenous fluids; poor lymphatic drainage; increased capillary permeability, as occurs with inflammation, burn trauma, and hypersensitivity reactions; and hypoproteinemia, in which plasma proteins create **colloid osmotic pressure** or **oncotic pressure,** which acts like a magnet that keeps fluid in the intravascular space. In hypoproteinemia, plasma proteins are low, pulling power is decreased and fluid escapes into interstitial space. This is often the basis for edema seen in such conditions as malnutrition, cirrhosis, congestive heart failure, and kidney disease.

- **Third spacing:** An accumulation of abnormal amounts of fluid in body spaces, where it is, in essence, trapped. Since it got there due to malfunction in fluid and electrolyte (F/E) regulation, mechanisms for returning it to normal fluid spaces are also severely hampered. Third

Table 27–4. Specialized IV Solutions

Solution	Common Therapeutic Uses
Alkalizing agents ⅙ Molar lactate Sodium bicarbonate	• Treatment of metabolic acidosis
Hyperalimentation	• Very special blend of electrolytes, proteins, vitamins, and glucose • Blend is based on individual client needs • Very hypertonic • Requires central IV route of administration • Requires blood glucose monitoring and insulin (even for nondiabetic patients)
Mannitol/Osmitrol	• Diuresis • Onset of acute renal failure • Onset of acute cerebral edema • Control of sudden increase in intraoccular pressure
Ethyl alcohol	• Calories
Dextran	• Plasma volume expander
Amigen	• Provides amino acids for tissue repair and calories
Intralipids (solution looks like thick milk)	• Provides calories and fatty acids • Often part of the nutritional therapy for the patient who is receiving hyperalimentation therapy • **This is the only IV fluid that is not clear**

spacing can occur in many body areas such as the peritoneal cavity (ascites), in intestines proximal to a bowel obstruction, and burns.

10. **What are some common IV fluids by tonic category and what are their therapeutic uses?** Intravenous fluids can be grouped into one of the three tonic groups. A solution is placed into a specific category based on its osmolarity, the measured pulling power of the solution based on its concentration of particles to solutes. Again, osmolarity values are basically the same as serum osmolality but are measured per liter, not per kilogram. Tables 27–1 through 27–3 present the most common IV fluids in each group along with the common uses for each. Table 27–4 presents information on specialized IV solutions. Table 27–5 has quick reference information for six common F/E imbalances. Students frequently try to simply memorize the common assessment findings seen in Table 27–5. However, the observations in this third column are part of the larger mosaic. It requires identifying the patient's status regarding the etiology column. For example, is your patient experiencing one of the common etiologies that commonly leads to hypernatremia? If the answer is "Yes," then your observations are probably indicative of increased serum sodium. On the other hand, if your patient does not fit any of the risk factors or etiologies for hypernatremia, what you are seeing may be due to another cause.

Table 27–5. Quick Reference for Six Common Electrolyte Imbalances

Imbalance	Common Etiologies	Common Assessment Findings
Hypervolemia	Excess oral fluid intake, renal failure, cirrhosis, fluid shifts following burns	• Tachypnea • Dyspnea • Edema • Weight gain • If not identified early may lead to low H&H, BUN, and sodium levels
Hyponatremia Serum sodium < 135 mEq/L Results in low serum osmolality	Excess water intake, vomiting, GI suctioning, diarrhea, excessive sweating, diabetic acidosis, renal failure, continuous IV infusion of D_5W	• Low-grade fever • Nausea • Abdominal cramps • Muscle twitching • If untreated and values continue to drop, can lead to changes in mental status as a result of the development of cerebral edema

(Continued)

Table 27–5. Quick Reference for Six Common Electrolyte Imbalances (Continued)

Imbalance	Common Etiologies	Common Assessment Findings
Hypernatremia Serum sodium > 145 mEq/L Results in increased serum osmolality	Renal failure with decreased sodium excretion, overuse of IV saline solutions, large number of blood transfusions, severe vomiting or diarrhea, congestive heart failure	• Thirst • Low-grade fever • Restlessness, agitation, weakness, and lethargy, especially when the patient is also hypovolemic • If untreated and sodium levels continue to rise, CNS changes will occur including coma and death
Hypokalemia[a] Serum potassium < 3.5 mEq/L Notify physician immediately if values fall near or below 2.5 mEq	Loop diuretics, vomiting, GI suctioning, large number of blood transfusions, severe vomiting or diarrhea, congestive heart failure	• Muscle weakness • Wear, irregular pulse • Anorexia, nausea, vomiting • If untreated and levels fall to critical, it can lead to cardiac and respiratory arrest
Hyperkalemia[a] Serum potassium > 5.3 mEq/L Notify physician immediately if values are near or > 7 mEq	Renal failure (oliguria or anuria), too rapid infusion of IV potassium, initial reaction to massive tissue damage (eg, trauma, burns, sepsis), metabolic acidosis, receiving potassium-sparing diuretics	• Muscle weakness • Nausea • Abdominal cramping • Diarrhea • ECG changes first as T wave abnormalities • If untreated and levels rise to critical, cardiac and respiratory arrest can occur

GI, gastrointestinal; H&H, hemoglobin and hematocrit; BUN, blood urea nitrogen; CNS, central nervous system; ECG, electrocardiogram.

[a] A few essential notes about potassium:

1. Do not administer potassium IV push.
2. Usual maximum concentration for IV use is 40 mEq/1,000 mL.
3. Usual maximum IV flow rate is ≤20 mEq/hr.
4. Current serum potassium levels should be known prior to IV administration of potassium chloride.
5. When administering IV potassium, urinary output should be at least 60 mL/hr.

Many nursing errors have been made (some fatal) in the administration of intravenous potassium.

IV Medication Administration

1. **Are there different ways to give a medication intravenously?** Yes. Common variations in IV drug administration techniques are:
   - Continuous peripheral venous administration with or without an infusion pump; IV piggy-back administration (IVPB); and IV push (IVP), or bolus administration.
   - Central venous (CV) access techniques such as subclavian entry, internal jugular entry, vascular access port, and peripherally inserted central catheter (PICC) lines. (PICC lines may be inserted by specially trained registered nurses.)
2. **Are there many medications that can be administered via IV route?** Yes. There are hundreds of medications that are suitable for administration via the IV route. Many medications have both intramuscular (IM) and IV forms. They cannot be interchanged!
3. **How do I know if a medication ordered IV can safely be given that way?**
   - Read the literature concerning the specific medication.
   - Read the label on the medication container.

     Once again, many medications have both IM and IV forms. They *cannot* be interchanged! The label will indicate if the form on hand is for IM or IV use. With few exceptions, errors occur because the nurse does not adequately read the label and literature!
4. **What precautions are necessary when giving a medication by one of the IV techniques?** Besides the standard information required for administering a medication by any route, knowing the length of time required to administer the medication is critical for IV meds. Since there are so many IV administration options, there is no one general rule except to remember that the medication is going directly into the circulatory system. The faster the medication enters the bloodstream, the faster its effect on the body. Administration rates, therefore, need to be known and followed. So if you have an order for a medication you are not familiar with, you need to find out about it before administration. No time to look it up? Well, a word to the wise: If an adverse reaction occurs, your "no time" excuse will not fly in court!

IV Complications

There are many complications associated with giving medications by the intravenous route. Basic guidelines and complications when giving IV medications are:

- If the medication is in a powder form, incompatibility may result if the medication is mixed with the wrong solution.
- Many IV medications come with their own diluent or have specific instructions regarding reconstitution.
- Mixing two IV medications that are physically incompatible can lead to color changes, gas formation, cloudiness, and precipitation formation. Do not use; discard.
- Many drug books contain compatibility charts that indicate information such as which drugs are compatible when administered at a "Y-site," and how long two drugs may be compatible in a syringe.
- Do not administer an IV medication into an IV line that has an incompatible fluid. For example, Dilantin is compatible in normal saline, but will precipitate if allowed to enter an IV line containing dextrose.
- Incorrect rate of administration, especially too fast a rate.
- Phlebitis, infiltration, occlusion.
- With central venous access devices all of the above are possible, plus additional complications such as pneumothorax, sepsis, and broken catheters.
- Follow directions.

This chapter has provided you with the highlights of three topics: basics of F/E IV medication administration, and IV complications. Although these are three separate topics, they are interrelated. From the section on "The Basics of Fluids and Electrolytes," the need for accurate intake and output records should be apparent. The basic theme in the "Intravenous Medication Administration" section centers on the fact that, although hand skills are important, safe administration of medication by this technique requires a strong knowledge base centered on the specific medication being given. The third topic, "Complications," looks at the major complications that can occur when medications are administered by intravenous techniques.

▊ Articles to Expand Your Knowledge Base

Macklin, D. (1997). How to manage PICC's. *American Journal of Nursing, 97*(9), 6–32.

Metheny, N. (1997). Focusing on the dangers of D_5W. *Nursing 97, 27*(10), 55–59.

Vonfrolio, L. G. (1995). Would you hang these IV solutions? *American Journal of Nursing, 96*(6), 37–39.

28

Laboratory and Diagnostic Studies

A complete health and illness assessment has three distinct portions: history, physical, and laboratory and diagnostic studies. This chapter will explore some of the basics of the latter. Most students tend to associate laboratory and diagnostic tests with patients who are in the hospital. In today's health care environment, however, these studies should be expected in all health care settings (clinics, long-term care, home health, etc).

Differences Between Lab and Diagnostic Studies

1. **What is the difference between laboratory and diagnostic studies?**
   Laboratory studies:
   - Involve analysis of body fluids collected through basic techniques of blood, urine, and feces samples.
   - May require food, fluid, and/or medication restrictions.
   - The sample collection does not require a separate consent form. (*Note:* The exception in most states is HIV testing, which requires a signed consent before blood can be drawn.)
   Diagnostic studies:
   - Involves analysis of body fluids or tissues collected through invasive techniques.
   - Includes viewing of various body structures using special equipment (x-ray, magnetic resonance imaging [MRI], computed tomography [CT] scans, electrocardiogram [ECG], oscopies, etc.).

- Usually require a signed consent form.
- Generally require food and fluid restrictions.

In actuality, although there is a difference between the laboratory studies and diagnostic tests, the terms are frequently interchanged. In the remainder of this chapter, they will be jointly referred to as lab tests.

Relatively new categories of lab tests are those done to monitor blood levels of medications that have a narrow therapeutic level. That is, the line between a therapeutic and toxic level of the medication is very thin. Some of these tests monitor the effects of medication rather than the blood level of the medication itself. For example, blood levels of heparin are not determined. What is measured, however, is the effectiveness of heparin therapy as determined by activated partial thromboplastin time (APTT) values. On the other hand, serum levels of many drugs are now being monitored. For example, orders to obtain serum levels of many anticonvulsants, antibiotics, and bronchodilators are common. At present, there are about 100 medications that are monitored for therapeutic levels and many lab books now include a chapter on this topic.

2. **How can you learn all of the material about lab tests?** Considering that most of the nursing books about lab tests are often 500 to 700 pages long, you cannot! However, the faculty will expect you to at least be able to do the following.
- Explain why your patient is having a specific test.
- Describe the nurse's role for the test—such as what the nurse should teach the client about the test, any special patient preparation, the nurse's role in sample collection, and documentation.
- Provide normal reference values for the test (normal reference values are almost always included on the test report).
- Explain the significance of your patient's test results.

How can nurses do all that? You will need to do your homework. Once you know your patient is having tests that you are not familiar with, look them up and make notes. Most instructors will allow you to refer to notes when discussing your patient's laboratory and diagnostic tests.

3. **Will you be expected to discuss laboratory tests without notes?** Yes. As you progress in school, you should know that faculty will expect you to discuss common tests without notes. The following are the lab tests you will probably be expected, at some point, to discuss without notes.
- Urinalysis (U/A)
- Complete blood count (CBC)
- Fasting blood sugar (FBS)
- Electrolytes: sodium, potassium, and chloride
- Blood urea nitrogen (BUN)
- Therapeutic drug levels

Your instructors may have additional lab tests without notes in mind. Be sure to ask.

4. **Where can you find this information about lab tests?** There are two main sources: your course textbook and a lab and diagnostic book. Although required nursing texts will have information about lab tests, a specialty book is recommended. Be sure you select a book that includes information on nursing implications for each test! In addition to the lab books, there are lab cards, which are boxes of index cards with one lab or diagnostic study per card. Since you can take out only the tests of interest, these cards are very convenient for use in clinical training. Again, if you are going to use these boxed sets, be sure the cards contain nursing implications.

5. **Are there some lab tests that are difficult for students to understand?** Yes. There are several tests that students have difficulty with.

   The difference between coagulation tests of PT and APTT:
   - **Prothrombin time (PT):** Used to monitor **oral** anticoagulant therapy.
   - **Activated partial thromboplastin time (APTT):** Used to monitor **heparin** therapy.
   - One way to remember the difference is PT (2 letters) matches the word with few letters (oral), whereas APTT (4 letters) matches the word with more letters (injection).

   Drug serum level terms:
   - **Steady state:** Indicates whether the plasma level of the drug is being maintained at the desired maintenance level.
   - **Peak level:** The time at which a drug is at its highest concentration in the blood. Blood to measure a peak level is drawn at **specific times** related to the drug administration time. Be sure to check with the lab for details.
   - **Trough level** (in some labs referred to as "residual level"): The time at which a drug is at its lowest concentration in the blood. Blood for trough levels is usually drawn 5 minutes before the next dose of the drug is to be administered. As with peak levels, be sure to check with the lab for specifics.
   - The accuracy of drug plasma levels depends on many factors under the nurse's control, including, in many settings, obtaining blood samples for testing. It is essential, therefore, that you know and follow protocol.
   - In addition to the timing for drawing the sample, drug plasma levels can be influenced by other factors such as other drugs the patient is receiving. Therefore, as with all lab and diagnostic tests, you need to be cautious when interpreting results.

6. **How have the normal reference values for the various lab tests been determined?** Over the years, data from individuals (usually men) who were considered "healthy" have been gathered and analyzed and a range for each lab test determined. Most lab values have a low and high range. Any values falling within that range are considered normal. It is interesting to note that over the years, most of these ranges remain unchanged. What have changed, however, are the number of new tests and the refinement of many older, established tests.

When comparing normal ranges between books and between institutions differences are often noted. These occur due to differences in equipment and techniques used to conduct the tests. These differences are usually small and the values all tend to be in the "ball park" with each other. The values used to report reference numbers, however, can create values that look very different. Older books report most values in mg% (milligram percent), which changed to mg/dL (milligrams per deciliter). With this change, the basic numbers remain the same. For example, a blood glucose of 80 mg% became 80 mg/dL. In an attempt to create more uniformity in reporting on a global basis, the World Health Organization (WHO) is encouraging the adoption of a new system. This system uses the International System of Units (SI). When values are calculated in SI they may or may not look familiar. For example, potassium ranges are 3.5 to 5.3 mEq/L and 3.5 to 5.3 mmol/L (SI). The numbers remain the same while the reporting unit changes. It is different with the hematocrit (Hct). Male values for Hct are generally 40 to 54% while the SI are 0.40 to 0.54. It is anticipated that with time, all values will be reported in SI units. Until then, many labs and books are presenting the current system followed by the SI.

7. **What are the traps that nurses fall into when looking at lab results?** Basically, there are two traps.
   - Lab reports are only one part of the picture. They must be evaluated in relation to other assessment data. No interventions should be made based on a lab report alone. A lab value that is outside the normal range, with all other test values inside the normal ranges and assessment findings basically normal, is suspect. Most of the time, the test will be repeated to verify the initial findings.
   - When you find a test result that falls well outside the reference values, you will generally find one or more companion tests that are out of range to some degree. Our physiology is very interconnected and interdependent.

8. **What will be my responsibilities as a graduate in relation to reported lab values?** You will be expected to quickly identify lab values that require immediate intervention. Most institutions have a list of critical lab values and the procedures to be followed when one occurs. The lists often include blood glucose (i.e., values below 40 and above 700 mg/dL), Na, Hct, and carbon dioxide combining power.

9. **Will I ever have to perform any lab tests?** Yes. Currently, the most common lab test conducted by the nurse, often called **point-of-care (POC) testing,** is blood glucose testing. It is anticipated that with advances in lab tests and the advent of simpler, more sophisticated equipment, nurses will be conducting more POC tests.

   In addition to actually conducting a diagnostic test such as blood glucose, nurses in many settings are collecting blood specimens. This requires

Table 28–1. Color Selection Guide for Blood Specimen Collection

Color of Tube Stopper[a]	Common Uses
Red stopper No additives to tube	Tests conducted on clotted blood such as electrolytes, proteins, enzymes, drug monitoring, serology.
Lavender stopper Additive: EDTA (ethylene-diaminetetraacetic acid)	Tests done for hematology studies such as CBC and platelet count, some chemistry studies, blood banking.
Green stopper Additive: heparin	Tests done for lupus erythematosus (LE), arterial blood gases (ABGs), ammonia levels.
Blue stopper Additive: citrate	Tests done for coagulation information such as prothrombin time (PT), activated partial thromboplastin time (APTT), hemoglobin.
Gray stopper Additive: sodium fluoride	Tests for glucose.

[a] Not sure what to use? Ask the lab. It is not fair to the patient to be "stuck" twice and charged twice because of faulty collection technique.

that the nurse know what diagnostic test is ordered so that proper specimen collection occurs (which includes factors such as collection site and technique, time of collection, labeling, and handling). In addition, blood specimens must be placed in the proper collection tube for test accuracy (Table 28–1).

As an example of how collection technique can influence test accuracy, Corbett (1996) identifies eight ways that accuracy of a blood specimen for potassium can be affected.

- Skin too wet with antiseptic.
- Moisture in the syringe or collection tube.
- Prolonged use of a tourniquet or clenching the fist.
- Use of a small-gauge needle to withdraw a large volume of blood.
- Use of a suction syringe.
- Vigorous shaking of the blood specimen.
- Not removing the needle from the syringe before expelling the blood into the collection tube.
- Vigorous expulsion of blood from the syringe into the collection tube.

You can anticipate having many responsibilities in relation to laboratory and diagnostic studies. These will include proper patient preparation, accurate specimen collection, and immediate recognition of critical values with appropriate nursing intervention.

29

ECG

Although many individuals still refer to this diagnostic test as an EKG, the abbreviation currently being seen for an electrocardiogram is ECG. Not too long ago, the only nurses who did cardiac monitoring were intensive care and cardiac care nurses. Today, however, cardiac monitoring is a nursing activity in many settings such as telemetry and progressive care units, medical–surgical units, labor and delivery units, postanesthesia units (both in- and outpatient), and oncology units. One of the easiest activities to learn about ECG is placement of the skin electrodes, whereas being able to interpret the resulting rhythm patterns requires knowledge of cardiac anatomy and physiology as well as interpretation of the displayed cardiac rhythms.

■ Understanding an ECG

Understanding an ECG requires several fundamental pieces of information. One of the basic pieces is normal blood flow through the heart. You should, therefore, be able to trace a drop of blood through the heart. One way to view this blood flow through the heart is to reshape the heart's anatomy into a straight line (Figure 29–1).

The second thing that needs to be understood is the heart's electrical conduction system. Think of this system as starting with a master switch that "turns" cardiac muscles on, rather like turning on the master fuse that all at once turns on all lights in the house. Except that in the heart, the lights come on in sequence, like a set of falling dominos, with the heart's master switch (the SA node) starting the cascade. This cascade is displayed in Figure 29–2.

286

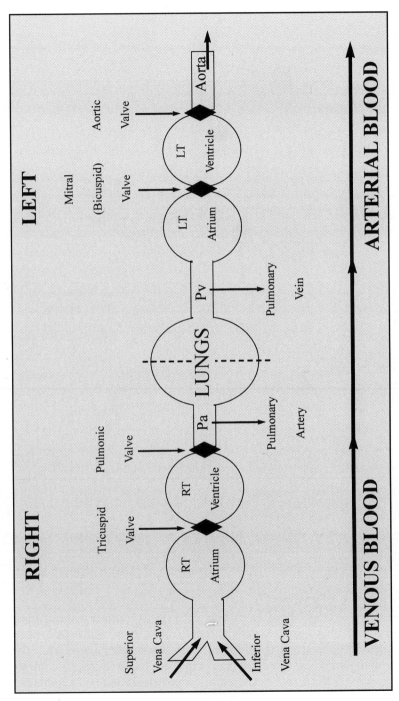

Figure 29–1. Heart structure in a straight line.

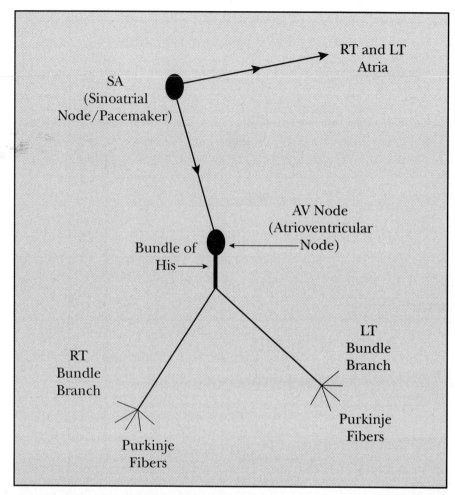

Figure 29–2. Electric cascade of the heart.

In addition to heart structure, there are several critical properties unique to heart muscle cells. The main properties are automaticity, irritability and excitability, contractility, conductivity, and rhythmicity. The basic definitions follow.

- **Automaticity:** The ability of specific cardiac cells to contract without stimulation by the SA node. For example, by itself, the atrioventricular (AV) node has the capacity to create 40 to 60 cardiac contractions per minute, while the Purkinje and ventricular fibers can independently create 20 to 40 contractions per minute. Beats that occur outside sinoatrial (SA) node stimulation are sometime referred to as **escape beats.**

- **Irritability and excitability:** The ability of cardiac cells to respond when exposed to an electrical stimulus.
- **Contractility:** The ability of cardiac cells to contract (get smaller) when exposed to an electrical stimulus.
- **Conductivity:** The ability of one cardiac cell to pass on an electrical impulse to another cardiac cell.
- **Rhythmicity:** The steady rhythm of normal cardiac cells as they repeat their cycle of stimulation–transmission–contraction–relaxation.

There are also several terms associated with the transmission of the impulse along cardiac cells: polarization, depolarization, repolarization, and refractory period.

- **Polarization:** Cardiac cells are in a resting state; the outside of the cells is covered with positive particles. The inside of the cells has negative particles.
- **Depolarization:** The cardiac cells respond to an electrical stimulus and the particles switch so that the cell surface now becomes negative (and the inside positive).
- **Repolarization:** The process of cardiac cells returning to their original resting state with the cell surfaces containing positive electrical charges.
- **Refractory period:** The time during which cardiac cells are not ready to respond to a new stimulus; occurs between repolarization and polarization time.

Thus, the sequence is P-D-R, over and over again. It is this repetitive sequence of ion exchanges between cell surface and cell interior that moves the electrical stimulus along cardiac cells. When the stimulus has completed the circuit, a heartbeat occurs with the atria contracting followed by the ventricles. One way to think of these terms is an old-fashioned fire line. One person receives the bucket with water (P), turns, passes it on to the next person (D), turns back and gets ready to receive a new bucket (R), gets the new bucket (P), passes it on, and so on. Can you see how the refractory period can influence how many buckets of water any one person can pass along? Or how many times the heart can beat per minute?

SPEED BUMP

Polarization—think P for positive (cell surface is positive and resting)

Depolarization—think D for denial (cell surface becomes negative and active)

Repolarization—think R for return (depolarized cells switch electrical charges and return to the polarized state)

This is the foundation for understanding an ECG, which is a record of the electrical impulse as it travels through cardiac cells. The ECG does not directly give any information about the heart's structure. However, analysis of the conduction system via the ECG can provide indirect information.

An ECG is obtained by placing electrodes on the skin that pick up the electric current that goes through cardiac cells. This current can be recorded on a TV-like monitor, telemetry, or recorded on special paper. In either case, the electrical activity is displayed as a series of waveforms. The wave pattern is analyzed in relation to the ECG paper and expected wave patterns. Figure 29–3 presents a sample of normal size and enlarged ECG paper.

As you can see, the standard paper is small. To accurately measure the time intervals, a set of ECG calipers is required (Figure 29–4). However, as technology progresses, there are some computer programs that do pattern interpretation. However, as with all technology, remember that this data must be correlated with the assessment of the patient.

ECGs come in 12 "forms." Although most of the time a single lead is used to analyze the heart's electric conduction system, there are times when the physician needs more information. In that case, a 12-lead ECG will be obtained. This simply means that the electrodes are repositioned several times on the patient to create 12 different views of the heart's electrical system. It is like having your picture taken from 12 different angles at one sitting. You remain sitting in the same chair and do not change your position, yet each frame presents you in a unique view. Thus, a 12-lead ECG views the electrical system of the heart from 12 different angles.

When you look at the 12-lead report, you will notice that each view has a specific name or label. Most of the time, however, you will only be using one of two common leads when monitoring the heart function of a patient. The two common leads that are used are lead II and modified chest lead (MCL_1). These leads present the basic cardiac cycle in a manner that allows analysis of each phase of the cycle.

Figure 29–5 on page 293 shows the basic electrical waveforms, P, QRS (known as the QRS complex), and T, which occur with every cardiac cycle (heartbeat). Note that each waveform has a *time limit*. That is, it occupies a specified distance on the grid of the ECG paper, which in turn represents time. Characteristics of the major portions of a normal cardiac cycle are summarized in Table 29–1 on page 294. When abnormalities are apparent, many other features of the wave formation are analyzed.

Interpreting an ECG rhythm strip requires a systematic approach. Table 29–2 on page 295 presents the basic elements to be analyzed in any ECG tracing. As you learn to analyze ECG tracings, one of the main points is to develop a consistent method of analysis.

Although there are many other parts of an ECG that can be analyzed, these basic elements can provide an enormous amount of information. As a

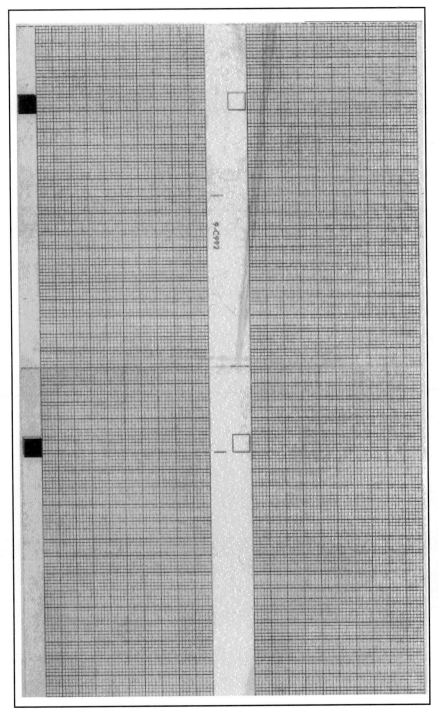

Figure 29-3. Normal size ECG tracing paper.

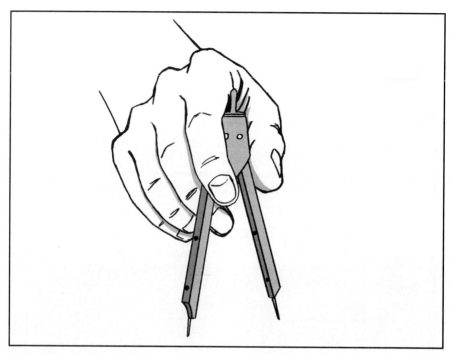

Figure 29–4. Cardiac calipers.

rule, cardiac problems that are in tissue above the bundle branches lead to P and PR changes. Pathology in or after the bundle branches leads to abnormalities in the QRS complex.

Before we leave the basics of an ECG, we look at a few terms that offer students a challenge, and then, a few cardiac rhythms that require immediate recognition.

ECG Basic Definitions

- **Preload:** Although preload concerns both the right and left ventricles, it mainly refers to the stretching of the left ventricle during filling with blood from the left atrium. Like a stretched rubber band has a strong snap when released, the more the left ventricle is stretched with blood, the more forcefully it will eject blood into the aorta on contraction (this is Starling's law of heart).

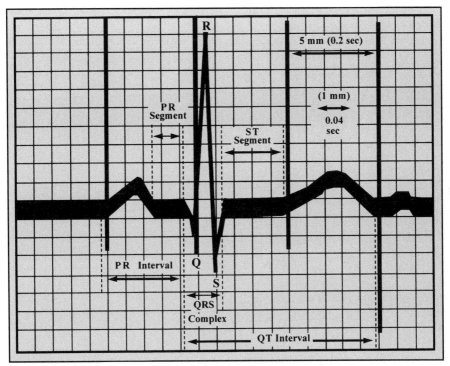

Figure 29–5. Normal ECG patterns with normal time intervals.

- **Afterload:** Represents the amount of tension or resistance the ventricles must overcome during contraction to open the pulmonic and aortic valves. Afterload for the left ventricle is frequently referred to as *systemic vascular resistance*. Afterload for the right ventricle is referred to as *pulmonary vascular resistance*.

Figure 29–1 (page 287) will help you visualize the effects of abnormal preload and afterload values. For example, if the muscles of the left ventricle become weak, they will fill with blood, but they will be unable to push the blood out through the aortic valve. Like a rubber band that is constantly overstretched and loses its elasticity, so do overstretched (or damaged) cardiac muscles lose their ejection power. The result is a back-up into the left atrium, and eventually the lungs, with development of pulmonary edema. This is a preload problem because the left ventricle is unable to empty completely, becomes overfilled, and blood backs up in the system. The same thing can happen in the right ventricle if it is unable to open the pulmonic valve. Eventually, many things can result from untreated right-sided abnormal preload values, such as edema and increased juggler pressure. Again, Figure 29–1 (page 287) will help you visualize these events.

Table 29–1. Normal Cardiac Cycle

Cycle Phase	Characteristics
P wave	• Time: < 0.12 sec • Indicates atrial depolarization
PR interval	• Time: < 0.12 to 0.20 sec • Indicates the impulse is traveling through the AV node, bundle of His, and the bundle branches
QRS complex	• Time: < 0.04 to 0.10 sec • Indicates depolarization of the ventricles (remember that once the ventricles depolarize they contract and eject blood, thus creating a heartbeat/pulse)
ST segment	• Time: not usually measured • Should be isoelectric; flat • Indicates ventricular refractory period
T wave	• Time: not measured • Evaluated by how it looks including amplitude (height) • Indicates repolarization of the ventricles

Prolonged abnormal afterload, on the other hand, will eventually result in damaged left ventricle muscles. Because the ventricle has to constantly overcome the increased force to open the aortic valve, the ventricle loses its contractility. The afterload problem is the *increased systemic force* (e.g., high blood pressure) not sick cardiac muscle. Left untreated, the left ventricle can become permanently damaged, leading to a combination of both preload and afterload pathologies.

The last topic is life-threatening arrhythmias. Although there are some very serious atrial arrhythmias, two abnormal ventricular rhythms require immediate recognition. They are ventricular tachycardia (V-tach) and ventricular fibrillation (Figures 29–6 and 29–7). In V-tach, the ventricular rate may be as high as 200 beats per minute. At this rate the ventricles cannot fill or empty properly, and the result is low cardiac output with a variety of consequences, such as weak or absent pulses, hypotension, and congestive heart failure. In ventricular fibrillation, the ventricles are in essence just vibrating like a bowl of gelatin. There is *no* cardiac output. If not treated *quickly*, death results. Because these two arrhythmias are so life-threatening, it is essential that you learn to recognize and take proper actions immediately. You will have many classes on the details of treatment including cardiopulmonary resuscitation (CPR), medications, and defibrillation.

Table 29-2. ECG Analysis*a*

1. Determine rhythm—regularity

Regular? Patterns? Measuring R-R interval provides information on ventricular rhythm. Using the same technique on the P-P intervals will provide information on arterial rhythm. It is possible for them to be different.

- On a piece of paper, mark two R waves (called the R-R interval). Move the marked paper along the strip. The rhythm is regular if all R-R intervals fall on the marks.
- Using calipers, place the points on the peaks of two consecutive R waves. Pivot the leg of the calipers to succeeding R peaks. The rhythm is regular if the caliper points always fall on the R-wave peaks.

2. Determine rate

There are several other methods for calculating rate. Calculated number of R waves will yield ventricular rate, while calculated number of P waves will yield arterial rate. It is possible for them to be different.
- Obtain a 6-second strip, count the number of R waves, multiple by 10.
- In the same 6-second strip, count the number of P waves, multiply by 10.
Note: This technique will provide a very quick estimate of rate. The actual rate may vary from the calculated.

3. Analyze the P waves

Some basic questions to ask.
- Are P waves present?
- Do they look normal in shape, direction, and duration?
- Are they all followed by a QRS complex?

4. Analyze the PR intervals

Locate the start of the P wave and the start of the QRS complex. Count the number of small squares between these two points. Multiply this number by 0.04. Results should be within the normal range of 0.12 to 0.20 seconds.

5. Analyze QRS complexes

Remember: The QRS complex has no horizontal parts. All parts of the wave are above and below the baseline.
- Locate the deflected peaks of the Q and S waves and count the number of small squares between these points. Multiply this number by 0.04. Results should be within the normal range of 0.06 and 0.10 seconds.
- Is there a QRS after each P wave?
- Does the complex look normal?

a Although there are many other parts of an ECG that can be analyzed, these basic elements can provide an enormous amount of information. As a rule, cardiac problems that are in tissue above the bundle branches lead to abnormalities in the QRS complex.

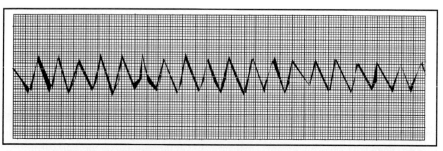

Figure 29–6. Ventricular tachycardia (V-tach).

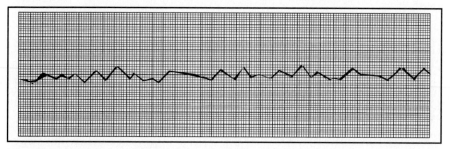

Figure 29–7. Ventricular fibrillation.

Today's nurses are doing more than nurses in the past ever dreamed of doing as far as nursing activities are concerned. One of those activities involves understanding and interpreting ECG patterns. This chapter has presented some basics. Use this foundation when you encounter in-depth classes on this important concept.

30

Nutrition

One of nursing's greatest challenges is helping individuals make changes in their dietary intake. Although the ultimate function of food is to sustain the body, an individual's background (culture, ethnic group, religion, knowledge about nutrition, lifestyle, financial situation, and food preferences) has a great influence on what foods are actually ingested. The forces on the individual to maintain the nutritional status quo are great. Therefore, before attempting to change someone's diet, the starting point must be determining the current dietary situation: What, when, and why does the patient eat? The answers to these questions will be the foundation for interventions aimed at creating new dietary patterns.

Nutritional Assessment

There are many nutrition assessment tools. However, some basic indicators of an individual's nutrition status are:

- General appearance
- Weight and height compared to weight and height tables
- History of recent unplanned weight gain or loss of 10% or more of body weight
- Serum albumin values (normal ranges: 3.5 to 5.0 g/dL)
- H&H (Remember: the first H always stands for hemoglobin, Hb, or Hbg, and is reported in g/dL; while the second H always stands for hematocrit, Hct, and is reported in percent; normal H&H ranges for men are 13.5 to 17 g/dL and 40 to 45%; for women, ranges are 12 to 15 g/dL and 36 to 46%)

297

Table 30–1. A Select Number of Therapeutic Diets

- High or low fiber
- Bland
- Dysphagia
- Renal
- Gastroplasty

- Lactose restricted
- Allergy
- Gluten controlled
- Purine restricted

▊Special and Therapeutic Diets

Currently the three most common therapeutic diets in use are ADA diabetic diets, sodium controlled diets, and fat and cholesterol controlled diets. However, there are at least 35 additional types of special diets. Table 30–1 presents a few of these.

As you assist patients adjust to new dietary patterns, one of your interventions will be teaching the patient two key things: the concepts in the Food Guide Pyramid, which in 1992 replaced the four food groups (Figure 30–1); and how to read the nutrition facts panel on food products (Figure 30–2). The material on this panel is established by federal mandate. For foods without labels, such as fruits and vegetables, meats, and fish, the buyer will find the information on a card or sign in the store. If not, the buyer can ask the store manager for the information. Along this same line, nutrition information on any item served in fast food and regular restaurants must also be available on request.

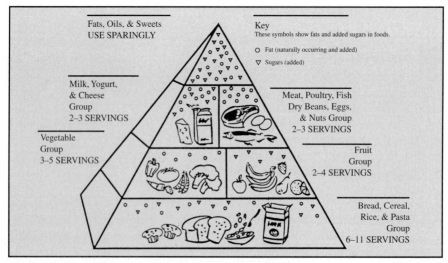

Figure 30–1. Food Guide Pyramid. *(Source: U.S. Department of Health and Human Services)*

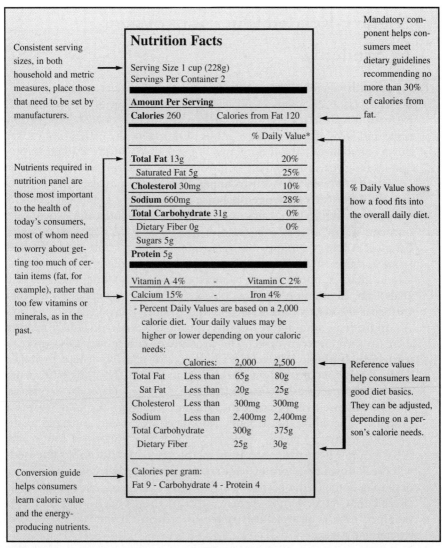

Consistent serving sizes, in both household and metric measures, place those that need to be set by manufacturers.

Nutrients required in nutrition panel are those most important to the health of today's consumers, most of whom need to worry about getting too much of certain items (fat, for example), rather than too few vitamins or minerals, as in the past.

Conversion guide helps consumers learn caloric value and the energy-producing nutrients.

Nutrition Facts

Serving Size 1 cup (228g)
Servings Per Container 2

Amount Per Serving

Calories 260   Calories from Fat 120

                                              % Daily Value*

Total Fat 13g	20%
Saturated Fat 5g	25%
Cholesterol 30mg	10%
Sodium 660mg	28%
Total Carbohydrate 31g	0%
Dietary Fiber 0g	0%
Sugars 5g	
Protein 5g	

Vitamin A 4%	-	Vitamin C 2%
Calcium 15%	-	Iron 4%

- Percent Daily Values are based on a 2,000 calorie diet. Your daily values may be higher or lower depending on your caloric needs:

		Calories:	2,000	2,500
Total Fat	Less than		65g	80g
Sat Fat	Less than		20g	25g
Cholesterol	Less than		300mg	300mg
Sodium	Less than		2,400mg	2,400mg
Total Carbohydrate			300g	375g
Dietary Fiber			25g	30g

Calories per gram:
Fat 9 - Carbohydrate 4 - Protein 4

Mandatory component helps consumers meet dietary guidelines recommending no more than 30% of calories from fat.

% Daily Value shows how a food fits into the overall daily diet.

Reference values help consumers learn good diet basics. They can be adjusted, depending on a person's calorie needs.

Figure 30–2. Standard nutritional label. *(Source: U.S. Department of Health and Human Services)*

You may also need two other resources for successful intervention. One is a **diet manual** that lists foods that are allowed and those not allowed on specific therapeutic diets (or has enough information about a specific food for you to determine how the food fits into the patient's therapeutic diet). Your second resource is a registered dietitian. This member of the health care team is essential, especially when dealing with patients who have complex dietary needs.

■ Dietary-Related Questions Asked by Students

1. **What is nitrogen balance?** Nitrogen is one by-product of protein break-down. Every 6.25 grams of protein will yield 1 gram of nitrogen that is excreted from the body via urine and feces. So, if in one 24-hour period, urine and feces analysis yields 8 grams of nitrogen, the patient has broken down (catabolized) about 50 grams of protein. When the amount of protein intake equals the amount of nitrogen lost from the body, the body is considered to be in **nitrogen balance.** When protein intake exceeds nitrogen output, **positive nitrogen balance** occurs. This is seen during periods of tissue growth (e.g., infancy and pregnancy). The opposite, when more nitrogen is lost than is consumed in food, results in **negative nitrogen balance.** A few conditions that can create a negative balance are massive injuries, burns, and infections. A negative balance will occur any time that caloric intake is not sufficient to meet energy needs—catabolism exceeds anabolism. In addition, one less obvious situation that creates a negative balance is the inactivity associated with bedridden individuals.

   Individuals who are in negative nitrogen balance obviously need to increase their protein intake. The proteins of choice are those proteins with **high biologic value (HBV),** also known as **complete proteins.** These foods contain all eight essential amino acids (those the body is unable to manufacture). Remember, there are 20 amino acids: 8 essential and 12 nonessential. It takes all 20 amino acids for the body to make proteins. Therefore, in patients who need to repair damaged tissue (postop, fractures, burns, wounds, etc.) dietary intake of foods with HBV is a must for tissue repair. If the protein is not available, the body will break down body proteins for repair and energy purposes. This is not desirable. Some of the best HBV foods are meats, eggs, cheese, and milk. (Recall that fat does not contain protein, therefore, low-fat and even skimmed milk is an excellent source of protein for individuals with restricted fat intake.)

2. **My patient is a vegetarian. Can he or she get a balanced diet?** Yes. Let's explore the highlights of vegetarians. First, being a vegetarian is not unique to any particular ethnic group; however, it may be associated with certain religions. Second, although there are many variations, there are basically four types of vegetarians based on which nonplant foods are allowed in the diet (Figures 30–3 through 30–6). Those four types are:
   - **Semivegetarian:** Included are dairy products, eggs, and fish; excluded are meat and sometimes poultry.
   - **Lacto-ovovegetarian:** Included are dairy products and eggs; excluded are meat, poultry, and fish.

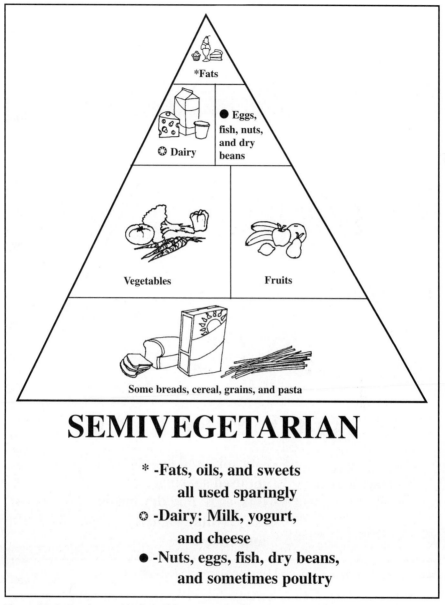

Figure 30–3. Food pyramid adjusted for a semivegetarian diet.

- **Lactovegetarian:** Included are dairy products; excluded are meat, fish, poultry, and eggs.
- **Vegan:** Excluded are all foods of animal origin.

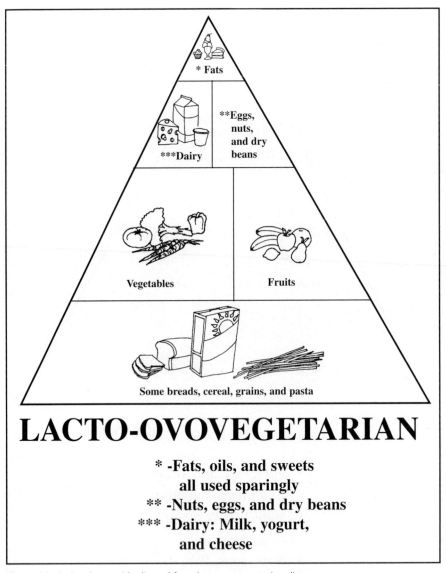

Figure 30–4. Food pyramid adjusted for a lacto-ovovegetarian diet.

As you can see, being a vegetarian has several interpretations. The first three groups can meet needs for HBV protein foods fairly easily. However, a practicing true vegan has a greater challenge to avoid deficiencies. But, it can be done. The key is to consume plants with different essential amino acids so that they complement each other. That is, foods lacking in specific essential amino acids are eaten with foods known to contain them.

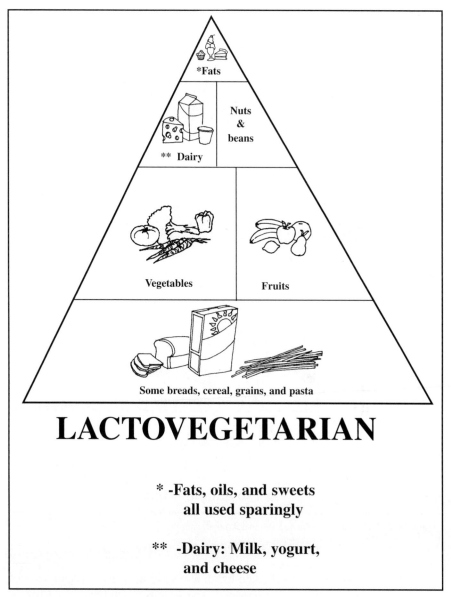

Figure 30–5. Food pyramid adjusted for a lactovegetarian diet.

For example, having baked beans with brown bread will provide all the essential amino acids. This practice requires, however, that the complementary foods, if not eaten at the same meals, be eaten throughout the day—every day. A greater challenge is a vegan who has a medical need for a clear liquid diet. Many of the traditional items on this diet have an animal

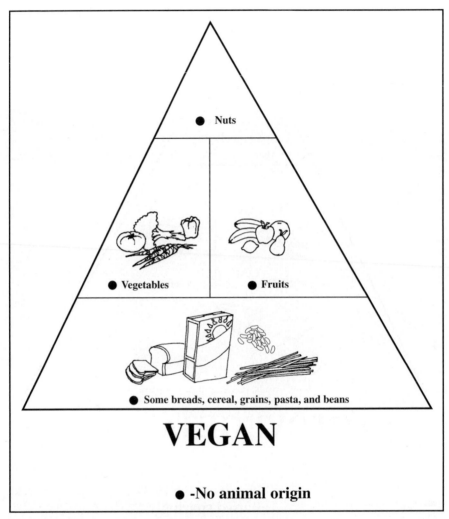

Figure 30–6. Food pyramid adjusted for a vegan diet.

base, including beef and chicken broth and gelatin, which a vegan will not eat. So if your patient has a need for clear liquids much beyond 24 hours, a consultation with a dietitian is essential.

Most vegetarians at any level know a great deal about how to maintain adequate nutrition. Their personal libraries usually include many books on the subject, and there are numerous vegetarian cookbooks. Problems, however, may occur during times of special physiological needs such as pregnancy, lactation, and injury. During these times, some individuals will supplement their vegetarian diets with foods they do not ordinarily eat; others will not. Therefore, your task is to do an in-depth dietary assessment and, along with the patient, come to a consensus on how to best meet the increased needs. In addition, it may be necessary for you to increase your knowledge base on vegetarian diets.

3. **What is the glycemic index (GI) value of a food?** For many years it was believed that 1 gram of carbohydrate (CHO), regardless of the source, always had the same effect on blood glucose levels. Research since the late 1980s has challenged this belief. The glycemic index represents how quickly 50 grams of CHO in a specific food will change the blood glucose level compared to 50 grams of CHO in white bread, which is used as the standard, with glycemic index values ranging from 1 to 150. Research indicates that there is a vast difference in the glycemic index of carbohydrate foods. For example, the 50 grams of CHO in the white bread has a GI of 100. The 50 grams of CHO in a new, white, boiled potato has a GI of 80, canned soy beans 22, and corn flakes 121 (Bloch & Shils, 1996). Foods with higher index numbers cause rapid increases in serum glucose; lower numbers cause slow increases.

   There are many factors influencing the GI of a food and much research needs to be done. However, the belief is that not too far down the road, GI information will become part of the dietary control for individuals with diabetes.

4. **What exactly do terms like fat-free, organic, and sugar-free mean?** Terms used in connection with foods have specific meanings that have been established by the Food and Drug Administration (FDA) as mandated by the Nutritional Labeling and Education Act of 1990. Table 30–2 summarizes the most common terms with their basic FDA definitions. These terms will have the same meaning regardless of which food label they appear on and are based on a single serving of the food.

RESOURCE WEB SITES

For more information on the glycemic index of foods, contact the Glycemic Research Institute:

> *www.anndeweesallen.com/dal_gly.htm*
> E-mail: *drallen@www.iocafe.net*
>   Or write:
> Glycemic Research Institute
> 601 Pennsylvania Avenue NW, Suite 900
> Washington, DC 20004

Table 30–2. Most Common Food Terms

Fat Terms

- **Fat-free:** Less than 0.5 g of fat.
- **Saturated fat-free:** Less than 0.5 g of fat and less than 0.5 g of trans-fatty acids.
- **Lowfat:** 3 g or less of fat per serving.
- **Low saturated fat:** 1 g or less per serving and not more than 15% of calories from saturated fatty acids.
- **Reduced/less fat:** At least 25% less fat per serving than the "regular" food.
- **Reduced/less saturated fat:** At least 25% less saturated fat than the "regular" food item.
- **Cholesterol-free:** Less than 2 mg of cholesterol and 2 g or less of saturated fats per serving.
- **Low cholesterol:** 20 mg or less and 2 g or less of fat per serving, and, if the serving is 30 mg or less or 2 tablespoons or less, per 50 g of the food.
- **Reduced/less cholesterol:** At least 25% less and 2 g or less of saturated fat per serving than the "regular" food.
- **Lean** (meat, poultry, seafood, game meats): Less than 10 g of fat, 4.5 g or less of saturated fat, and less than 95 mg of cholesterol per serving and per 100 g (3½ oz).
- **Extra lean:** Less than 5 g of fat, less than 2 g of saturated fat, less than 95 mg of cholesterol per serving and per 100 g (3½ oz).

Sodium Terms

- **Sodium-free:** Less than 5 mg of sodium.
- **Low-sodium:** Less than 140 mg of sodium for serving.
- **Very low-sodium:** Between 5 and 35 mg of sodium.
- **Reduced or less sodium:** Food has at least 25% less sodium than regular food.

Sugar Terms

- **Sugar-free:** Less than 0.5 mg of CHO per serving.
- **No added sugar, without sugar added, no sugar added:**

  No sugar added during processing or packing, including ingredients that contain sugars (e.g., fruit juices, applesauce, or dried fruit).

  Processing does not increase the sugar content above the amount naturally present in the ingredients.

  The food that it resembles and for which it substitutes normally contains added sugars.

  If the food does not meet the requirements for a low- or reduced-calorie food, the product bears a statement that the food is not low calorie or calorie reduced and directs the customers' attention to the nutrition panel for further information on sugars and calorie content.
- **Reduced sugar:** At least 25% less sugar per serving than the "regular" food.

Table 30–2. Most Common Food Terms (Continued)

Fiber Terms

- **High fiber:** 5 g or more per serving (foods making high-fiber claims must meet the definition for low fat, or the level of total fat must appear next to the high-fiber claim).
- **Good source of fiber:** 2.5 to 4.9 g of fiber per serving.
- **More or added fiber:** At least 2.5 g more per serving than the "regular" food.

Lite/Light Terms

- Food contains ⅓ less calories and half the fat of the "regular" food.
- The sodium content of a low-calorie, low-fat food reduced by 50%.

The following terms have no standard government definition. Therefore, their use in relation to food items is not always clear.

- **Dietetic:** Pertaining to diet or proper food. A very general term. Sometimes used to indicate foods with low caloric content. Patients often mistake the dietetic section of the grocery store for diabetic foods. There is no such thing as diabetic foods. With proper guidance, almost any food can be part of a diabetic diet.
- **Natural or organic:** Although there is no consensus on this phrase, it generally means that the food (plant or animal) was grown without antibiotics, pesticides, fertilizer, and herbicides. The U.S. Department of Agriculture is developing definitions for the organic food industry. It is anticipated that at some time during 1998, these definitions will be finalized. Once this happens, the word *organic* will have a specific meaning like the terms in Table 30–2.

5. **How do I evaluate the many claims made about certain foods and supplements like vitamins and minerals?** Now this is a truly challenging question! Claims that specific foods or substances have remarkable curative or health powers are not new; there are still a large number of health claims surrounding specific foods and supplements. However, the scientific research supporting many of these claims is usually very limited. The major task in examining these claims is to separate the wheat from the chaff. Here are a few basic rules to help you do that.

   - **Do not take all claims seriously.** This, however, may be difficult because so many of the products have exaggerated claims that are promoted with very elaborate, sophisticated, glittery promotions. If you are not careful, you may be convinced that this item is the answer to cure all that ails the human body. Therefore, how can companies make these claims if they are not supported by facts? First, not all of the holes have been filled by the FDA labeling rules. Second, some individuals and companies make false claims until they are caught. They may then elect to fight the law several ways, including going to court. Thus, it may take years for issues regarding a product's advertising claims to be settled.

- **Look for the small print.** Be aware of a claim such as: "These statements have not been evaluated by the FDA. This product is not intended to diagnose, treat, cure, or prevent any disease." This does not automatically mean the claims are false. It only means that the FDA does not have enough research to support or refute the claims.
- **When the advertisement states that the product claims are backed by research, write or call and ask for copies of the research.** If you do not receive any response, be wary. If you do receive a response, use your critical thinking skills to analyze the information. In addition, critically analyze claims that the "established medical community does not want you to know about or use this product because . . ."
- **Currently, the best advice for you and your patient is to accept the dietary information from reputable, known sources until research supports the claim.** A few examples of reliable nutritional information are registered dietitians, colleges and universities, the FDA, and organizations such as the American Cancer Society, the American Diabetes Association, and the American Heart Association.

Finally, a few words about food taboos. Just thinking about someone eating worms makes most of us groan. However, analysis of such "nonfoods" reveals that the items are good nutrition sources. The psychology behind why we do not consider them legitimate foods is very complex. An interesting article by Milton (1997) provides one theory that food is one way to establish cultural identity. When we encounter a group whose food intake includes food we would never consider putting past our lips (versus foods we find different or do not like), Milton proposes that we are claiming a superior status. Somehow, individuals eating these "nonfoods" are envisioned to be less civilized than other individuals.

One recent example of a nonfood is the state of Louisiana's attempt to get its citizens to eat nutria (Cobb, 1997). The nutria is a very destructive water animal in the rodent family that lives in coastal wetlands of the state. For many reasons, their numbers are vast and control measures are failing. Thus, Louisiana is launching a $2 million campaign to encourage individuals to eat nutria. Eating nutria would help control their numbers and provide a lean, high-protein meat source. Are you ready to eat nutria? So far, most individuals in Louisiana are not.

The role of nutrition in maintaining health and preventing and controlling specific problems is an emerging science. Research may, in time, support many of the claims surrounding current nutrition fads. Until then, be vigilant and stick with information that you know has a sound research base.

31

Epidemiology and Infectious Diseases

Although the word *epidemiology* may seldom be used in class, much of what you are learning about health and illness is rooted in the science of epidemiology. **Epidemiology** is the area of study that identifies "causal relationships between health problems and the multitude of etiological factors that initiate them" (Berger & Williams, 1999). The focus of epidemiology is public or community health issues that look at groups of individuals that share a common health problem or specific condition. This specific group is called a **population.** The size of the population is not important. What is significant is the fact that all the members of this special group share an illness or health problem. The characteristics of the population, therefore, change for each health problem. The results of epidemiologic studies usually play a major role in the formulation and implementation of public health policy.

Some Basic Elements of Epidemiology

Epidemiologists are often considered medical detectives. When a problem is identified, they probe every nook and cranny looking for clues that identify a cause and effect relationship. Among the facts gathered are data concerning the time and place of a specific health problem, as well as characteristics of the population affected such as physical, biologic, social, cultural, and behavioral factors.

- Epidemiologists study communicable diseases; acute, chronic, and congenital illnesses; and environmental health hazards.

309

- When analyzing a community health problem, the epidemiologist breaks it down into three major areas of investigation: the host, the agent, and the environment (Berger & Williams, 1999), with each part being analyzed in as much depth as possible.

Three Areas of Epidemiologic Investigation

1. **Host:** The individuals involved—age, gender, culture, place of residence, ethnicity, occupation, etc.
2. **Agent:** The cause of the specific health problem; there are two main categories of agents
   - *Infectious agents* such as parasites, bacteria, or viruses
   - *Noninfectious agents* such as smoking, cholesterol, or radiation
3. **Environment:** The surrounding conditions
   - *Physical environment* includes climate, terrain, atmospheric conditions, chemicals, or physical agents
   - *Biological environment* includes the agent's reservoir, methods of transmission of the agent, and elements in the environment that block the disease development
   - *Social environment* includes public policies, housing conditions, cultural habits, and family health practices

Therefore, the development of a disease or community health problem is the result of many factors interacting, not a single, isolated factor. It is through the analysis of the interplay of these three factors that strategies to control the problem are developed.

Although local and state health departments carry out epidemiologic investigations, many investigations are conducted by the Centers for Disease Control and Prevention (CDC), which is a federal agency. The CDC is the leader in epidemiologic studies and, with a knowledgeable and specialized staff, often identifies factors associated with a problem relatively quickly; other times a great deal of time is required. (Note that in 1993, the name of the CDC was expanded to the Centers for Disease Control and Prevention. However, the acronym, CDC, has not changed.)

A few examples of the hundreds of health problems that have been solved or understood as a result of epidemiologic research include:

1. Toxic shock syndrome and use of specific tampons
2. Smoking and various health consequences
3. The connection between human immunodeficiency virus (HIV) infection and the development of acquired immune deficiency syndrome (AIDS)
4. Source of a staphylococcal infection in a newborn nursery
5. Connection between fat intake and heart problems
6. Effect of lead ingestion by children and IQ development
7. Legionnaires' disease and air conditioning systems

There are two points that need to be made about the work of epidemiologists. As items numbers 1, 2, 5, and 6 in the previous list indicate, the current scope of investigations goes far beyond traditional communicable diseases. Second, epidemiology is not directly concerned with curing or treating a specific disease or condition. However, because epidemiology identifies the interplay of causative factors, it is often the foundation for actions aimed at treatment or control. For example, once we learned the mode of transmission of the virus that leads to AIDS, programs were developed to educate people on how to control or prevent the spread of HIV infection.

The tools that epidemiologists use to describe their findings are described through various epidemiology statistics.

Important Epidemiologic Statistics

1. **Demographic statistics:** These numbers describe what individuals with the disease look like—age, gender, occupation, geographic location, etc.
2. **Vital statistics:** These are events in a community that are officially recorded into the government records—births; deaths, including the causes of each death; adoptions; marriages; divorces; etc.
3. **Health and disease statistics:**
   - Mortality figures are the number of deaths in a specific population due to a specific cause. These numbers are usually broken down into very specific subgroups. Examples are the number of suicides among men between the ages 75 to 80 and the number of women who died of breast cancer in 1997 in a specific state.
   - Morbidity figures are the number of people in a given population who are ill with a certain condition. Two terms that often are confused, which are part of morbidity numbers, are *prevalence* and *incidence*. *Incidence* is the number of new cases of a specific health problem that has occurred during a specified period of time. *Prevalence* is the total number of cases existing in a given population at a specific period in time.

For example, if a state recorded 35 new cases of HIV in the year 1996, this is the annual incidence rate. However, if on July 1, 1996, there were a total of 95 HIV cases in the state, 95 is the prevalence rate.

A common error made by many individuals is taking prevalence data and making invalid conclusions. For example, suppose that investigators were interested in knowing the relationship between headaches after eating at Restaurants A and B. Over 2 days, the investigators interviewed 50 people who ate at both restaurants and placed the data in a prevalence or cross-section table (Table 31–1).

Looking at the table, many individuals will draw the erroneous conclusion that eating at Restaurant A caused the headaches. However, prevalence tables provide only the number of cases of a disease in a specific population and no

Table 31–1. Prevalence Data for 50 Individuals Who Ate at Two Restaurants and Developed Headaches

	Restaurants	
Outcome Type	A	B
Headache	41	15
No headache	9	35

conclusion about causation can be drawn. The table does indicate a relationship between headaches and the two restaurants. Further research may find a cause and effect correlation. So once again, prevalence data cannot be used to make a cause and effect conclusion.

Communicable Diseases and Immunity

Although current epidemiologic research includes a variety of health concerns, its main component is communicable diseases. One of the main mechanisms for control of many of these diseases is development of immunity. When considering immunity, it is essential to understand the two major types: active and passive. These terms indicate how the body obtained its immunity. If the body had to work at it, it is known as **active immunity.** On the other hand, if the body did nothing to get the protection, it is known as **passive immunity** (Figure 31–1).

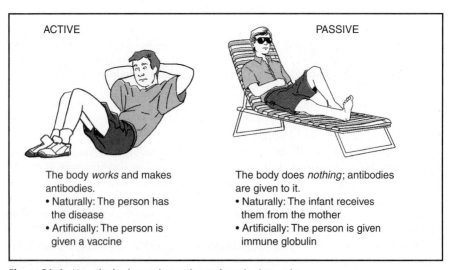

ACTIVE

The body *works* and makes antibodies.
• Naturally: The person has the disease
• Artificially: The person is given a vaccine

PASSIVE

The body does *nothing*; antibodies are given to it.
• Naturally: The infant receives them from the mother
• Artificially: The person is given immune globulin

Figure 31–1. How the body acquires active and passive immunity.

Key Terms Associated with Immunity

- **Immunity:** Protection against an infectious disease as a result of the functioning of a healthy immune system.
- **Antigen:** A substance that the body does not recognize as self. Almost all antigens have a protein component. In the healthy immune system an antigen will cause the body to create a defense against it (called an antibody).
- **Antibody:** A protein created when the body is exposed to an antigen. The antibody makes the antigen incapable of causing harm. Antibodies are specific. That is, they only work when they are paired up with their specific antigen. Antibodies against polio will not protect someone exposed to chickenpox.

The two ways of becoming immune have different characteristics that can be seen in Table 31–2. Let's take a few examples and see how they fit into the table.

Table 31–2. Two Ways of Developing Immunity

Terminology	How the Body Develops Immunity	Length of Time the Body Is Protected
Natural		
Active	Natural contact with the antigen (you are near an individual who has the disease). You develop a clinical or subclinical[a] case of the disease.	Permanent. The individual is considered immune to the specific disease for life.
Passive	Natural contact with the antibody through placenta, colostrum, and/or breastmilk.	Temporary. Protection lasts 6–8 weeks. Then the antibodies are gone and the body no longer has protection.
Artificial		
Active	The body is inoculated with the antigen, called vaccinations.	Permanent. Some diseases require a periodic booster to ensure continued protection.
Passive	The body is injected with a specific antibody, immune globulin (old term: gamma globulin).	Temporary: 6–8 weeks.

[a] Subclinical case occurs when the individual is exposed to small amount of an antigen but, although the body makes antibodies, shows no outward signs of being sick with the disease.

- A child is vaccinated against diphtheria, tetanus, and pertussis. The type of immunity is active, artificial immunity. The child's body has been given antigens (in this example, three specific antigens) and must work to create the corresponding specific antibodies.
- A mother has immunity (antibodies) to measles and is breast feeding her newborn. The type of immunity is passive, natural immunity. The infant's body is receiving ready-made antibodies from its mother.
- A high school student develops a case of chickenpox. The type of immunity is active, natural immunity. The student's body is exposed to the chickenpox antigen and must work to create antibodies.
- An adult is exposed to hepatitis B and the physician orders an injection of an immune globulin preparation. The type of immunity is passive, artificial immunity. The adult's body is receiving is ready-made antibodies in the immune globulin injection.

Understanding the type of immunity an individual possesses influences nursing interventions, especially patient education issues. For example, the CDC recently recommended beginning immunization of all newborns against hepatitis B before the newborn leaves the hospital. This will require that the parent be taught not only the reason for the immunization, but also the importance of following the immunization schedule after discharge.

Nurses have several major responsibilities in relation to vaccine-preventable diseases.

- **Be sure that the reference vaccine schedule used for children and adults is current.** As of the printing of this book, such charts should have a November 2000 date for children and a May 1998 date for adolescents and adults. If you are in doubt, call the CDC for updates.
- **Teach parents the importance of having their children immunized on schedule.**
- **Know and follow specific administration techniques.** For example, in adults, hepatitis B vaccine should be administered in the deltoid muscle.
- **Know the specific vaccine storage and handling requirements.**
- **Be aware of myths associated with vaccinations.** The CDC publication (1995) cited at the end of the chapter is an excellent source of information on the most prevalent myths. For example, it lists 10 reasons that are often given as contraindication to vaccination, such as someone in the household is pregnant. In fact, the CDC states that pregnancy in the household is not a valid reason to delay vaccinating a child in that household.
- **Spend time with patients who do not follow vaccination recommendations for infants, children, or adults.** Is their action based on religious or cultural reasons? If so, then attempts to convince them to receive vaccinations may be unethical. If, however, they have other reasons, you may be able to help them realize the benefits of vaccinations. Be cautious with advice to

parents that there are no dangers with vaccinations. Although very small in number, problems do occur.

Another issue related to communicable diseases is the frequently misunderstood role of standard precautions and the spread of various diseases. **Standard precautions** is the term created to describe techniques to prevent the spread of pathogens that are bloodborne. Differentiating bloodborne spread of infections from respiratory spread requires some remembering from microbiology regarding the major factors influencing the transmission of a communicable organism.

Six Major Factors Associated with the Spread of Communicable Diseases

The six major factors associated with the spread of communicable diseases form a vicious circle, and are listed as follows:

1. Characteristics of the infectious agent
2. The agent's reservoir—where it lives and multiplies
3. Portal of exit from the reservoir
4. Mode of transmission away from the reservoir
5. Portal of entry into a new host
6. Susceptible new host

In control of communicable diseases, the major goal is to break the cycle at one of the six points. One of the most important breaking points is immunization of susceptible populations, which breaks the chain at susceptibility of the new host. In patient care, handwashing is so crucial because it intercepts transmission away from the reservoir. Antibiotics interfere with certain physiological functions of an organism preventing it from multiplying, thus breaking the transmission chain at the first listed point. Figure 31–2 shows in more detail the linking nature of these six factors.

So, we go back to standard precautions. When you look at the transmission elements, you see that standard precautions are aimed at intercepting transmission at points 3, 4, and 5 on the list for organisms that leave and enter the body via blood and body fluids that contain blood. The most prevalent of these bloodborne organisms are HIV, which leads to AIDS, and the virus that causes hepatitis B. Standard precautions, therefore, do not interrupt the cycle for diseases that are airborne or organisms that enter the body through the mouth. You must understand many things about a pathogen in order to know where to break the chain.

Before we close, let's look at two specific infectious diseases of special concern to health care workers. Although HIV, the blood- and body fluid–borne disease that leads to AIDS, is always high on the list, there are two other dis-

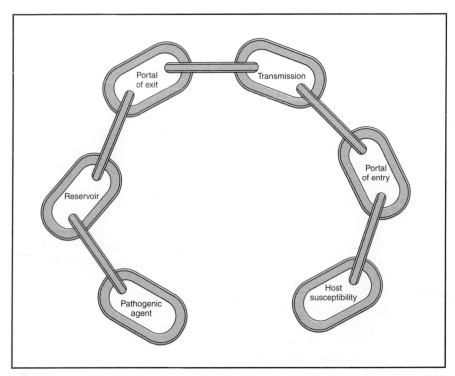

Figure 31–2. Chain of infection. (*From Ball, J., & Bindler, R. [1999]. Pediatric nursing: Caring for children [2nd ed.]. Reprinted by permission of Pearson Education, Inc. Upper Saddle River, NJ 07458.*)

eases that are of concern. One is tuberculosis (TB). In the early 1900s, TB was a major health problem. It was frequently referred to as *consumption,* and there were no effective treatments. By the middle of the century, however, effective antibiotics were developed and with time TB was no longer considered a major public health problem. However, tuberculosis is resurfacing as a global health concern. The problem is not the disease per se. It is the fact that a large number of the new emerging cases are multidrug resistant; current drugs are not effective in controlling the infection and individuals are again dying of TB. Remember, the main mode of transmission of TB is the respiratory system. In addition, the organism is ubiquitous—it can be found *everywhere.* It is not confined to a specific country, part of a city, or certain socioeconomic groups, thus the need for you to always practice good medical asepsis, especially, not letting patients cough or sneeze in your face. (As an aside, TB is not an easily acquired disease. When you maintain your own health with adequate sleep, exercise, and diet, you are creating excellent protection when exposure to the organism occurs.)

Another group of infectious diseases that are of concern to health care workers is hepatitis. Although many individuals consider HIV their major occupational hazard, it is not. Hepatitis is a much greater threat! There was a time when hepatitis had only two classifications: infectious hepatitis and serum hepatitis. Starting in the 1960s, diagnostic technology led to improved viral identification and the development of the current classification system of five types of hepatitis: A, B, C, D, and E. Each is referred to by three letters, such as HAV—hepatitis A virus, HBV—hepatitis B virus. You are encouraged to study the various charts found in your texts that compare the types of hepatitis. These charts point out differences in such important areas as incubation period, mode of transmission, and risk factors.

Of the five forms of hepatitis, the one of great concern for health care workers is HBV. This form of hepatitis is much more infectious than HIV and, like HIV, its mode of transmission is bloodborne, especially needle sticks. Because HBV is such an occupational hazard, many schools require their students take the now available vaccine. Like all vaccines, it is not 100% effective, therefore the need for constant caution when handling sharps and blood contaminated items.

On a small scale, infection control nurses in hospitals practice the principles of epidemiology every day. For example, these nurses receive notices of postoperative infections. One of the many activities the nurse will have related to these reports is looking for patterns by answering questions such as: What day of the week did the surgery occur? Which operating room was used? What type of surgery did the patient have? What staff were on duty? In other words, can a common thread be found so that the chain of infection can be broken?

This chapter has provided highlights of epidemiology, which is seldom a separate course topic. Our current knowledge about relationships between smoking and respiratory illness, cholesterol and cardiovascular disease, food poisoning and the degree to which hamburgers are cooked, blood and HIV transmission, has its foundation in the science of epidemiology.

Books to Consider Adding to Your Personal Library

Grimes, D. E., Grimes, R. M., & Hamelink, M. (1991). *Infectious diseases.* St. Louis: Mosby-Yearbook.

Preston, R. (1994). *The hot zone.* New York: Random House.

Stolley, P. D., & Lasky, T. (1995). *Investigating disease patterns: The science of epidemiology.* New York: Scientific American Library.

RESOURCE WEB SITES

American Liver Foundation: *www.sadieo.ucsf.edu/alffinal/homepagealf/html*
Hepatitis Foundation International: *www.hepfi.org/hepinfo/grid.htm*
Centers for Disease Control and Prevention:
  www.cdc.gov/ncidod/dieseases/hepatitis/h96issue.htm

32

Challenging Concepts

There are a number of terms that tend to be difficult to understand and remember. We will look at a few that tend to offer the greatest challenges.

■ Terms Associated with the Nervous System That Also Are Used in Pharmacology

The autonomic division of the nervous system has two divisions. One division is the sympathetic; the other division is the parasympathetic. Table 32–1 is an overview of how major organs respond when stimulated by each of the systems.

Although the two systems are independent, they complement each other's actions to maintain balance, or homeostasis, like two children on a teeter-totter. However, once stimulated into action, responses of the sympathetic system are on an all or none basis. You cannot have just one organ respond without all of them responding. When the bear is after you, your heart rate will not increase without all of the other responses occurring. However, this is not true of the parasympathetic system. It is possible to have parasympathetic stimulation of the salivary glands without a corresponding change in cardiac rate.

A few words about the subsystems of the sympathetic system, the alpha and beta receptors. The sympathetic nervous system (SNS) has multiple struc-

319

Table 32–1. Organ Response to Stimulation by the Autonomic Nervous System

Organ	Sympathetic Nervous System	Parasympathetic Nervous System
• Heart	Increases rate	Decreases rate
• Blood vessels	Constricts	Dilates visceral and brain vessels
• Lungs (bronchi)	Dilates	Constricts
• Gastrointestinal	Decreases peristalsis	Increases peristalsis
• Eyes	Dilates pupil	Constricts pupil
• Gastric and salivary secretions	Decreases	Increases
• Liver	Stimulates glycogen	
• Adrenal medulla	Stimulates production of epinephrine	

tures on various tissues known as alpha and beta receptors. These receptors are further divided into alpha$_1$ or alpha$_2$ and beta$_1$ and beta$_2$ sites. Each site has a distinct effect on cell function. For example, beta$_1$ receptor sites of the heart influence the heart's rate, automaticity, impulse conduction, and force of contraction. Knowing the actions of the alpha$_1$ and alpha$_2$ and beta$_1$ and beta$_2$ receptors leads to understanding of how and why specific medications work. For example, when epinephrine reaches the beta$_2$ receptors of the bronchi, it causes the smooth muscles to relax and the bronchi to dilate. A medication classified as a beta blocker would, therefore, prevent (block) this action and, in essence, allow the parasympathetic action on bronchi to occur—the bronchi constrict. Table 32–2 contains common terms associated with medications and the autonomic nervous system.

Terms Associated with Medications and the Autonomic Nervous System

- **Neurotransmitter:** A chemical that allows a nerve impulse to bridge the gap (synapse) between nerve cells. The autonomic nervous system has two major neurotransmitters: norepinephrine (NE) and acetylcholine (ACh).
- **Norepinephrine:** Neurotransmitter that is stored in parts of specific tracts of the nervous system, as well as the adrenal medulla. The body releases NE as a response to hypotension and stress. It is also known as *noradrenaline.*

Table 32–2. Common Terms Associated with the Autonomic Nervous System

	Sympathetic Nervous System (SNS)	Parasympathetic Nervous System (PNS)
Also Known As	Thoracolumbar	Craniosacral
Primary chemical/ neurotransmitter	Norepinephrine (NE)	Acetylcholine (ACh)
Terms given to nerves transmitting the impulses	Adrenergic	Cholinergic
System subtypes	Alpha₁ and alpha₂ Beta₁ and beta₂	(None)
Common terms used in pharmacology related to the two systems	• Adrenergic agonist, also called sympathomimetic (creates the flight or fight response) • Sympatholytic, also called adrenergic receptor blockers; these are artificial and generally react to a specific alpha or beta receptor site; these agents will decrease or block the action of NE	• Cholinergic • Parasympathomimetic • Acetylcholinesterase inhibitor; all three will mimic the effects of ACh; each in a different way, thus the different terminology • Anticholinergic, also called parasympatholytic • Parasympatholytic; these two reduce/block the actions of ACh

- **Acetylcholine:** Neurotransmitter that is released from many points along the ganglia of the sympathetic and parasympathetic nervous systems.
- **Sympathomimetic and parasympathomimetic:** Both terms are usually used when describing the action of a medication. They indicate that the action of the medication mimics, or has actions, that look like the respective system that has been stimulated.
- **Sympatholytic and parasympatholytic:** Both terms are usually used in relation to actions of medications and indicate that the medication will lyse, or block, the respective neurotransmitter.

We will place some of this information into an activity that you will do almost every day, look up information about a specific medication. You are looking up a medication and read the following: Autonomic nervous system agent; beta-adrenergic antagonist (sympatholytic, blocking agent); cardiovascular agent; antihypertensive, antianginal; selectively blocks beta₁-adrenergic receptors located in cardiac tissue. Don't panic! Just break it down into its parts.

- **Autonomic nervous system (ANS) agent:** The medication involves action of the autonomic nervous system. Note that it does not indicate which branch of the ANS is involved.
- **Beta-adrenergic antagonist** (sympatholytic, blocking agent): We now learn that it is the sympathetic nervous system that is involved, since the parasympathetic system does not have an alpha and beta subsystem. It also tells us "adrenergic," which is the term associated with the sympathetic system. In addition, the medication's target is the beta site versus alpha sites. The phrase also tells us that the medication is an "antagonist," a medication with an opposing action.
- **Sympatholytic, blocking agent:** The medication acts to inhibit (sympatholytic) the effects of the SNS or occupy (block) the site. These two terms are just another way of saying beta-adrenergic antagonist.
- **Cardiovascular agent:** The medication will have its desired action on the cardiovascular system versus, say, the respiratory system. As you read the details of the medication, you also find that it selectively blocks beta$_1$-adrenergic sites in heart muscle.
- **Antihypertensive; antianginal:** The focus of the medication's use is high blood pressure and anginal pain.

What looked incomprehensible at first is now understandable. This is a drug that will have actions such as reducing heart rate and decreasing the force of the heart's contractions.

Pharmacodynamics and Pharmacokinetics

Pharmacodynamics and pharmacokinetics are two words that seem to jump out at you when you look up information about a medication.

- **Pharmacodynamics:** Describes how a medication acts at the target cells (point where it does "its thing") to produce the desired therapeutic results.
- **Pharmacokinetics:** Describes what happens before and after the medication acts at the target cells. It includes how the medication is absorbed into the body, distributed to target cells, metabolized into other compounds, and excreted from the body.

Negative and Positive Feedback

Students frequently have difficulty with the concepts of negative and positive feedback. A question that is frequently asked by students is, "What keeps your blood pressure within normal limits, your temperature okay, and your blood pH in a narrow range?" The answer: balance of the body's regulating mechanisms. In most of your books you see this balance referred to as **adaptation** or **homeostasis.** It is the continuous interaction of physiological actions that keeps body functions in a state of equilibrium. Two frequently used terms associated with this balancing act are negative and positive feedback.

- **Negative feedback:** An action that returns a system back to a preset standard or norm. It restores homeostasis, or balance. The healthy body functions on the basis of negative feedback.
- **Positive feedback:** An action that moves the system away from the preset standard or norm. Unchecked, positive feedback actions lead to disequilibrium with death as the undesired outcome.

(We know! We think of negative things as bad or undesirable and positive things as good or desirable. However, as far as the body is concerned, bad is good and good is bad.)

Negative feedback is in essence a series of events that occur in a circular sequence. Three major steps in this loop are:

1. At least one organ or tissue identifies an impulse or signal. This step is often referred to as the **receptor component** because the message is received.
2. Once received, another organ or tissue then judges how well the impulse or signal matches the preset standard. Often referred to as the **comparator component,** it is the step that compares how well the signal matches the norm.
3. When the identified signal is considered outside the established limits, messages are sent to organs and tissues to do something to bring the signal back into the normal, acceptable range. This is often referred to as the **effector component.** This portion of the loop effects, or brings about changes, in organ and tissue functioning so that the undesired signal returns to the desired preset condition.

One of the most common examples of negative feedback is the way a thermostat maintains a house at a desired temperature. To start, someone determines that the most comfortable temperature for the house is 75°F. This temperature corresponds to the preset standard in the feedback loop. Once the standard has been determined, the sequence looks like the sequence in Figure 32–1. If you substitute various body actions in this loop—for example, how the healthy body maintains a constant blood level of hormones—you will have

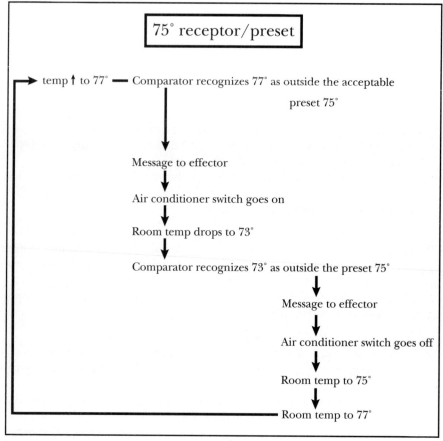

Figure 32–1. House thermostat as an example of negative feedback.

negative feedback as it occurs in the body. Figure 32–2 is an example of one of the body's many negative feedback loops.

Afferent, Efferent

Two terms are used in connection with anatomy that are easy to confuse: *afferent* and *efferent*.

- **Afferent:** The flow (nerve impulse; blood flow) is toward the central structure.

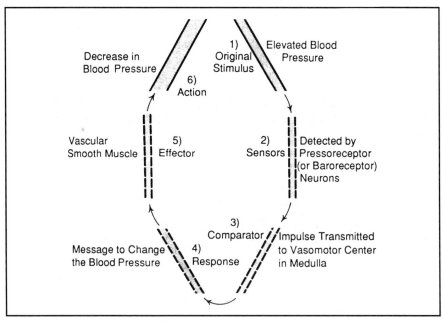

Figure 32–2. Example of a negative feedback loop in the body. (*From Burrel, L. O., Gerlach, M. M., & Pless, B. S. [1997]. Adult nursing: Acute and community care. [2nd ed.]. Reprinted by permission of Pearson Education, Inc. Upper Saddle River, NJ 07458.*)

- **Efferent:** The flow (nerve impulse; blood flow) is away from the central structure.

Remember that they always refer to some central point or structure such as a nerve or blood vessel. For example, Bowman's capsules in the kidneys have afferent and efferent arterioles. The afferent arterioles carry blood into the capsules and the efferent carry blood out of the capsules.

There are many terms and concepts that are discussed throughout nursing textbooks. This chapter highlights some of the common ones that seem to present students with the most difficulty. When you come across a term that is tough to remember, try to create your own memory tricks such as the afferent and efferent tips.

SPEED BUMP

Remember: Afferent structures have an Affinity for the center.
Efferent structures Exit from the center.

Another example is the following mnemonic for remembering the name of each of the 12 cranial nerves.

SPEED BUMP

On Old Olympus's Treeless Top A Finn And German Viewed Some Hops.

	Cranial Nerve	**Word**
I	Olfactory	On
II	Optic	Old
III	Oculomotor	Olympus's
IV	Trochlear	Treeless
V	Trigeminal	Top
VI	Abducens	A
VII	Facial	Finn
VIII	Acoustic	And
IX	Glossopharyngeal	German
X	Vagus	Viewed
XI	Spinal	Some
XII	Hypoglossal	Hops

We still remember the 12 nerves in their numerical order by the mnemonic learned in school many years ago. So, if you are struggling to remember some specific information, try creating your own mnemonic!

One of the challenges of nursing school is learning a new language. This chapter has presented some of the terminology most students frequently find difficult to learn. When studying these, and other challenging concepts and terminology, use all of your study skills. Remember that reading and looking up definitions is only the first step. You will need to add other activities such as creating flash cards, discussing the terms with classmates, asking specific questions in class, and creating mnemonics. One thing is sure. This knowledge will not come by osmosis. You are going to have to be an active learner.

33

Research

■ Research

Most nurses cringe when they hear the word *research*. For some reason, they tend to think that research is something that is done far away in a lab by people who have never set foot near a patient. Nothing could be further from the truth. Research occurs on a daily basis in most facilities. Research of a clinical nature requires constant contact with patients. You may have been involved in research as a data collector, or perhaps as a subject.

There is nothing intimidating about research. Most of us apply some form of research in our daily lives. How many of you travel out of your way to shop at a particular grocery store? Why? Most likely, over time you have learned that the store you choose to shop at has lower prices, better quality, or both. How did you figure this out? Did you go to several stores and check prices on the same items? If you did, you were doing some basic research. Through the process of elimination and trial and error, you were able to determine which store you wanted to patronize.

Is choosing the best store much different than determining the best antibiotic for a specific bacterium? Although it took several years for researchers to discover which antibiotics work on which bacteria, the basic process was the same. So, if you are one of those nurses who harbors great fear about research, forget it! Research goes on around us every day. Our job is to help our pa-

tients reap the rewards of research. To help patients understand and use the results of research, we have to be able to discern which research is valid and applicable to their specific patient situations.

Using Research to Guide Patients

Several important things to remember when guiding patients in the use of
research are as follows.

- It is important to remember that some of your patients will have already
  done some information gathering on their own, but remember that nearly all
  of your patients will require some assistance with interpreting research results
  (Figure 33–1). For example, some patients will swallow anything they read
  with the words "proved to be" or "significant."
- It is necessary for you to help patients put significant information into perspective. For example, you might ask the patient, "What did the study find?"
- It also helps to know if the research was conducted on a group that the
  patient is a part of. For example, if the patient is past menopause, was the
  research done on postmenopausal women?

What You Need to Know About Research

To help your patients and to determine whether or not specific research findings should be implemented in a clinical setting, you need to know some basics
about research use. Whether or not you ever decide to become a nurse
researcher, it is important for you to be able to incorporate the knowledge
gained from nursing research into your clinical practice. Once again, the terminology may seem foreign to you, but do not let that dissuade you. We are sure
you can recall when medical terminology seemed foreign, and you mastered
that! To help you learn to understand research reports (a must if you are going
to benefit from them) and find something of interest to yourself, we have
included the following information.

Understanding Research Reports

Some ideas to follow when gathering infomation through research reports are:

1. Review some guidelines for critiquing research reports.
2. When you encounter a clinical problem that is of interest to you, go to
   the library.

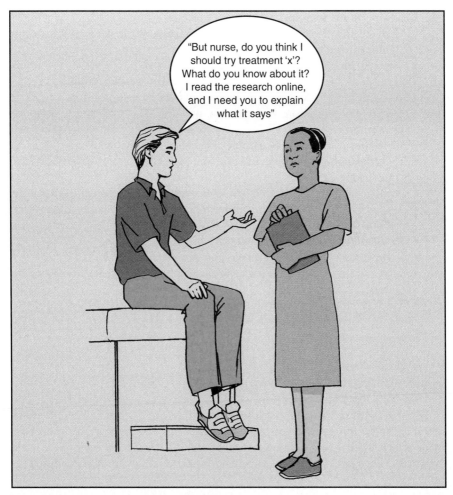

"But nurse, do you think I should try treatment 'x'? What do you know about it? I read the research online, and I need you to explain what it says"

Figure 33–1. Patients will need help understanding research.

- Ask the reference librarian to help you find information from CINAHL or another database about the problem.
3. Look in other areas outside your specific practice area.
   - Many nursing problems are common across practice settings.
4. As you learn to read research articles, remember to be patient with yourself.
   - Read the topic and see if it is of interest to you and then skim the article.
   - If you need help, find a nurse who has some research expertise to join you.

5. Read the results section.
   - Look at how the authors interpret the results of the study and note any significant findings.
   - The statistics should be explained as well.
6. Determine if the findings are applicable to your practice setting.
   - Was the sample similar to your patients? For example, if you work in cardiac rehabilitation with female patients, was the study done on women or men?
   - Were they in the same age range as most of your patients?
   - Use common sense to decide how much of the research is applicable to your setting.
7. Consider setting up a research group at your practice setting.
   - Find other nurses who are interested in sharing research information and start a brown bag lunch group once a month.
   - Read and share research articles.
   - Invite a nurse researcher to help you decipher an article.
   - Invite someone who has participated in research to share his or her experiences.
   - Make it a fun time.

(Beyea & Nicholl, 1997)

Research Red Flags

In reading research on your own, or in helping your patient interpret results, there are some things that you need to watch out for. New health claims are made every week and sometimes the "research" appears to contradict other "research." Be suspicious when you cannot find the following research information.

- Number of subjects who participated in the study
- Gender, ethnicity, or age of subjects
- Whether the subjects were paid (by whom)
- Whether a control group (nontreatment) group was used
- The condition of subjects before the study took place (did they have a recorded illness, or specific lab values, etc.)
- Whether a double-blind study design was used (this is the best type because neither the subjects nor the researcher knows who is receiving the experimental treatment)
- Whether significant differences were found between the control and treatment group results
- Funding sources
- The benefactor of the study's results (e.g., a specific drug manufacturer)

Red Flags That Should Alert You to Potentially Fraudulent Claims

1. Recommendations that promise a quick fix
   - Be wary of the "new" drug or "new" treatment that will cure everything that ails you.
2. Dire warnings of danger
   - Research in the past few years has told us to "not drink coffee," to "drink coffee," to "not eat butter," and to "eat butter."
   - When research tells us to avoid a specific thing, it is often interpreted in a vacuum.
   - In other words, only one research study is examined without the benefit of examining all the results of other studies about the same thing. For example, one study might suggest that smoking does not cause lung cancer, but if that study is examined in conjunction with all the other studies about smoking and lung cancer, one might conclude that smoking does indeed relate to lung cancer. The first study that concluded that smoking does not cause lung cancer may in fact be a valid study; however, there are many other valid studies that concluded something far different.
   - It pays to review all the studies on a particular topic, not just one.
3. Recommendations that are based on a single study.
   - Many times the press, or some researchers, will make conclusions based on just one study.
   - An important aspect of research is that the same conclusions can be reached time and time again.
   - Be sure that the study results recommended have been shown to occur more than once.
4. Recommendations made to help sell a product.
   - Be sure that you notice who funds research studies.
   - Frequently, the pharmaceutical company that just happens to make that drug funded studies that support the use of a specific medication.
   - Many fiascoes have occurred due to this type of research.
5. Recommendations from studies that have not been peer-reviewed.
   - Most reputable nursing journals use a peer-review system.
   - In other words, before a study can be published in a journal, other researchers in a similar specialty area review it.
   - In this way, the journal can be relatively sure that the research has merit and that research principles were followed.
6. Research results that sound too good to be true.
   - Sometimes you will read that treatment "X" has been found to cure disease "Y."
   - Be wary of this type of claim, especially if you know that the disease in question is chronic in nature and treatments are still being investigated.

- Once again, patients will bring you all kinds of information (some of it computer generated) touting various cures.
- We have found cures for cancer, multiple sclerosis, amyotrophic lateral sclerosis, and schizophrenia all on the Internet.
- Rarely will you be able to access formalized research to support these claims.
- You need to instill in yourself, and in your patients, a healthy dose of skepticism.

SPEED BUMP

Research-Associated Glossary

Assumptions: Beliefs that are held to be true but have not necessarily been proved

Conceptual framework: A background or foundation for a research study that is less well developed than a theoretical framework

Demographic variables: Characteristics of subjects such as age, gender, marital status, and education level

Hypothesis: A statement of the predicted relationship between two or more variables

Instruments (research tools): Devices used to collect data in research studies (e.g., questionnaires)

Limitations: Weaknesses of a study

Reliability: The consistency of an instrument to measure a variable over time

Sample: A subset of the population that is selected to represent the population and is used for data collection

Theoretical framework: A study framework based on relationship statements (showing the relationship between two or more concepts) that are taken from a theory

Validity: The ability of an instrument to measure what it is supposed to measure

Variable: A characteristic or attribute of a person or object that varies, for example, age, weight, height, and blood type

Source: Nieswiadomy, R. M. (1998). Foundations of nursing research *(3rd ed.). Stamford, CT: Appleton & Lange. Used with permission.*

We would like to add a personal note here. One of us has multiple sclerosis (MS). She considers herself to be well informed about the disease and about available treatments. As someone who regularly uses a computer to surf the Internet, she has been appalled at some of the fraudulent information available. About twice a month she receives e-mail solicitations informing her of a "cure" for MS that also contains "testimonials" from people who have been cured of the disease. Although she is a health care provider and nurse researcher, her curiosity is often piqued by these claims. In her head she realizes that a "cure" is not available for MS at this time; however, in her heart she wishes there were. So each time that she reads about a "cure," she wonders if this "treatment" is the answer. So, if your patient wants to believe in a "cure" that he or she found, be gentle! Our desire to hope and believe needs to be encouraged, but we also require a healthy dose of reality at times. Help patients to understand the information that they bring you, and help them to understand why specific research may or may not apply to their situation.

34

Theory

Many nurses and students regard nursing theory as something that is only understood at the graduate level. Nursing theory is not really that hard to understand. Theory is a way of guiding nurses in practice, education, and research. This means that nursing schools and clinical facilities have some type of model that guides their education or practice. The same holds true for nursing research. All research articles should refer to a theoretical model or base.

Conceptual Models

While you are in nursing school, you will discover that your school has a conceptual model or theory that it follows. You have probably been exposed to this model or theory in a fundamentals or concepts course. Do you know what model your school uses? For example, Dorthea Orem developed a theory that focuses on a person's ability to perform self-care. If your school uses a model based on Orem's self-care theory, you might study self-care deficits and how to correct them through nursing care (Figure 34–1; Fitzpatrick & Whall, 1996). On the other hand, if your school uses a model based on Sr. Callista Roy's theory of adaptation (1999), you will be familiar with terms such as adaptation level and focal, contextual, and residual stimuli. The model or theory that your school uses may be so commonplace to you that you have not really thought about its origin. Let's use these two models to examine a patient situation.

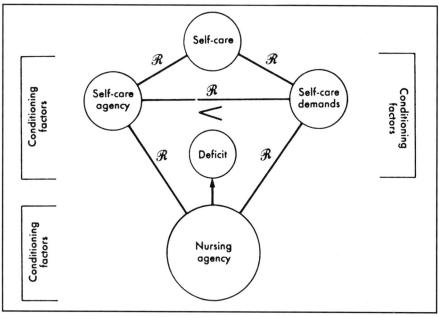

Figure 34–1. Orem's self-care theory. *(From Orem, D. E. [1991]. Nursing: Concepts of practice. St. Louis, MO: Mosby. Used with permission.)*

A CASE IN POINT

> Dottie is a 15-year-old girl who just discovered that she is pregnant. Dottie is unmarried and currently living with her divorced mother. Dottie has been raised in a strict Catholic home and attends church regularly. Dottie is unsure of who the father of the baby is and does not plan to include him in her decision making. Dottie is attending school and is in the top one-third of her class. Her mother works full time at the police department as a dispatcher.

Using Orem's model, the nurse would look for alterations in universal, developmental, or health-deviation self-care requisites. Dottie's pregnancy during adolescence would be considered an alteration in **developmental self-care requisites.** The nurse would then determine the ability of the patient to fulfill **self-care** by looking at **self-care demands, self-care agency,** and calculating **self-care deficits.**

Since Dottie is healthy overall, she is still able to meet most of her self-care demands. However, the nurse would need to assist her in meeting some of the self-care demands (partially compensatory nursing system) as well as provide support and education. The nurse would focus on determining what specific needs Dottie has with regard to:

- Food
- Shelter
- Physical needs
- Financial concerns
- Focusing on ways the above needs could be met
- What her options are in relation to the pregnancy
- Psychological support
- Guiding the decision-making process
- Information about prenatal planning, exams, etc.

(Fitzpatrick & Whall, 1996)

Using Roy's model, the nurse would examine **focal and contextual stimuli** and adaptation in the four modes: **physiological, role function, interdependence,** and **self-concept.** In Dottie's situation, pregnancy is the **focal stimulus.** The nurse would also examine **contextual** and **environmental stimuli,** which would include things such as housing, food, and finances. **Physiological adaptation** would be examined in relation to Dottie's current physical condition. The nurse would also be concerned with Dottie's **self-concept mode** in that pregnancy would effect both psychological and spiritual factors (her belief in Catholicism and what to do about the pregnancy) (Roy, 1999). Another concern would be her **role-function mode** because Dottie is attending school and being pregnant may effect her role as a student. To help Dottie, the nurse would focus on the following steps:

- Assessment of Dottie's behavior
- Assessment of stimuli
- Establishing a nursing diagnosis
- Setting goals with Dottie
- Intervention (what the nurse will do to assist Dottie)
- Evaluation (whether Dottie has adapted or not)

As you can see, although the two theories are very different, at times they are similar. There are many nursing theories and models that are based on development, needs, adaptation, and other components.

If you are already working in a hospital, your hospital also may use a conceptual model or theory. All hospitals have a mission statement, which may give you clues as to what model they use. It is important for you to familiarize yourself with your facility's philosophic beliefs, mission statement, and model.

Your beliefs and that of your institution need to be similar. For example, if you have strong Catholic religious beliefs, you might not want to work for an institution where birth control and abortion are practiced. Your belief system would more likely be congruent with a religious-based facility.

All nursing theories and models have four paradigms (or rules) that they address. These paradigms are a guide for nursing practice, nursing research, and nursing education by giving a consistent basis to work from.

The Nursing Paradigms

There are four areas that any theory or model will speak to in an attempt to guide nurses.

* Individual/Person
* Environment/Society
* Health
* Nursing Practice and Nursing Process

It is important to read the definitions of how each theory or model describes these four paradigms. These descriptions provide an understanding of each paradigm and how it is used in a particular theory or model.

Theories and models are made up of smaller building blocks called concepts. **Concepts** are ideas or phenomena such as stress, hunger, caring, pain, depression, or empathy. In theories and models, concepts are related to one another. A **relationship statement** describes the bond between concepts. For example, a relationship statement might state that when someone is under *stress* (concept 1) they need more *caring* (concept 2). Another example of a relationship statement would be that when a person is undergoing diagnostic testing, the more *accurate information* (concept 1) the person has, the less *anxiety* (concept 2) they will have.

All theories are also based on assumptions. **Assumptions** are statements that are supposed to be true without having to prove them. For example, Roy's nursing model (1999) is based on eight assumptions, one of which is "In humanism, it is believed that humans, as individuals and in groups, share creative power" (p. 34). Although at first glance this statement seems rather hard to decipher, all it is saying is that each of us has creative powers that we are born with, or learn, which can be used individually or in groups. When trying to understand theory, it is important for you to break it down into smaller pieces. Read through a paragraph once, then return and look for words that you recognize. First look for the major concepts and then see how they relate to one another.

All theories and models will also have operational definitions. An **operational definition** is a definition of a term that can be measured. For example, if one of the terms in a nursing model or theory is anxiety, there are many ways to measure anxiety. How would you measure anxiety? Can you think of more than one way to measure the concept of anxiety? There are many. Perhaps one way to measure anxiety would be a score on the uptight anxiety scale. Another way to measure anxiety might be the number of times a person is observed leaving a chair to pace up and down a room. Both of these examples are measurable; therefore, they could serve as an operational definition. It can be very difficult to develop operational definitions for abstract terms, but each theory or model will present a list of terms that are operationally defined.

From these basic components of a theory (concepts, assumptions, operational definitions, and relationship statements), it would be possible to use the theory to develop a hypothesis. A **hypothesis** is a basic component of research. It is important to note here the direct correlation from theory and model to research. Nursing theory guides nursing research, and nursing research can help support further development of a nursing theory or model (Figure 34–2). Let's put together a fictitious model.

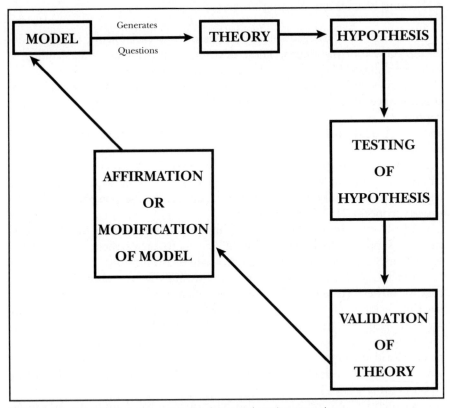

Figure 34–2. Relationship between nursing theory and nursing research.

A Fictitious Model

You and your sister are always arguing about the fastest way to get to your parent's house. You claim that by going down Main Street you can avoid the freeway on and off ramps, slowing down for poor drivers, and that Main Street is a more direct route. Your sister claims that the freeway is a much quicker route even though it is a longer distance because there are no traffic lights and she does not have to stop for people turning into various gas stations and retail stores. A conceptual model used to represent this disagreement might look like a typical road map.

1. The concepts in this model would include:
   - Time
   - Speed
   - Distance
   - Number of stops
2. The relationship statements for this model would be:
   - The shorter the distance, the shorter the time.
   - Increased number of stops equals increased amount of time.
   - Increased speed equals decreased time.
3. Assumptions for this model would be:
   - Both cars would be in good working order with equal amounts of engine power, approximately the same weight, and full tanks of gas.
   - There would be no road construction, accidents, or delays on either road.
   - There would be no rain, snow, fog, or other hazardous road conditions.
   - Both parties would comply with the posted speed limit.
4. An example of an operational definition for this model is:
   - Number of stops is the number of times a vehicle must come to a complete stop for any reason.
   - Amount of time is equal to the time calculated from the moment a car crosses the end of either driver's driveway until the time that a car crosses the end of the driveway at their mother's house.
5. A research hypothesis that could be developed from this basic information is:
   - There is a relationship between going a shorter distance with more stops and arrival time at a destination.

This is just one rather silly example of how the components of a theory or model fit together (Figure 34–3). A true nursing theory or model requires much thought and many years of experience prior to development.

6. Why is nursing theory important?
   - Nursing theory gives us the ability to define and direct the profession.

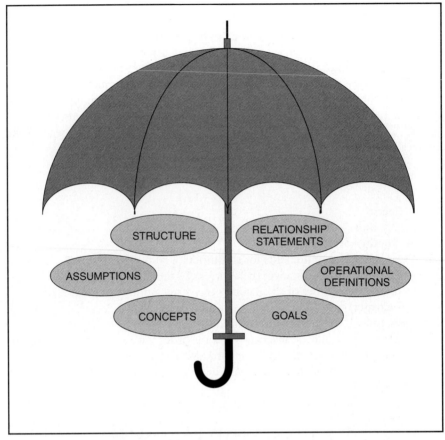

Figure 34–3. Nursing theory or model components.

- It gives nursing a unique body of knowledge.
- By providing nurses with a unique body of knowledge, we are able to develop professional autonomy.
- Theory helps all nurses to be more purposeful and more congruent in their actions whether they are in a clinical setting, education, or research.

To fully comprehend nursing theory, one must be willing to read more about nursing theory and its development.

- Pull out your school catalog and look for a mission statement.
- Find out what your college or department's philosophy is and what theory or model is used as a basis for your curriculum.

- When you are at work or in clinical, look for the facility's mission statement and philosophy.
- Determine if your personal philosophy is congruent with the philosophy of your educational institution.

Nursing theory may seem a bit overwhelming at first, but if you break it down into smaller pieces, it is very easy to understand.

35

Accessing Health Information via the Internet

Consumer Knowledge

Many years ago health professionals knew a great deal of information and shared very little of it with their patients. Most consumers accepted that the doctor was supposed to know everything, and the general public was to follow the doctor's recommendations. Today, with the advent of new technology and the Internet, patients frequently know as much as or more than their physicians and other health care professionals. Nurses can no longer be assured that they know more than the patient does. Consumers are questioning their treatment protocols and nurses are expected to have some answers.

Many consumers are also now able to communicate with their health care provider via computer. Some patients are able to access their physicians via e-mail, request prescription refills online, make doctor's appointments, and view lab and x-ray reports. This technology will provide patients much more control in their health care decision making, but it also will lead them to seek more and more information via other avenues.

Consumers have access to numerous sources of information. Today, mainstream bookstores (Barnes & Noble, Borders, etc.) carry many books on health as well as specific books for health professionals. It is likely that any magazine you pick up will have at least one article that relates to health

342

and provides data, symptoms, treatment, and various resources. Most newspapers also have a health feature on a weekly basis if not on a daily basis. The television provides health information on most channels and some cable/satellite channels are devoted solely to the topic of health. Who would have thought even 15 years ago that one would be able to turn on the TV and watch someone have his or her appendix removed? TV also has been inundated with various drug commercials that encourage consumers to contact their health care provider in order to get a prescription for everything from allergy medicine to Viagra! The consumer today is extremely well informed and can easily access information whether accurate or not. The nurse needs to be prepared to provide health information and answers to health-related questions.

The Internet and Nursing

To keep abreast of the information, health care professionals must stay current in their profession and knowledge base. It is important for nurses to be informed and to be able to provide consumers with knowledgeable feedback regarding all aspects of their health care. One of the primary ways to stay ahead is to use the information offered on the Internet via the World Wide Web (WWW). To make use of the Internet, one must have a computer, a modem (allows your computer to communicate via telephone lines), and some type of online service (America Online, CompuServe, Prodigy) or Internet service provider (ISP) (Strauch, 1997). (Check your telephone book for local service providers.) You will also need some type of software to connect with and view the various Web sites. Most online service providers and ISPs will provide you with the necessary software free of charge or you may wish to purchase a Web browser such as Netscape Navigator or Microsoft Explorer. Antiviral software is recommended so that you will not pick up viruses when you download files to your personal computer.

After you have connected your service and can access online information, you will need to learn how to access various Web sites. Typing in a Web address or uniform resource locator (URL) will allow you to access Web sites. It is extremely important that you type in addresses exactly as they appear. Some Web addresses are very long but you must type them character by character (Levine & Young, 1994). An example of a URL or Web address might be *http://www.personnell/groups.brs.net/479832/bcusc.org.* The following are actual URL addresses of some health-oriented Web sites:

- *http://www.rheumatology.org*
- *http://www.nimh.nig.org*

Search Engines

Most Web sites or Web pages allow you to travel from one site to another via **links.** A link is usually highlighted in a color that is different from the main text of the page. By clicking on the highlighted area you can travel to that Web page or Web site and continue your search. To assist you in your search for information on the WWW, it is important to locate either a *Web directory* or *search engine* (Strauch, 1998). These two items allow you to search the WWW for the desired information (Figure 35–1). One way to think of this is to consider looking for a specific book in a huge library. It would be possible, but it might take a long time. On the other hand, if you had some type of computerized card file you could easily cross-reference and find the desired book. A web directory or search engine is similar. It can wade through the mass of WWW information to find what you are looking for.

When using a search engine you type in the word or words that you are looking for in the search blank. For example, if you were interested in learning more about multiple sclerosis, you would type in the words *multiple sclerosis.* After a short time, the search engine would tell you how many Web sites match your query. Depending on which search engine you choose, you may receive 100 matches (hits) or 10,000. Be aware that the search engine is retrieving all the associated Web sites that use the words multiple sclerosis, and any other combination thereof. To narrow your search, you might want to use apostrophes—since the Web site will return only an exact match. For example, you would type in "multiple sclerosis." Most search engines will provide a listing of the better-matched sites first. Some search engines provide you with a short list of recommended sites (see Figure 35–2).

Once you receive the links for Web sites that match your search words, make note of the URL addresses. Remember that .edu is from an educational

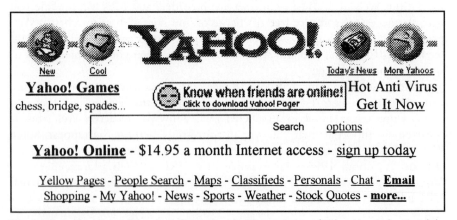

Figure 35–1. Yahoo! search engine. *(Reproduced with permission of Yahoo! Inc. Yahoo! and the Yahoo! logo are trademarks of Yahoo! Inc.)*

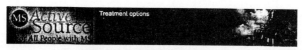

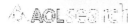 Enter words below and click Search.

Multiple sclerosis [**Search**]

Home | Search Options | Help

Search Results for "Multiple sclerosis"

Web Sites   Web Pages   Related News

SEARCH HERE:

RECOMMENDED SITES
- **National Multiple Sclerosis Society** - Official site
- **Multiple Sclerosis Chats** - Find scheduled chats and discuss with others
- **Multiple Sclerosis** - Symptoms, conditions, treatments, resources and info

- MULTIPLE SCL...
- Buy Books Here
- SEARCH AMAZON!

SPONSORED LINKS
The search results below are provided by a third party and are not necessarily endorsed by AOL
- MSActiveSource.com

Search books:
MULTIPLE SCL...

- **The Raj Natural Health Center**
- **Hyperbaric Therapy Multiple Sclerosis**

BARNES&NOBLE

MATCHING SITES
(1 - 10 of 1349) next >>

Show Me: AOL and the Web | AOL Only | Most Popular Sites
Results from the WorldWideWeb may contain objectionable material that AOL doesn't endorse.

RELATED HOT
SEARCHES
- multiple sclerosis symptoms
- symptoms of multiple sclerosis
- national multiple sclerosis society
- stiff neck in multiple sclerosis
- multiple sclerosis society

The National Multiple Sclerosis Society
Dedicated to ending the devastating effects of multiple sclerosis.
http://www.nmss.org
Show me more like this

Rotorua & District Multiple Sclerosis Society
With information on Multiple Sclerosis, Field Officer services, activities, and links.
http://www.cole.gen.nz/MS
Show me more like this

MSOhio Online Multiple Sclerosis Support Group
MSOhio is sponsored by the Northeast Ohio Chapter of the National Multiple Sclerosis Society. MSOhio offers weekly online support chats, an "E-mail Pal Program" and has an extensive "Links" page. The Cleveland Clinic has linked directly to the MSOhio site.
http://www.msohio.org
Show me more like this

Multiple Sclerosis, University of Chicago Medical Center
Information on multiple sclerosis for patients, physicians, medical students, and health care professionals. Information on clinical trials for newer treatments.
http://ucneurology.uchicago.edu/Neurological_Disorders/...
Show me more like this

Doctor's Guide to Multiple Sclerosis
The latest medical news and information for patients or friends/parents of patients diagnosed with Multiple Sclerosis.
http://www.pslgroup.com/MS.HTM
Show me more like this

Multiple Sclerosis (MS) Support
Infosci's Information about Multiple Sclerosis is available from this Server

Figure 35–2. Search engine results showing number of terms and percentages. *(Copyright 1998, America Online, Inc. All rights reserved. Used with permission.) (Continued)*

http://www.infosci.org
Show me more like this

Healthology Multiple Sclerosis Focus
A comprehensive resource for patients and families living with multiple sclerosis.
http://www.healthology.com/focus_index.asp?f=m_sclerosi...
Show me more like this

Help for Multiple Sclerosis
A Scientifically Safe, Patented, and Natural Non-Drug Alternative for Multiple Sclerosis.
http://naturalessentials.com/ms.htm
Show me more like this

Multiple Sclerosis - Suite101.com
Unique, starting-point website in a banner-free community. Offers monthly discussions, articles, and links to
reputable web sites that inform, enlighten, and support those seeking reliable information on MS.
http://www.suite101.com/welcome.cfm/multiple_sclerosis
Show me more like this

National Multiple Sclerosis Society, Delaware Chapter
A one stop information source for people with Multiple Sclerosis and those that support them.
http://skyconsulting.com/mssdel
Show me more like this

Next 15 Sites (of 1349) for Multiple sclerosis >>

MATCHING CATEGORIES   (1 - 5 of 67) next >>
1. Health > Conditions and Diseases > Neurological Disorders > Demyelinating Diseases > **Multiple Sclerosis**
2. Regional > Oceania > New Zealand > Health > Conditions and Diseases > **Multiple Sclerosis**
3. Regional > North America > United States > Delaware > Health > Conditions and Diseases > **Multiple Sclerosis**
4. Health > Conditions and Diseases > Neurological Disorders > Demyelinating Diseases > Multiple Sclerosis > **Support
Groups**
5. Health > Conditions and Diseases > Neurological Disorders > Demyelinating Diseases > Multiple Sclerosis >
Associations

Search Again for "Multiple sclerosis" Using These Search Services:
Picture Search Preview • News Search • Web Search • Personal Home Pages • Message Boards
Newsgroups • Health • Kids Only

Additional Search Resources:
People • ClassifiedPlus • Movies • White Pages
Yellow Pages • International Directories

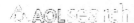

Enter words below and click Search.

| Multiple sclerosis | **Search** |

Home | Search Options | Help

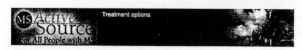

Link to Us | About AOL Search | How to Add Your Site | Advertise with Us | Sherlock Plug-in
Questions? Comments? Send us feedback.

Figure 35–2. *(Continued)*

site, which is more likely to provide you with accurate information than a .com or commercial site. It is also important to note the description of the site—for example, refer to Figure 35–2 and you will notice that the first site listed is the National Multiple Sclerosis Society with a URL address nmss.org (organization). However, further down the page you will see a site called "Help for multiple sclerosis," which talks about a "scientifically safe, patented and non-drug alternative for MS." This site has a .com (commercial) forum, and you might want to question the information provided there. Note that when doing a search, you are pretty much on your own as far as gathering valid up-to-date information.

When using a search engine, it is important to note what its capabilities are. For example, Yahoo! is a general search engine that searches by category and is good for basic searches. If you request a search through Yahoo! and yield little results, Yahoo! will direct you to AltaVista, which provides a more detailed search. Lycos is helpful when you want to do a more detailed search, although they have recently added some categories for a more basic search (Strauch, 1998).

Although search engines can assist you with finding the information you need, it is important to note that no search engine will provide you with all of the possible Web pages on a particular topic. As a matter of fact, recent research has found that even the best search engine will index only about 40% of all Web pages (Beaumont Enterprise, 1998). Steve Lawrence and C. Lee Giles of the NEC Research Institute (1998) found that due to the vast amount of information on the Web even the most sophisticated search engines have a difficult time sorting through it. The main problem is that hundreds of Web pages are added daily to the approximate 325 million Web pages that already exist. Lawrence and Giles found that HotBot covers about 34% of existing pages and AltaVista covered about 28%. Lawrence and Giles found that using five search engines on one topic produced three times as much information as using just one search engine (Beaumont Enterprise, 1998).

This research has shown that it is worthwhile to use two or three search engines to try to find the best possible answers to your questions. You may get some overlapping Web pages or links, but your search will be much more thorough. It is also recommended that when searching for medical information you consider a search engine that searches only health or medical information. Although search engines are not 100% thorough, they are still better than the alternative of trying to sift through Web information on your own.

During the last decade many search engines have been developed that focus on more specific areas. For example, there are specific engines that search only government sites, business sites, health sites, and so on. You may find that when you have an idea of where a specific topic can be found, using a specific search engine might help you narrow your search. Web directories differ from search engines in that they are often much smaller so their results tend to be more narrowly focused. Be sure to use a search engine if you are looking for hard to find information or conducting comprehensive research.

If you want to search for health information, you might choose to use Health A to Z or Achoo. As you become more familiar with the Internet and the various search engines, you will probably find one or two that you rely on for most of your searching. Also note that most search engines offer advanced searches that can help you streamline your search even further. There are a number of search engines and Web sites listed at the end of this chapter.

Search Problems

Every once in awhile you will run into problems when attempting to search using a search engine. Before you give up, consider the following:

- If your search ended up with few results, consider trying a different term. For example, if you are searching for information on *hyperlipidemia,* you may need to use the word *cholesterol* to get started.
- If your search ended up with too many results, consider narrowing it. For example, if you searched for *medications,* you might need to search for heart medications or diabetes medications.
- Be sure that you spell the search terms correctly.
- If you are searching for *diabetes treatments,* it helps to write the search as *diabetes and treatments;* this way, the search will include both terms together, not just one and then the other.

Other Search Options

ASK JEEVES
This service helps you search by asking a question rather than searching for specific terms. All you do is type in your question (Figure 35–3). You will then be shown similar questions with "go to" buttons leading to the answer (Strauch, 1998). For example, we asked Jeeves, "What are the symptoms of diabetes?" Follow-up questions are found in Figure 35–4. We think that Jeeves did an excellent job of answering this question. It also helped provide a number of sites for further investigation. Be sure to remember Jeeves when you are doing all of that homework! Ask Jeeves is located at *http://www.askjeeves.com.*

E-mail

Once you are connected to the Internet, you will most likely want to take advantage of electronic mail, or e-mail. With e-mail you can communicate with anyone else in the world who is connected to the Internet as long as you know his or her e-mail address. E-mail addresses are always configured in the same manner *(screenname@place.domain).*

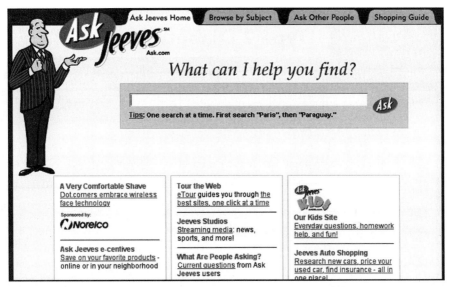

Figure 35–3. Questions for an Ask Jeeves search. *(Ask Jeeves is a trademark of Ask Jeeves, Inc., Copyright 2001, Ask Jeeves, Inc.)*

The place is where the e-mail is sent from, usually a service provider or ISP such as *aol.com, compuserv.com,* or *juno.com.* For example, if you received e-mail from *Ishdoc@aol.com,* Ishdoc is the screen name of the person sending the mail, aol is the service provider, and .com means that it is a commercial agency. Another example would be *P.Jones@twu.edu,* in this case, P.Jones is the person sending the mail, twu is Texas Women's University, and .edu means that it is a college or university.

When you connect with a service provider, they will assist you in setting up an e-mail address. Once connected, you can send and receive e-mail as well as forward files, documents, and photographs! Once you are comfortable with the Web, and if you decide that you want to be adventuresome, some providers will also allow you to set up a Web page of your own.

Common Domain Endings	
Educational Institution	.edu
Government Agency	.gov
Commercial Agency	.com
Network	.net
Organization	.org
Military Site	.mil

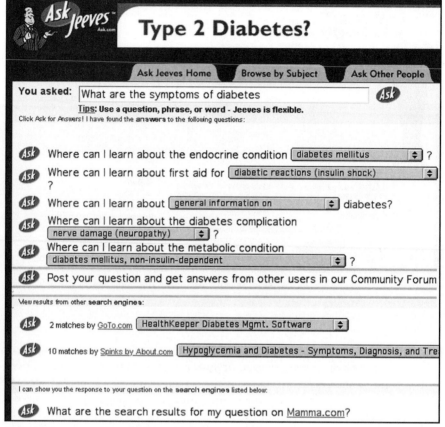

Figure 35–4. Health care consumers will need your assistance. *(Ask Jeeves is a trademark of Ask Jeeves, Inc., Copyright 2001, Ask Jeeves, Inc.)*

It is important to remember that access to the Internet is not just fun and games. You need to be aware of security and privacy issues and become a responsible Internet consumer. The following are some things that you need to consider.

Internet Privacy Issues

1. Never give your password to anyone! All reputable sites will *not* request it!
2. While surfing the Internet you may be subjected to "cookies."
   - Cookies are used by various sites to track your surfing so that commercial sites can develop a profile of your interests.
   - Cookies embed themselves on your hard drive and have positives and negatives. For example, if you like to browse the Amazon.com bookstore (they use cookies), when you return to the site, they will suggest books that might be of interest to you based on your previous selections.

- You need to decide whether you want to accept cookies or not.
- Most browsers allow you to accept or reject cookies, or limit the amount of time they are stored on your hard drive.
- Once you decide what you want to do, examine the security settings on your browser and set it to meet your privacy needs (Hinton, 1997).

3. Be careful of sending personal information over the Internet!
   - Look for the Lock symbol in the lower righthand corner of the screen.
   - Do not give out credit card numbers unless using encryption software, or unless your browser uses encryption.
   - Decide whether you want to share your address, telephone number, and other information when asked to register at various Web sites. If you tend to guard this personal information, you need to remember that once you share it, the potential is for millions of people to have access to it.
   - If you hesitate to discuss personal or business information on a cellular or portable telephone, then you should think twice before discussing it on the Internet.
   - Remember that if you send or receive e-mail at work, it is considered company property and may be accessed by others. People have been fired for sending and receiving e-mail that was derogatory to a boss or a business.
   - Remember that your Internet surfing is recorded on the hard drive in the "history" file. You can change your "history" settings so that sites are deleted after a certain number of days. Your employer can look at the sites that you visit and decide whether or not they are appropriate. There have been cases of people losing their jobs because they surfed pornography sites at work.

4. Spam mail:
   - Spam mail is mail that is sent to you from various sources.
   - It is mail that you did not request and do not want.
   - The majority of spam is sent in an attempt to get you to purchase something.
   - Do not answer spam! Delete it! If you respond to spam, more information will be sent to you!
   - Your ISP may have rules about spam mail. Check them out. We need to work together to eliminate unwanted e-mail. Follow the ISP's wishes regarding reporting spammers.
   - Some spam is pornographic in nature.
   - If you have children, be sure that you set privacy settings so that they do not have access to certain Web sites and spam mail.

5. Downloading files:
   - Be certain that you have virus protection before downloading any files.
   - Do not download files from someone that you do not know.
   - Set your antivirus software to check all e-mail attachments automatically.
   - Some files have been known to carry viruses that can destroy your computer.
   - Be sure that you are downloading information from a reputable site.

Common File Format	
Databases	.DBF
File Compression	.ZIP
Fonts	.FNT
Graphics	.BMP, .GIF, .JPG, .TIF.
Presentation	.PDF
Sreensavers	.SCR
Spreadsheets	.XLS
Text Documents	.DOC, .TXT
Video Clips	.MPG, .MPEG
Web Content	.HTM, .HTML

Listserves

Another way to communicate with others is to join a mailing list or "listserves." There are thousands of mailing lists available for nearly any interest you might have. Once you become a list member, you can send messages to others on the list that share your interests. For example, if you are interested in IV therapy nursing, there is a listserve for IV therapy nurses. You would join by sending e-mail to: *listserve@netcom.com* requesting to subscribe to Ivtherapy-1. You will receive a return e-mail acknowledging your request. Be sure that you print and keep a copy of the original welcome message, as it will tell you how to stop your subscription from the list. You will begin receiving e-mail messages from other list members immediately. Be prepared—some lists generate almost 100 messages per day. You may want to limit the number of lists that you join or your e-mail box may be inundated!

If you are interested in learning more about what listserves are available the following addresses will help.

- List select at *http://www.liszt.com.*
- Several addresses can be found at *http://www.tile.net/listserv/index.html.*
- Another option is to send e-mail to *listserv@listserv.earn.net.*

Newsgroups

Another way to communicate with others who share your interests is by Usenet newsgroups. Usenet groups are online discussion groups in which people with common interests read and post messages. Newsgroups are similar to listserves except that messages are posted to a message board that is open for all to read in a public location, while listserve messages are sent to you as an individual. Some newcomers choose to lurk for awhile before posting any messages.

Lurking is reading messages that are posted without adding a message of your own. Deja news at *http://www.deja.com* allows you to search for newsgroup names. Most online services also maintain a smaller listing of available groups. Health on the Net Foundation (HON) is a nonprofit group in Geneva, Switzerland. This Web site, located at *http://www.hon.ch/home.html*, includes a list of hospitals on the World Wide Web as well as medical support groups, newsgroups, and mailing lists.

Chess

CHESS (Comprehensive Health Enhancement Support System) is a new computerized tool developed by the University of Wisconsin at Madison. Currently available in Web site format, it can be accessed by 17 different hospitals and a few health maintenance organizations (HMOs) that have licensed it or helped fund it. This new software helps breast cancer patients to make decisions about treatment. CHESS is a comprehensive and reliable interactive tool that can answer patients' specific concerns by:

- Allowing patients to access successive steps in treatment
- Providing the pros and cons of decisions such as breast-sparing surgery versus mastectomy
- Keeping detailed records of changes in physical and emotional health by answering daily questionnaires
- Helping patients prioritize their concerns and rank options from least to most suitable
- Providing audio and video clips
- Answering e-mailed questions

(Landro, 2000)

It is certain that more such tools will continue to be developed in the future that will allow patients not only more decision-making capabilities, but also instant access to answers to health care problems in a controlled environment.

Health Information

It is important to remember that there are all kinds of information available on the WWW and at this time there is no quality control mechanism in place. Some information is accurate; other information is false. It is often difficult to separate the two because the false information may look quite plausible. This is the primary area in which health care professionals must be well versed. Consumers may not have the ability to sort through all kinds of medical information to determine which information is accurate. However, the health care professional must be able to provide guidance in making decisions based on the information obtained.

A CASE IN POINT

We would like to provide a personal example of how the Internet was used to access health information. A colleague called and explained that her nephew had been diagnosed with Berger's disease. She had diligently searched the textbooks and could discover only that it was some form of chronic kidney disease. She called knowing that we have access to the Internet. To find out more about Berger's disease, the health search engine Health A to Z at *http://www.healthatoz.com* was used (Figure 35–5). We discovered that another term for Berger's disease is IgA nephropathy, so in the search blank, we typed in the term IgA Nephropathy. Health A to Z came up with 28 related sites (Figure 35–6) that had some information about IgA nephropathy. We clicked on the first site entitled IgA nephropathy and were rewarded with a great deal

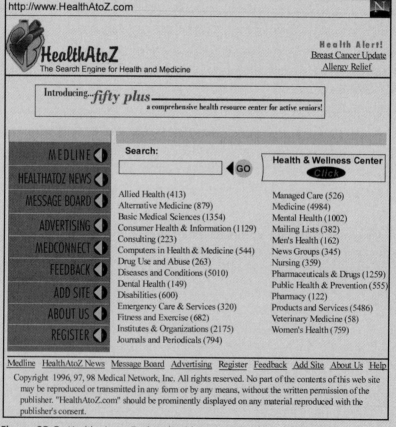

http://www.HealthAtoZ.com

HealthAtoZ
The Search Engine for Health and Medicine

Health Alert!
Breast Cancer Update
Allergy Relief

Introducing... *fifty plus*
a comprehensive health resource center for active seniors!

MEDLINE
HEALTHATOZ NEWS
MESSAGE BOARD
ADVERTISING
MEDCONNECT
FEEDBACK
ADD SITE
ABOUT US
REGISTER

Search:
[   ] GO

Health & Wellness Center
Click

Allied Health (413)
Alternative Medicine (879)
Basic Medical Sciences (1354)
Consumer Health & Information (1129)
Consulting (223)
Computers in Health & Medicine (544)
Drug Use and Abuse (263)
Diseases and Conditions (5010)
Dental Health (149)
Disabilities (600)
Emergency Care & Services (320)
Fitness and Exercise (682)
Institutes & Organizations (2175)
Journals and Periodicals (794)

Managed Care (526)
Medicine (4984)
Mental Health (1002)
Mailing Lists (382)
Men's Health (162)
News Groups (345)
Nursing (359)
Pharmaceuticals & Drugs (1259)
Public Health & Prevention (555)
Pharmacy (122)
Products and Services (5486)
Veterinary Medicine (58)
Women's Health (759)

Medline   HealthAtoZ News   Message Board   Advertising   Register   Feedback   Add Site   About Us   Help

Figure 35–5. Health A to Z. *(Used with permission from Medical Network, Inc., www.healthatoz.com.)*

A CASE IN POINT

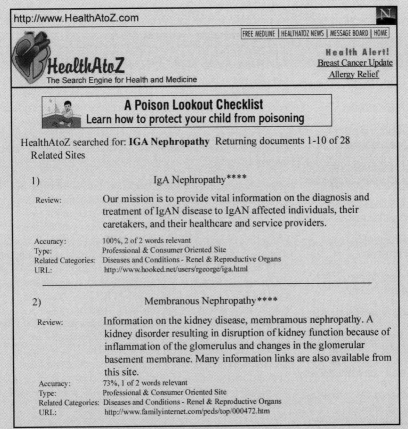

Figure 35–6. Health A to Z IgA nephropathy. *(Used with permission from Medical Network, Inc., www.healthatoz.com.)*

of information about the disease, treatment, and research protocols (Figure 35–7). The pertinent material was printed and a hard copy mailed to our colleague. We then called her to give her some basic information. Upon receipt of the information, she contacted her nephew. He was able to take the information about current treatment to his physician for his next appointment. The physician was familiar with some of the treatment but not all, and was willing to try some of the newer treatments suggested by the Web site. Not only has my colleague's nephew improved considerably, but he and his physician have also been able to keep his condition under control with some of the treatment protocols suggested by the Web site. My colleague was not only grateful for the information, she also decided that she needed Internet access as well!

IgA Nephropathy Home Page

Home of the IgAN Foundation and IgAN E-Mail List

Site Contents

What's New

What is IgA Nephropathy?

IgAN E-Mail List subscriber information

Illustrated Kidney Function and IgAN

Kidney Disease in Perspective

Hypertension / High Blood Pressure

IgAN and Pregnancy

Current treatments for IgAN

Alternative Heatlhcare

Help us find a cure by understanding ourselves. Add your personal medical data

Click here for the On-line IgAN Internet Research Project Questionnaire

Make a contribution to the IgA Nephropathy Foundation

IgA **Nephropathy** or Berger's Disease is the most common non-diabetic kidney disease. Included in the diagnosis of IgAN is Henoch Schonlin Purpurea (where it involves the kidney) and sometimes other forms of glomerulenephritis. Available evidence suggests that IgA nephropathy occurs from either increased production or reduced clearance of the immune protein IgA and associated antigen complexes that are ultimately deposited within the kidney.

Many sources categorize IgAN as a rare disease afflicting 1:100,000 - 1:200,000. It seems that this esitmated level of incidence for IgAN is not accurate as a large proportion of patients who present with IgAN symptoms have mild disease which is not diagnosed via the accepted biopsy diagnosis. Some published research of random diagnostic kidney biopsies suggests IgAN may be vastly more common and may affect up to 2-4% of the human population at large. Certainly there is a dramatic variance in the prevalence of diagnosed IgAN. In Japan and France where testing for the condition is part of regular preventative medical care the disease incidence is twice that found in the USA where testing for IgAN is rarely performed as preventative medicine. Most people probably never realize they have the disease or at least do not realize it until a late stage. Amongst those diagnosed as having IgAN as many as 20%- 30% will suffer eventual kidney failure within 10-20 years. They will require life saving dialysis and/or a kidney transplant.

There are no "widely accepted" western medical treatments for IgAN save in the latest stages of the disease. There is however growing evidence that a number of therapies can be effective in delaying the deterioration of kidney function for many years. Most nephrologists with an active awareness of IgAN prescribe ACE inhibitors and fish oil at a minimum. In some cases powerful steroid treatment is utilized. For about half of those with IgAN tonsillectomy, which treats part of the underlying immune disorder, is effective. There are additional new treatments that show the promise of being a start on finding a cure for the disease.

Figure 35–7. IgA nephropathy home page. *(Used with permission from Russ George of the IgAN Foundation, Palo Alto, California, www.igan.org.)*

SPEED BUMP

Practice Searches

1. You want to know if a new obesity drug that you read about has received FDA approval.
   - Which search engine would you use (if any)?
   - What Web site would you go to?
   - Hint—don't forget the U.S. government has a number of Web sites.
   - Hint—the FDA is a government agency.
2. You have a patient who has a disease that you have never heard of before.
   - You can't find the disease in any of your textbooks.
   - Which search engine would you use (if any)?
   - What Web site would you go to?
   - Hint—if it isn't in any textbooks that you have, or in a textbook at the library, chances are it is a rare disease.
   - Hint—there is an organization that specializes in rare disorders (listed at the end of this chapter).
3. You want to learn more about multiple sclerosis.
   - Which search engine would you use (if any)?
   - What Web site would you look for?
   - Hint—you will probably find a number of sites from various search engines.
   - Hint—look for an agency that specializes in this disease such as the National MS Society.

Here are some guidelines to help you determine the accuracy of information presented on the Internet; unfortunately, they are not foolproof!

Internet Information Guidelines

1. Be certain that you check when the Web site was last updated. This author recently found a great Web site, but it had last been updated in 1996. You can be certain that this information is now out of date.
2. Until legislation sets standards for content, sponsorship, and privacy of online health information, check to see if a site conforms to the Health

on the Net Foundation's Code of Conduct. Sites that do are allowed to display the HON code symbol. The foundation allows Web surfers to search for reputable health sites through its site at *www.hon.ch.*

3. Be wary of Web sites that offer things for sale. You can bet that whatever information they provide will include the need for something that they are trying to sell. On the other hand, you may see many advertising banners that are placed there in order to raise funds for the site itself. There is nothing wrong with this practice.

4. If in doubt, visit more than one Web site! If you get the same information on two or more, chances are the information is safe.

5. Check out the author of the material that you are reading.
   - Does the author have credentials?
   - Is the author an expert in this area?
   - There is some feeling that group-maintained Web sites might be more accurate than individually maintained sites, for example, the American Heart Association versus John Doe's heart page. However, there are a number of excellent sites that are individually maintained and have much more information than group-maintained sites.

6. Check the author's affiliation.
   - Is the author associated with a government agency, professional organization, or major national disease-specific nonprofit organization?
   - Is the author located at an educational facility?

7. If the author refers to a study or research article, check to see if the article exists.
   - See where the research is published and if it is in a reputable source.
   - Find out if the study is funded and by whom.
   - Can the information presented be validated?

8. It is important that you watch your "domain" and see if in surfing you have left the original domain.
   - For example, if you access a university site with a domain of .edu, and you link to other sites, when you find the information that interests you, has the domain changed to .com (commercial)?
   - If such a change has occurred, you will know that you are no longer at an educational site, you are now at a site that is business owned. This may or may not be reflected in the information provided. For example, Harvard University might have conducted a study on use of hypertensive medication in postmenopausal women. As you surf, you may access the site of a pharmaceutical company that is touting their latest antihypertensive medication.

9. Avoid sites that offer to treat a long list of diseases or have a cure to offer for money.
   - Do you believe everything you see on infomercials?
   - There are a number of Web sites that are just like infomercials!
   - Remember that there is no quality control on the Web.

10. One Web page is available that provides information on other pages that may provide questionable advice.
    - Check it out at *http://www.quackwatch.com.*

Internet Search Engines and General Information

To get a description of all available search engines, go to:

www.home.netscape.com/home/internet-search.html

Library Reference and Library Recommended Sites

Internet Public Library: *www.ipl.org*
Online Computer Library Center: *www.olcl.org*
Electronic Newsstand: *www.enews.com*
Libraries Index to the Net: *wunsite.berkeley.edu/internet-index/*
St. Joseph County Public Library Hot List: *www.sjcpl.lib.in.us/homepage /reference/internetlinks.html*
National Library of Medicine: *www.nim.nih.gov/medlineplus*

Search Engine Review Sites

www.searchenginewatch.com
www.notess.com/search

Find a Directory or the Best Search Engine for Your Search

Government Documents and Information: *www.gpo.lib.purdue.edu/*
Health Information: *www.healthweb.org*
Business Information: *www.northnlight.com*
Federal Web Locator: *www.law.vill.edu/fed-agency/fedwebloc.html*

Use a Human-Constructed Directory (Instead of Computer-Generated) for More Detailed Information and More Topic Branches

www.snap.com
www.yahoo.com

General Information and Search Engines

All In One Search: *www.albany.com*
All the Web: *www.alltheweb.com*

AltaVista: *www.altavista.com*
Excite: *www.excite.com*
Google: *www.google.com*
Hot Bot: *www.hotbot.com*
Infoseek: *www.infoseek.com*
Magellan: *www.mckinley.com*
Netlocator: *www.nln.com*
Savy Search: *www.cs.colostate.edu:2000*
Search: *www.search.com*

Encyclopedia

www.britannica.com

Health Information

Hardin Meta Directory: *www.lib.uiowa.edu/hardin/me* (massive but extremely well-organized site aimed mainly at physicians, reviews, and sorting medical links)
National Institutes of Health: *www.nih.gov* (health info, research links, health hotlines—very reliable)
Government Search Engine for Health Topics: *www.healthfinder.gov*
Medline (more professional based): *www.medscape.com*
Medscape (more for consumers): *www.cbs.healthwatch.com*
Run by Former U.S. Surgeon General: *www.drkoop.com*
Mayo Health Organization: *www.mayohealth.org*
Medicine on the Net: *www.medicinenet.com*
Johns Hopkins & Aetna Insurance Co.: *www.intellihealth.com*
National Woman's Health Information Center: *www.4women.gov*
Columbia University: *www.goaskalice.columbia.edu*
National Health Information Center: *www.nhic-nt.health.org/*
Annotated Health Links: *www.slackinc.com/matrix*
Achoo: *www.achoo.com*
Health A to Z: *www.healthatoz.com*
Healthweb: *www.hsinfo.ghsl.nwu.edu/healthweb*

Nursing

Student Nurses: *www.nursing.net.org*
Student Nursing Links: *www.free.websight.com/miller5/*
American Journal of Nursing: *www.ajn.org*

Nurseweek: *www.nurseweek.com/ahwhome.html*
Journal of Nursing Jocularity (health humor): *www.jocularity.com/index.html*
Springhouse: *www.springnet.com*
Nursingworld: *www.nursingworld.org*
The Nursing Student WWW page: *www.csn.net/~tbracket/htm*

Medicine

American Medical Association: *www.ama-assn.org*
American Medical Woman's Association: *www.amwa-doc.org*
New England Journal of Medicine: *www.nejm.org*

To Check a Physician's Credentials

www.certifieddoctor.com
www.docboard.org

Prescription Medication Information

www.pharminfo.com

To Find Self-Help Newsgroups and Mailing Lists

www.healthy.net/selfcare
www.selfhelpgroups.org

Other Professional Organizations

American Physical Therapy Association: *www.apta.org*
American Public Health Association: *www.apha.org*
American Association for Respiratory Care: *www.aarc.org*

Guide to Health Information Resources

It is important for you to know whether a site conforms to the Health on the Net Foundation's code of conduct. Sites that do conform are allowed to display the HON code symbol. The Foundation allows surfers to search for reputable health sites through its site at *www.hon.ch.*

It is important to note that some of these Web sites or addresses may have changed. Should you be unable to access a particular address, try using a search engine to locate it. Occasionally, a site is particularly busy and you will get the following "URL not accessible or unavailable." When this happens, do not give up—wait and try again. Some sites are much easier to access during off hours, very early in the morning, or very late at night.

We also want you to be aware that we are not validating that all of the information provided on these Web sites is true or accurate. Some of these sites may provide misinformation or erroneous information. We are in no way suggesting that you follow any of the information provided by these sites. These sites are provided to assist you in gaining information and making your own decisions.

RESOURCE LISTINGS

Abuse

National Resource Center on Domestic Violence: 800-537-2238
National Council on Child Abuse Hotline: 800-222-2000
National Clearinghouse on Child Abuse and Neglect: *www.caliber3calib.com/nccanch*
National Child Abuse Hotline: 800-422-4453

Addiction

National Clearinghouse for Alcohol and Drug Information: 800-729-6686
Cocaine Hotline: 800-262-2463
Habit Smart: *www.habitsmart.com/* (information about addiction and recovery, various links related to addiction and recovery)
Alcoholism: Another Empty Bottle: *www.alcoholismHELP.com/help/* (contains links, help groups, hotlines, a kids section, information, and personal stories related to alcoholism.
Med Help—The Addiction Medicine Forum: *www.medhelp.org/forums/addiction/index.htm* (ask-the-doctor open forum for addiction issues, including an extensive searchable archive of addiction articles)
Alcoholics Anonymous Active Resource Project: *www.aaresources.org* (a national database project of daily Alcoholics Anonymous meetings, AA events, and recovery-related information)
Parallel Paths of Recovery: *www.parallel-paths.virtualave.net* (dual-diagnosis support group for individuals diagnosed with a mental/emotional illness as well as an addictive disorder and their significant others)

Sober Times—Dedicated to sobriety: *www.sobertimes.com* (Web site on recovery from alcohol and drug addiction, free monthly newsletter, literature and Sober Nuggets; personal experience stories)

Aging

American Association of Retired Persons: *www.aarp.org*
Seniors Online: *www.seniors-on-line.com*
For grandparents: *www.grandparenting.org*
Seniors who want to continue learning: *www.circleoflearning.com*

AIDS

AIDS Hotline: 800-342-AIDS; in Spanish: 800-342-SIDA
CDC National AIDS Clearinghouse: 800-458-5231 or *www.cecnac.org*
AIDS Caregivers Support Network:
  www.vive.com/connect/acsn/acsnhome.htm
National Institute for Allergies and Infectious Diseases: 800-822-ASMA or
  www.niaid.nih.gov
HIV/AIDS site law library, publications, and patient support:
  www.aegis.com

Alcoholism

National Clearinghouse for Alcohol and Drug Information: 800-729-6686
National Council on Alcoholism: 800-NCA-CALL
Al-Anon Family Group: 800-356-9996; in New York: 212-245-3151
American Council on Alcoholism: 800-527-5344

Allergies

American Academy of Allergy, Asthma, and Immunology Information:
  800-822-2762 or *www.execpc.com/~edi/aaai.html*
Allergy Information Center Hotline: 800-727-5400
Food Allergies: *www.healthtrek.com/ifdaller.htm*
National Institute for Allergies and Infectious Diseases: 800-822-ASMA or
  www.niaid.nih.gov

Alternative Health

Alternative Health Information: *www.healthy.net*
Wellness: *www.wellweb.com*
Alternative Medicine: *www.pitt.edu/~cbw/altm.html*

Alzheimer's Disease

Alzheimer's Association: 800-272-3900 or *www.alz.org*
Alzheimer's Disease Education and Referral Center (ADEAR): *www. alzheimers.org*
Alzheimer's Resource Center: *www.mayohealth.org/mayo/common/htm/alzh eimers.htm*
Alzheimer.com: *www.alzhemiers.com*
Alzheimer Web Home Page: *www.alzweb.org*

Anxiety Disorders

Anxiety Disorders Association of America: *www.adaa.org/* (complete information on anxiety, as well as a special section on teen anxiety)
Panic/Anxiety Disorders: *www.panicdisorder.about.com/* (a guide to exploring panic/anxiety disorders, from About.com)
Anxiety Network International: *www.anxietynetwork.com/* (Social anxiety disorder (social phobia), panic, and generalized anxiety disorder are comprehensively covered. Many articles on anxiety, a social anxiety mailing list, chat room, bookstore, question-and-answer pages, and related links)

Arthritis

Arthritis Foundation: *www.arthritis.com*
Arthritis Research: *www.arthritis-research.com* (journal providing the arthritis research community with updates on the latest developments in the field; also available in print)
Arthritis—Doctor's Guide to Internet: *www.pslgroup.com/ARTHRITIS. HTM* (the latest medical news and information for patients or friends/ parents of patients diagnosed with arthritis and arthritis-related disorders)
Arthritis Web site: *www.arthritiswebsite.com* (arthritis portal with information, resources, news, and community)

Asthma

Asthma and Allergy Foundation of America Information Clearinghouse: 800-727-8462 or *www.aafa.org/*
American Academy of Allergy, Asthma, and Immunology Information: 800-822-2762 or *www.execpc.com/~edi/aaai.html*
American Lung Association: *www.lungusa.org/*
The Canadian Lung Association: *www.lung.ca/*

Back Pain

BackCare: *www.backpain.org*
Spine Health: *www.spine-health.com* (written by a multispecialty group of medical professionals, this site covers a broad range of topics about back pain, including prevention, diagnosis, and treatment)
Back Pain Information: *www.BackPainAnswers.com* (information about chronic back pain with useful advice about exercise and self-help)
Spine Universe: *www.spineuniverse.com* (currently operates the most encyclopedic Web site on back pain and spinal disease. This portal delivers a comprehensive interactive tool for the consumer to understand all elements of spinal care.)

Birth Control

Birth Control Information links: *wwwlbynpages.com/ultimate*
Birth Control Information Hotline: 800-468-3637
Birthright (Right to Life): 800-848-5683; in New Jersey: 609-848-1819
Abortion Hotline: 800-772-9100; in the District of Columbia, Alaska, and Hawaii: 202-667-5881

Breast Cancer

Y-Me National Breast Cancer Hotline: 800-221-2141
Breast Cancer Clearinghouse: *www.nysernet.org/bcic*
Breast Cancer Answers: *www.medsch.wisc.edu/bca/bca.html* (offers news and research, clinical trial information, and questions to ask your doctor [University of Wisconsin Comprehensive Cancer Center])
Inflammatory Breast Cancer Research Foundation: *www.ibcresearch.org* (Inflammatory breast cancer [IBC] is an advanced and accelerated form of breast cancer, first diagnosed as Stage IIIb, which usually does not show up in mammograms or ultrasounds.)
Dr. Susan Love's Breast Cancer Web site for Women: *www.susanlovemd.com*

Breast Cancer: *www.healthlink.mcw.edu/breast-cancer/* (information from the Medical College of Wisconsin's HealthLink Web site; searchable index for other health and medical topics)

Breast Cancer Education Network: *www.healthlink.com/bcen/* (links to discussions between leading medical specialists and breast cancer patients plus support information)

Breast Feeding

La Leche League International: 800-LA-LECHE

Cancer

American Cancer Society Response: 800-ACS-2345

American Cancer Society: *www.cancer.org* (types of cancer/treatment/trials etc.)

National Cancer Institute: 800-4-CANCER or *http://rex.nci.nih.gov/*

Make Today Count Inc.: 800-432-2273

Oncolink (cancer information links): *www.oncolink.upenn.edu*

Information Data Base of the National Cancer Institute: 800-422-6237 or *www.icic.nci.nin.gov/patient.htm*

National Marrow Donor Program: *www.marrow.org/*

Childhood Leukemia Center: *www.patientcenters.com/leukemia/* (created especially for parents and others caring for a child with leukemia or other cancer)

Drug Information Center for Cancer Patients: *www.pharminfo.com/disease /cancer_db.html* (cancer drug information, health and medial resources, case studies, discussion threads, and treatment FAQs)

CancerEducation.com: *http://www.cancereducation.com* (improving cancer care through the dissemination of up-to-date and accurate educational programming (MedClips™) and information for health care professionals, cancer patients, and their family members)

CancerSource.com: *www.cancersource.com*

Cancer Page: *www.cancerpage.com/*

Caregivers

American Association of Retired Persons—Elderly Advice: *www.aarp.org* (hot line information on caregiving)

Chats, Resource Guides, Newsletter, Articles: *www.ec-online.net*

Family Caregiver Alliance: *www.caregiver.org* (information on memory loss/brain injury)

National Family Caregivers Association (tips, surveys): *www.nfcacares.org*
Well Spouse Foundation (support groups and chats): *www.wellspouse.org*

Children's Health

Children's Health Information @ Parent's Place: *www.parentsplace.com*
National Immunization Hotline: 800-232-2522

Chronic Fatigue Immunodeficiency Syndrome

CFIDS National Chronic Fatigue Syndrome Association: 816-931-4777
Association for Chronic Fatigue Syndrome: *http://weber.u.washington.*
  edu/~ndedra/aacfsl.html
CDC Chronic Fatigue Syndrome Home Page: *www.cdc.gov/ncidod/dis-*
  eases/cfs/cfshome.htm
About.com on CFS and Fibromyalgia: *www.chronicfatigue.about.com/*
  health/diseases/chronicfatigue/
Links to information on CFIDS/ME and Fibromyalgia: *www.cfids-me.org/*
  (collection of links to information and references of use to people with
  chronic fatigue syndrome and fibromyalgia)

Clinical Trials

www.clinicaltrials.gov
www.centerwatch.com (lists trials by condition and geographical location)

Cystic Fibrosis

Cystic Fibrosis Online Resources: *www.vmsg.csd.mu.edu/~5418/ukasr/*
  syctic/html
Cystic Fibrosis Foundation: 800-FIGHT-CF or *www.cff.org*
Cystic Fibrosis Mutation Database: *www.genet.sickkids.on.ca/cftr/*
Cystic Fibrosis Genetic Testing: *www.phd.msul.edu/cf/fam.html*
FAQ on Cystic Fibrosis: *www.cf-web.mit.edu/cystic-l/index.html*
Cystic Fibrosis Research Inc.: *www.cfri.org/*

Depression

National Mental Health Association: 800-969-6642 or *www.worldcorp.*
  com/dc-online/nmha/
National Foundation for Depressive Illness: 800-248-4344 or *www.depres-*
  sion.org/

Mental Health Net: Depression: *www.depression.cmhc.com/*

Depression: PharmInfo Drug Information Center: *www.pharminfo.com/disease/mental/dep_info.html*

Depression.com: *www.depression.com/*

Diabetes

American Diabetes Association: 800-969-6642 or *www.diabetes.org*

DiabetesLine: *www.diabetesline.com*

Diabetes Digest Magazine: *www.diabetesdigest.com*

MyDiabetes: *www.mydiabetes.com* (includes a personal daily diary for tracking blood glucose levels, medication usage, diet, and exercise. Advice, support, and encouragement are available.)

Diabetes News: *www.diabetesnews.com/* (provides the latest breaking news relating to diabetes and related subjects; as well as information hyperlinks of particular interest to diabetics)

Disabilities

Links to Disabilities Web sites: *www.VTEP.edu/dsso/links.htm*

National Organization on Disabilities: 800-248-ABLE

National Rehabilitation Information Center: 800-346-2742

Wellness and Aging with Disability: *www.jik.com/hwawd.html*

Eating Disorders

Bulimia–Anorexia Self-Help Information: 800-227-4785

Eating Disorders Awareness and Prevention: *www.edap.org*

Overeater's Anonymous: *www.overeaters.com*

Anorexia Nervosa and Related Eating Disorders: *www.anred.com*

The American Anorexia Bulimia Association: *www.aabainc.org/* (a national nonprofit organization of concerned members of the public and health care industry dedicated to the prevention and treatment of eating disorders)

National Association of Anorexia Nervosa and Associated Disorders (ANAD): *www.anad.org/*

Epilepsy

Epilepsy Foundation of America: 800-EFA-1000 or *www.efa.org*

Epilepsy Surgery Unit: *www.neurosurgery.mgh.harvard.edu/epilepsy.htm* (Massachusetts General Hospital/Harvard. Research and surgical treatment; links to support organizations)

American Epilepsy Society: *www.aesnet.org/* (promotes research and education for professionals dedicated to the prevention, treatment, and cure of epilepsy)

Fibromyalgia

Fibromyalgia Network: 800-631-1950 or *www.fmnetnews.com*
Sapient Health Network: *www.shn.net*
American Fibromyalgia Syndrome (FMS) Association, Inc.:
  www.afsafund.org/
Oregon Fibromyalgia Foundation: *www.myalgia.com*
National Fibromyalgia Research Association (NFRA):
  www.teleport.com/~nfra/

Headache

National Headache Foundation: 800-843-2256; in Illinois: 800-523-8858
  or *www.headaches.org*
Migraine Foundation: *www.niagara.com/migraine/*
American Council for Headache Education: *www.achenet.org/*
The Electronic Headache Support Group: *www.medsupport.com/survival/*
  (offers insights via neurologists and nurses who treat headache disorders)

Head Injuries

Traumatic Brain Injury: *www.neuro.pmr.vcu.edu*
National Head Injury Foundation: 800-444-6443
Perspectives Network: *www.tbi.org*
Traumatic Brain Injury Resource Guide: *www.tbiguide.com*

Hearing

Association for Hearing and Speech: 800-638-8255
Hearing Helpline: 800-327-9355
Hereditary Deafness: *www.boystown.org/hhirr/*

Heart

American Heart Association: 800-AHA-USA-1 or *www.americanheart.org/*
National Heart, Lung, and Blood Institute High Blood Pressure Hotline:
  800-575-WELL

British Heart Foundation: *www.bhf.org.uk*

Heart and Stroke Foundation: *www.hsf.ca/* (research, education, and promotion of healthy lifestyle; A–Z glossary; also in French)

Hospice

Hospice Hands: *www.gator.net/~jnash/hospice.html*

National Hospice Organization Hotline: 800-658-8898

Hospice Link/Hospice Education Institute: 800-331-1620

Partnership for Caring (formerly Choice in Dying): 800-989-9455

Bereavement Resources Online: *www.funeral.net/info/brvres.html*

Infectious Diseases

Centers for Disease Control: 404-332-4555 or *www.cdc.gov*

National Foundation of Infectious Diseases: 301-656-0003

Infertility

American Society for Reproductive Medicine: 205-933-8494 or *www.asrm.com*

Internet Health Resources: Infertility: *www.ihr.com/infertility/index.html* (extensive information on IVF, GIFT, and other assisted reproductive technologies; listing of clinics, pharmacies, and donor egg/sperm and surrogacy services, infertility medications; male factor infertility; and social, legal, and psychological issues)

Atlanta Reproductive Health Centre: *www.ivf.com/*

RESOLVE: *www.resolve.org/* (provides support and information to individuals who are experiencing infertility issues through advocacy and public education)

INCIID—International Council on Infertility: *www.inciid.org/*

Kidney

American Association of Kidney Patients: 800-749-2257

National Kidney Foundation: 800-622-9010 or *www.ivf.com//index.html*

Liver

American Liver Foundation: 800-223-0179 or *www.sadieo.ucsf.edu/alf/alf final/homepagealf.html*

Hepatitis Central: *hepatitiscentral.com/hepweb/websites.html*

Lupus

Lupus Foundation of America: 800-558-0121

Lupus Homepage: *www.hamline.edu/lupus/*

American Lupus Foundation: 800-331-1802

The Lupus Site—About.com: *http://lupus.about.com* (original feature articles and collection of links written and assembled by a health professional who is also a lupus patient)

Lupus at Suite101.com: *www.suite101.com/welcome.cfm/lupus* (tons of lupus information, with articles written by a nurse who has lupus. You can ask questions, have discussions, and get the information that you need.)

Lyme Disease

American College of Rheumatology: *www.rheumatology.org*

The Lyme Disease Network: *www.lymenet.org/*

American Lyme Disease Foundation: *www.aldf.com*

The Lyme Disease Foundation: *www.lyme.org/index2.html* (The Lyme Disease Foundation [LDF] is a nonprofit medical health care agency dedicated to finding solutions to tickborne disorders.)

Mental Health

National Institute of Mental Health: 800-421-4211 or *www.nimh.nih.gov/*

National Mental Health Association: 800-969-6642 or *www.worldcorp.com/dc-online/nmha/*

National Mental Health Consumers Self-Help Clearinghouse: 800-553-4539 or *www.libertynet.org~nmha/cl.house.html*

Crisis Hotline: 800-762-3334

Minority Health

Office of Minority Health Resource Center: 800-444-6472

Multiple Sclerosis

National MS Society: 900-FIGHT-MS or *www.nmss.org/home/html*

MS Foundation: *www.msfacts.org*

Consortium of Multiple Sclerosis Centers: Leadership in MS Care and Research: *www.mscare.org*

MS-Network: *www.ms-network.com/* (features news, interviews with patients and care-partners, and treatment information)

MS Education Network: *www.htinet.com/msen.html* (interactive resource for people with multiple sclerosis and the people in their lives)

MS Information Gateway: *www.ms-gateway.com/*

Nutrition

American Dietetic Association: *www.eatright.org*

National Center for Nutrition and Dietetics Consumer Hotline: 800-366-1655

Organ Transplantation

American Council on Transplantation: 800-ACT-GIVE

Living Bank: 800-528-2971

Organ Donor Hotline: 800-243-6667

Transplants and Organ Donation Information: *www.asf.org*

Ostomy

United Ostomy Association: 800-826-0826 or *www.uoa.org* (a volunteer-based health organization dedicated to providing education, information, support, and advocacy for people who have had or will have intestinal or urinary diversions)

Parkinson's Disease

American Parkinson Disease Association: 800-223-2732

National Parkinson Fund: 800-327-4545

National Parkinson's Foundation, Inc.: *www.parkinson.org/* (The NPF has created an extensive Web site that includes information about Parkinson's disease, articles from their newsletters, online tests for tremor and clinical depression, as well as an Ask-the-Doctor forum.)

Michael J. Fox Foundation for Parkinson's Disease Research: *www.michaelfox.org/*

Premenstrual Syndrome (PMS)

PMS Access: 800-222-4PMS

Premenstrual Syndrome Web sites: *www.healthlinkusa.com/premenstrual.syndrome.htm*

Rare Disorders

National Organization for Rare Disorders: 800-999-6673 or *www.nord-rdg.com/~orphanpcnet.com/~orphan/*
National Center on Orphan Drugs and Rare Diseases: 800-456-3505

Rehabilitation

National Rehabilitation Information Center: 800-346-2742
Selected Rehabilitation and Assistive Technology Web sites:
www.lib.usf.edu/virtual/internetrefs/index.php?s=rehab

Sexually Transmitted Diseases (STDs)

Centers for Disease Control and Prevention STD Hotline: 800-227-8922
or *www.medtext.com/std.htm*
STD Health Online: *www.homestead.com/chrisloga/stdhealth.html*
STD Prevention: *www.stdprevention.com*

Sickle Cell

National Association for Sickle Cell Disorders: 800-421-8453
Sickle Cell Anemia: *www.sunsite.unc.edu/asha/*
Sickle Cell Information Center: *www.emory.edu/PEDS/SiCKLE*
Sickle Cell Disease Association of America: *http://sicklecelldisease.org*

Spinal Cord Injuries

Spinal Injury Information Network: *www.spinalcord.uab.edu/*
Spinal Cord Network International: 800-548-2673
National Spinal Cord Injury Hotline: 800-526-3456 or *www.spinalcord.org*
National Spinal Cord Injury Foundation: 800-962-9629

Stroke

Stroke Connection of American Heart Association: 800-553-6321 or
www.strokeassociation.org/
National Stroke Association: 800-367-1990 or *www.stroke.org/index/html*
Internet Stroke Center at Washington University: *www.neuro.wustl.edu/stroke/* (a comprehensive Web resource for stroke patients, family members, and health professionals; includes a database of stroke clinical trials, listings of more than 100 U.S. stroke centers, meetings calendar, stroke guidelines, and links to teaching sites)

Heart and Stroke Foundation: *www.heartandstroke.ca* (Canadian oragniza-tion offering healthful tips and recipes, news items related to stroke, and information on provincial resources for survivors)

Sudden Infant Death Syndrome (SIDS)

Sudden Infant Death Syndrome Institute: 800-232-SIDS
SIDS Network: *www.eskimo.com/~pageless/home/sids.net*
Sudden Infant Death Syndrome Network: *http://sids-network.org*
Sudden Infant Death Alliance: *http://sidsalliance.org/*
Foundation for the Study of Infant Deaths (FSID): *www.sids.org.uk/fsid/*
  (The United Kingdom's leading cot death [SIDs] charity, supporting bereaved families, providing information to the public, and funding research into infant health and infant death)

Ulcerative Colitis and Crohn's Disease

Inflammatory Bowel Disease: *www.qurlyjoe.bu.edu/chuchome.html*
Crohn's Disease Resource Organization: *www.crohnsawareness.com*
Pediatric Crohn's & Colitis Association, Inc.: *www.pcca.hypermart.net*
Crohn's & Colitis Foundation of America: *www.ccfa.org*
United Ostomy Association, Inc.: *www.uoa.org* (a volunteer-based health organization dedicated to providing education, information, support, and advocacy for people who have had or will have intestinal or urinary diversions)

Urinary Incontinence

Help for Incontinent People: 800-BLADDER
Agency for Health Policy and Research: *www.text.nim.nih.gov/ftrs/dbac-cess/ahcpr*

Vision

National Center for Sight: 800-221-2004
Links to Information on Blindness: *www.nyise.org/eye/htm*
Association for Research in Vision and Ophthalmology: *www.arvo.org/arvo/* (deals with research in various fields of ophthalmology)
Macular Degeneration Foundation: *www.eyesight.org/*
Vitreous Society: *www.vitreoussociety.org/* (exchange of scientific informa-tion regarding diseases of the retina and vitreous)

Wellness

Training and Nutrition Logs: *www.asimba.com*

American Heart Association—Weight/Exercise Program: *www.choosetomove. org*

Workout Schedules/Fitness Calendar: *www.getfit.com*

Women's Health

Women's Health Resource Center at the Mayo Clinic: *www.mayo.ivi.com/ mayo/common/htm/womenpg.htm*

Women's Health Web sites: *www.ohsu.edu/women*

References

Allen, C. (1997). *Nursing process in collaborative practice: A problem-solving approach* (2nd ed.). Stamford, CT: Appleton & Lange.

Andrews, M. M., & Boyle, J. S. (1996). *Transcultural concepts in nursing care* (2nd ed.). Philadelphia: Lippincott-Raven.

Atkinson, W., Furphy, L., Gantt, J., & Mayfield, M. (Eds.). (1995). *Epidemiology and prevention of vaccine preventable diseases* (2nd ed.). Rockville, MD: US Department of Health and Human Services.

Bacon, J. (1995). Healing prayer: The risks and rewards. *Journal of Christian Nursing, 15*(3), 14–17.

Barren, M. (1995). Take charge of your pain. *Modern Maturity,* 35–37, 80–81.

Barsch, J. (1996). *Barsch learning style inventory.* Novato, CA: Academic Therapy Publications.

Berger, K. J., & Williams, M. B. (1999). *Fundamentals of nursing: Collaborating for optimal health.* Stamford, CT: Appleton & Lange.

Besdine, R. N. (1990). Introduction. In W. B. Abrams, & R. Berkow (Eds.). *The Merck manual of geriatrics.* Rahway, NJ: Merck, Sharp & Dohme Research Laboratories.

Beyea, S. C. (1996). *Critical pathways for collaborative nursing care.* Menlo Park, CA: Addison-Wesley.

Beyea, S. C., & Nicoll, L. H. (1997). Research utilization begins with learning to read research reports. *AORN Journal, 68*(3), 402–403.

Beyer, B. K. (1987). *Practical strategies for the teaching of thinking.* Boston: Allyn & Bacon.

Brookfield, S. D. (1987). *Developing critical thinkers: Challenging adults to explore alternative ways of thinking and acting.* San Francisco: Jossey-Bass.

Burgess, A. W. (1997). *Psychiatric nursing: Promoting mental health.* Stamford, CT: Appleton & Lange.

Burke, M., & Walsh, M. (1992). *Gerontological nursing care of the frail elderly.* St. Louis, MO: Mosby-Year Book.

Burrell, L. O., Gerlach, M. M., & Pless, B. S. (1997). *Adult nursing: Acute and community care* (2nd ed.). Stamford, CT: Appleton & Lange.

Byrd, R. C., & Sherrill, J. (1995). The therapeutic effects of intercessory prayer. *Journal of Christian Nursing, 2*(1), 21–23.

Chaffee, J. (1985). *Thinking critically*. Boston: Houghton Mifflin.

Clark, C. C. (1978). *Assertive skills for nurses*. Wakefield, MA: Contemporary Publishing.

Cobb, K. (November 2, 1997). A nutria in every pot? *Houston Chronicle,* 10A–11A.

Corbett, J. V. (1996). *Laboratory tests and diagnostic procedures with nursing diagnoses* (4th ed.). Stamford, CT: Appleton & Lange.

Dossey, L. (1994). The science of prayer. *Natural health.* March/April.

Drug Watch (2000). *American Journal of Nursing 100*(8), 37.

Erwin, B., & Dinwiddie, E. T. (1983). *Test without trauma*. New York: Grosset & Dunlap.

Farrell, J. (1990). *Nursing care of the older person*. Philadelphia: Lippincott-Raven.

Fitzpatrick, J. J., & Whall, A. L. (1996). *Conceptual models of nursing practice* (3rd ed.). Stamford, CT: Appleton & Lange.

Fontaine, K. L. (2000). *Healing practices: Alternative therapies for nursing*. Saddle River, NJ: Prentice Hall.

Fretwell, M. D. (1990). Comprehensive functional assessment. In W. B. Abrams, & R. Berkow (Eds.). *The Merck manual of geriatrics*. Rahway, NJ: Merck, Sharp & Dohme Research Laboratories.

Gallup Poll. (February 1, 1997). Religion Survey Results.

Grant, E., Newton, M., & Moore, S. (1995). Keeping patients on the right track. *Nursing 95, 27*(8), 57–59.

Guido, G. W. (1997). *Legal issues in nursing* (2nd ed.). Stamford, CT: Appleton & Lange.

Habel, M. (1997). Stroke rehabilitation: What you need to know. *Healthweek-Houston/San Antonio, 2*(16), 18–19.

Hayflick, L. (1994). *How and why we age*. New York: Ballantine Books.

Herman, S. J. (1978). *Becoming assertive: A guide for nurses*. New York: Van Nostrand.

Hinton, W. D. (1997). Are cookies crumbling our privacy? *PC Novice, 8*(4), 83–85.

Hughes, C. E. (1997). Prayer and healing: A case study. *Journal of Holistic Nursing, 15*(3), 318–324.

Humphrey, M. A. (1986). Effects of anticipatory grief for the patient, family member, and caregiver. In T. A. Rando (Ed.). *Loss and anticipatory grief*. Lexington, MA: Lexington Books.

Humphry, D. (1991). *Final exit*. Eugene, OR: Hemlock Society.

Kee, J. L. (1999). *Laboratory & diagnostic tests with nursing implications* (5th ed.). Stamford, CT: Appleton & Lange.

Keithley, J. K., Keller, A., & Vazquez, M. G. (1996). Promoting good nutrition: Using the food guide pyramid in clinical practice. *Medsurg Nursing, 5*(6), 397–403.

Kohn, L. T., Corrigan, J. M., & Donaldson, M. S., (Eds.). *To err is human: Building a safer health system*. Washington, DC: National Acadamy Press.

Kübler-Ross, E. (1969). *On death and dying*. New York: Macmillan.

Levine, J. R., & Young, M. L. (1994). *More Internet for dummies*. San Mateo, CA: IDG Books Worldwide.

Mainelli, T. (1996). Internet search services show the way. *PC Novice, 7*(10), 77–79.

Marriner-Tomey, A. (1994). *Nursing theorists and their work.* St. Louis, MO: Mosby.

Matteson, M. A., McConnell, E. S., & Linton, A. D. (1997). *Gerontological nursing: Concepts and practice* (2nd ed.). Philadelphia: Saunders.

Melzack, R. (April, 1992). Phantom limbs. *Scientific American,* 120–126.

Melzack, R. (February, 1998). Phantom limbs. *Discovery, 19*(266), 20.

Milton, K. (1997). Real men don't eat deer. *Discover, June 18*(6), 46–49.

Murray, R., & Zetner, J. (1997). *Health assessment & promotion strategies through the life span* (6th ed.). Stamford, CT: Appleton & Lange.

Nieswiadomy, R. M. (1998). *Foundations of nursing research* (3rd ed.). Stamford, CT: Appleton & Lange.

O'Toole, M. T. (Ed.). (1997). *Miller-Keane encyclopedia & dictionary of medicine, nursing, and allied health.* Philadelphia: Saunders.

Orem, D. E. (1991). *Nursing: Concepts and practice.* St. Louis, MO: Mosby.

Pauk, W. (1988). *How to study in college* (4th ed.). Boston, MA: Houghton-Mifflin.

Paul, R. W. (1993). *Critical thinking: How to prepare students for a rapidly changing role.* Santa Rosa, CA: Center for Critical Thinking.

Rando, T. A. (1993). *Treatment of complicated mourning.* Champaign, IL: Research Press.

Roy, C., & Andrews, H. (1999). *The Roy adaptation model: The definitive statement* (2nd ed.). Stamford, CT: Appleton & Lange.

Siegel, K., Mesagno, F. P., Karus, D., Christ, G., Banks, K., & Moynihan, R. (1992). Psychosocial adjustment of children with a terminally ill parent. *Journal of American Academy of Child Adolescent Psychiatry, 31*(2), 327–333.

Spector, R. E. (1996). *Cultural diversity in health and illness* (4th ed.). Stamford, CT: Appleton & Lange.

Strauch, J. (1997). I spy a good ISP. *Smart Computing, 5*(8), 71–74.

Strauch, J. (1998). Search service secrets. *Smart Computing, 5*(9), 81–84.

Sullivan, E. J., & Decker, P. J. (1992). *Effective management in nursing.* Redwood City, CA: Addison-Wesley.

The Associate Press. (April 3, 1998). Internet world is too wide for software engine to search. *Beaumont Enterprise.* 8C and 7C.

Togno-Armanasco, V., Hopkin, L. A., & Harter, S. (1995). How case management really works. *AJN, 95*(6), 24I–24J.

US Bureau of the Census. (1996). *Statistical abstract of the United States: 1996.* (116th ed.). Washington, DC.

US Department of Commerce, Bureau of Census. (1993). *1990 census of population-social and economic characteristics.* Washington, DC: Government Printing Office.

Varcarolis, E. M. (1994). *Foundations of psychiatric-mental health nursing.* Philadelphia: Saunders.

Vincent, C., Young, M., & Phillips, A. (1994). Why do people sue doctors? A study of patients and relatives taking legal action. *Lancet, 343,* 1609–1613.

Wilkinson, J. M. (2000). *Nursing diagnosis handbook with NIC interventions and NOC outcomes* (7th ed.). Upper Saddle River, NJ. Prentice Hall Health.

Suggested Reading

Agency for Health Care Policy and Research (1992). *Clinical practice guidelines: Urinary incontinence in adults* (AHCPR Pub. No. 92-0038). Rockville, MD: U.S. Department of Health and Human Services, Public Health Service.

Alfaro-LeFevre, R. (1995). *Critical thinking in nursing*. Philadelphia: Saunders.

Ashby, D. A. (1997). Medication calculation skills of the medical-surgical nurse. *Medsurg Nursing, 6*(2), 90–94.

Egbert, L. A. (1990). The spectrum of suffering, *AJN* (8) 35–39.

Eschleman, M. M. (1996). *Introductory nutrition and nutrition therapy*. Philadelphia: Lippincott-Raven.

Hill, S. S., & Howlett, H. A. (1993). *Success in practical nursing*. Philadelphia: Saunders.

Kirtzweil, P. (1993). "Nutritional facts" to help consumers eat smart. *FDA Consumer, 27*(4), 22–27.

Lilley, L. L., & Guanci, R. (1997). Persistent potassium problems. *American Journal of Nursing, 97*(6), 14.

McClelland, C. (October, 1997). Personal communication.

Nornhold, P. (1997). Nursing on trial. *Nursing 97, 6*(7), 33.

Plum, S. D. (1997). Nurses indicted. *Nursing 97, 6*(7), 35–36.

Rubenfeld, M. G., & Scheffer, B. K. (1995). *Critical thinking in nursing: An interactive approach*. Philadelphia: Lippincott-Raven.

Short, M. S. (1997). Charting by exception on a clinical pathway. *Nursing Management, 28*(8), 45–46.

Simpson, R. L. (1997). Point-of-care technology: A new perspective. *Nursing Management, 28*(8), 16.

Stehlin, D. (1993). A little "lite" reading. *FDA Consumer, 27*(5), 12–16.

Tomky, D. (1997). Taking a new look at an old adversary: Diabetes. *Nursing 97, 27*(11), 41–45.

Valanis, B. (1999). *Epidemiology in health care* (3rd ed.). Stamford, CT: Appleton & Lange.

Index

A

Abuse, elder, 150–152
Abuse resource listings on the Internet, 362
Acceptance and the dying process, 224, 226
Accommodation phase and mourning process, 228
Accountability, 80
Acculturation-assimilation continuum, 173–175
Acetylcholine, 321
Achoo, 348
Acid-base imbalances, 249
Acidosis, 245, 247, 249
Activated partial thromboplastin time (APTT), 283
Active immunity, 312–314
Active transport, 273
Activities of daily living (ADLs), 135, 147
Acupuncture, 194
Adaptation, Roy's theory of, 334, 337
Addiction and pain control, 125
Addiction resource listings on the Internet, 362–363
Admission histories, 89, 90
See also History, patient
Adrenal cortex, 253
Adult Protective Services (APS), 150

Advanced health care directives
directive to physicians, 219, 222
do not resuscitate, 219
durable power of attorney for health care, 218, 220–221
living wills, 214–216
medical durable power of attorney, 218, 220–221
natural death act, 214, 217
Patient Self-Determination Act (PSDA) of 1992, 213
Advocacy, 79–80, 199–200
Afferent, 324–325
African Americans, 174, 176–177
Afterload, 293–294
Ageism, 142–143
See also Elderly population
Agency for Health Care Policy and Research (AHCPR), 41, 42, 127, 129
Agent and epidemiology, 310
Aggressive behavior, 50
Agnostics, 207
Agriculture, United States Department of (USDA), 307
AIDS (acquired immune deficiency syndrome), 154, 310–311, 315
Alcoholism, 166, 363
Aldosterone, 269
Alkalosis, 245, 247, 249
Allergy resource listings on the Internet, 363

B

Back pain, 365
Backup data and computers, 37–38
Baclofen, 170
Baltimore Longitudinal Study of Aging (BLSA), 145–146
Baptists, 204
Bargaining and the dying process, 224, 225
Barsch Learning Style Inventory, 3–4
Behavior change, asking for, 54
Beneficence, 68
Benign prostatic hypertrophy (BPH), 149
Berger's disease, 356
Beta-adrenergic antagonist, 322
Beta carotene, 189
Beta receptors and sympathetic nervous system, 319–320
Bicarbonate (HCO$_3$), 243–245
Bill of Rights, pain patient's, 126–127
Biofeedback, 194
Biological age, 142
Biological environment and epidemiology, 310
Biologic programming and aging, 144
Biomedical-scientific view of health/ illness, 175
Birth control, 365
Black Muslims, 201
Bowman's capsules, 325
Brain and pain, 118
Breast cancer, 365–366
Brethren, 205
Buddhism, 201
Burnout, 113

C

Calendar, nursing school and keeping daily/weekly, 21–24
Calipers, cardiac, 290, 292
Camp nursing, 57
Cancer, 166, 366
Capsaicin, 188, 190–191
Carbohydrates, 305

Carbon dioxide (CO$_2$), 243–249
Carbonic acid (H$_2$CO$_3$), 243–245
Cardiovascular agent, 322
Caregiver resource listings on the Internet, 366–367
Care plans, 91, 93–96
Case management, 96–101
Centers for Disease Control (CDC), 41, 310, 314
Central nervous system (CNS), 170
Central venous (CV) access, 279
Certification, 58–60
Chain of infection, 315, 316
Chamomile, 190–191
Charting. *See under* Documentation
Cheating on exams/paper writing, 12, 31–32
Checklists, 86–88
CHESS (Comprehensive Health Enhancement Support System), 353
Children and death and dying, 210, 227–228, 231
Children of Aging Parents, 157
Children's health resource listings on the Internet, 367
Chiropractors, 194
Choice in Dying, 239
Chondroitin, 190–191
Christianity, 203
Christian Scientist, 205
Chrone's disease, 374
Chronic fatigue immunodeficiency syndrome, 367
Chronic illness, 131–133
Chronological age, 141–142
Church of Christ, 205
Church of God, 205
Church of Jesus Christ of Latter Day Saints, 205
Civil law, 68
Class preparation, 8–9
Clinical trials, resource listings on the Internet for, 367
Clofibrate, 170
Colloquialisms, 181, 184
Communicable diseases and immunity active/passive immunity, acquiring, 312–314

M

N